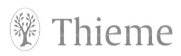

# Physical Therapy Examination and Assessment

Antje Hueter-Becker
Physical Therapy Teacher
and Physical Therapist
Neckargemünd, Germany

Mechthild Doelken
Physical Therapist
School for Physical Therapists
Mannheim, Germany

360 illustrations

Thieme
Stuttgart · New York · Delhi · Rio

*Library of Congress Cataloging-in-Publication Data* is available from the publisher.

This book is an authorized translation of the 2nd German edition published and copyrighted 2011 by Georg Thieme Verlag, Stuttgart. Title of the German edition: Untersuchen in der Physiotherapie.

Translator: Stephanie Kramer, Berlin, Germany
Illustrator: Martin Hoffmann, Elchingen, Germany

**Important note:** Medicine is an ever-changing science undergoing continual development. Research and clinical experience are continually expanding our knowledge, in particular our knowledge of proper treatment and drug therapy. Insofar as this book mentions any dosage or application, readers may rest assured that the authors, editors, and publishers have made every effort to ensure that such references are in accordance with **the state of knowledge at the time of production of the book**.

Nevertheless, this does not involve, imply, or express any guarantee or responsibility on the part of the publishers in respect to any dosage instructions and forms of applications stated in the book. **Every user is requested to examine carefully** the manufacturers' leaflets accompanying each drug and to check, if necessary in consultation with a physician or specialist, whether the dosage schedules mentioned therein or the contraindications stated by the manufacturers differ from the statements made in the present book. Such examination is particularly important with drugs that are either rarely used or have been newly released on the market. Every dosage schedule or every form of application used is entirely at the user's own risk and responsibility. The authors and publishers request every user to report to the publishers any discrepancies or inaccuracies noticed. If errors in this work are found after publication, errata will be posted at www.thieme.com on the product description page.

© 2015 Georg Thieme Verlag KG
Thieme Publishers Stuttgart
Rüdigerstrasse 14, 70469 Stuttgart,
Germany, +49 [0]711 8931 421
customerservice@thieme.de

Thieme Publishers New York
333 Seventh Avenue, New York, NY
10001, USA, 1-800-782-3488
customerservice@thieme.com

Thieme Publishers Delhi
A-12, second floor, Sector-2, NOIDA-201301,
Uttar Pradesh, India, +91 120 45 566 00
customerservice@thieme.in

Thieme Publishers Rio
Thieme Publicações Ltda.
Argentina Building, 16th floor, Ala A,
228 Praia do Botafogo, Rio de Janeiro
22250-040 Brazil, +55 21 3736-3631

Cover design: Thieme Publishing Group
Typesetting by primustype Robert Hurler GmbH,
Notzingen, Germany

Printed in India by Replika Press Pvt. Ltd.
ISBN 978-3-13-174641-2

Also available as e-book:
eISBN 978-3-13-174651-1

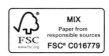

Some of the product names, patents, and registered designs referred to in this book are in fact registered trademarks or proprietary names even though specific reference to this fact is not always made in the text. Therefore, the appearance of a name without designation as proprietary is not to be construed as a representation by the publisher that it is in the public domain.

# Contents

## 1   The Physical Therapy Process: Examination, Clinical Reasoning, and Reflection

*Elly Hengeveld*

## 2   Examination of Structures and Functions of the Locomotor System

## 3   Examining Posture and Muscle Balance

*Salah Bacha*

## 4    Pain as the Chief Symptom

*Mechthild Doelken*

## 5    Examining Cardiopulmonary Functions

# Preface

"Physiotherapy without careful examination is like a tree without roots."

Often—almost always in Germany—a patient is referred for or "prescribed" physical therapy by a doctor following a medical diagnosis. The physical therapist should certainly scrutinize this biomedical diagnosis but under no circumstances can the diagnosis replace the physical therapist's own careful examination. That is to say, only the examination can accurately define this particular patient's individual combination of symptoms, their intensity and expression.

The focus of observation is not only on objectively verifiable data and dysfunctions, but also on the significance of these dysfunctions for the patient's quality of life and living conditions. In other words, physical therapists not only adhere to the rules of biomedical thinking customary in clinical medicine, they also base their intervention on a biopsychosocial view such as that expressed in the International Classification of Functioning, Disability, and Health (ICF). Just as important as the extent to which movement is restricted, and how this restriction could be reduced or even resolved, is the issue of everyday activities for which the patient urgently requires unrestricted movement. Does restriction mean incapacity for employment or is it, despite being inconvenient, of secondary importance to quality of life? The motivation and cooperation of the patient are influenced quite decisively by such subjective factors and finding out about them is therefore an indispensable step in the examination and treatment process. All this applies equally, if not even more so, if the patient accesses the physical therapist directly without a referral or "prescription."

The experienced therapist succeeds in maintaining a constant interplay between the examination and treatment process because the results of the one determine the form of the other, and at certain points of the treatment a re-examination becomes necessary. For the therapist who is still learning, this is too ambitious—he or she must first learn and practice the steps and techniques of careful physical therapeutic diagnosis, just as he or she also learns and practices the steps and techniques of the therapeutic process. Then, with increasing practice and experience, he or she will be able to bring them both into line and structure the transitions smoothly.

The contents of this book contribute to this gradual development of therapeutic competence. First, the complex process is described and then individual techniques for the examination of structures and functions of the musculoskeletal system, including posture and muscle balance, as well as cardiopulmonary functions, are explained. Particular attention is paid to pain as a principal symptom of numerous dysfunctions and as one of the main reasons for seeking medical and therapeutic assistance in the first place.

The overall aim of this book is to clarify that a physical therapeutic diagnosis is a prerequisite for treating patients individually and effectively in order to help them to enjoy the best possible participation in life in the best-case scenario. Careful examination ensures that treatment starts with the patient's main problem, takes advantage of the patient's own resources and—in the best-case scenario— leads to the intended result.

The editors are delighted to be able to present this approach to physical therapy examination to the English-speaking world and we have the Thieme Publishing Group to thank for this, in particular Angelika Findgott and Jo Stead from Thieme Publishers.

*Antje Hueter-Becker*
*Mechthild Doelken*

# Contributors

**Salah Bacha, PT**
Nürnberg, Germany

**Jan Cabri, PT, PhD**
Professor
Nowegian School of Sport Sciences
Department of Physical Performance
Oslo, Norway

**Mechthild Doelken, PT**
School for Physical Therapists
Mannheim, Germany

**Andreas Fruend**
Head of the Department of Physical Therapy
Heart Center North Rhine Westphalia
Bad Oeynhausen, Germany

**Elly Hengeveld, MSc, BPT, OMT svomp,
Clin Spec Fisioswiss/MSK**
Senior Teacher OMT Maitland-Concept (IMTA)
Oberentfelden, Switzerland

**Antje Hueter-Becker**
Neckargemünd, Germany

**Petra Kirchner**
Teacher of Physical Therapy
Frankfurt am Main, Germany

**Brigitte Tampin, PT, Grad Dip Manip Ther, MSc, PhD**
Advanced Scope Physiotherapist,
Sir Charles Gairdner Hospital
Adjunct Research Fellow,
Curtin University
Perth, Australia

**Barbara Trinkle**
School for Physical Therapists
Mannheim, Germany

# 1 The Physical Therapy Process: Examination, Clinical Reasoning, and Reflection

# 1 The Physical Therapy Process: Examination, Clinical Reasoning, and Reflection

*Elly Hengeveld*

## 1.1 The Physical Therapy Process

Physical therapy is a process during which the therapist assumes different roles. The physical therapist must accompany, lead, teach, and advise the patient during the process of rehabilitation, usually of movement dysfunction.

Within this process, examination and clinical reasoning, together with therapeutic interventions, form an inseparable unit with no formally defined boundaries. Many examination methods can also be used as treatment techniques. Generally speaking, treatment should never be performed without a prior examination, and no treatment should be performed without regularly assessing its effects (Maitland 1986; Hengeveld and Banks 2014a,b). Thus, in addition to treatment interventions, various forms of *assessment* are used in all physical therapy sessions to monitor the therapeutic process as closely as possible (**Fig. 1.1**). It is essential during various critical phases of the overall therapeutic process to regularly reflect on hypotheses, interactions, and actions, including the explicit planning of subsequent procedures.

### 1.1.1 The Physical Therapy Examination

Since the early years of the physical therapy profession in the late 19th century, the examination has played a central role in all physical therapy procedures. However, professional associations have not always made it clear that therapists themselves must perform an examination in order to draw up an individualized treatment plan together with a patient. Even now, those outside the profession frequently assume that physical therapists can plan their treatments on the basis of a biomedical diagnosis alone. This is often reflected in physician referrals, patients' expectations, and health insurance policies that often fail to reimburse physical therapists for their specific examination procedures.

However, for several decades now it has been suggested that physical therapists should clinically assess a patient's problem with a biomedical diagnosis from the physical therapy–specific perspective before embarking on the treatment process (Maitland 1968). This process of emancipation is based on the growing recognition that, as a result of their specialized knowledge base, physical therapists use their own problem-solving processes and that these differ from the way other clinicians, for instance, physicians, think (Parry 1991). The current definition of the World Confederation for Physical Therapy (WCPT) clearly states that the specific examination is an essential part of the physical therapy process for achieving satisfactory treatment results (WCPT 1999).

In order to develop a comprehensive treatment plan with a patient, the specific physical therapy examination must identify any precautions and contraindications to examination and treatment procedures. Treatment goals are formulated in collaboration with the patient before appropriate interventions (and possible alternatives) are chosen.

The physical therapy process is a hypothesis-guided process (Payton 1985) similar to the problem-solving processes applied in other fields such as medicine and physics (Elstein et al 1978; Larkin et al 1980). During the patient interview, physical examination tests, and also while applying therapeutic interventions, therapists constantly formulate different hypotheses that will be modified by further information and the patient's response to the therapy (Grant et al 1988). Most experienced physical therapists group their hypotheses into categories to enhance the efficiency of the examination and treatment process (Thomas-Edding 1987). These categories of hypotheses are discussed later on in this chapter on pages 18–19 (**Fig. 1.2**).

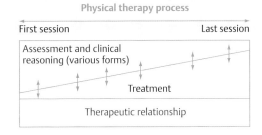

Fig. 1.1 Examination and treatment are two distinct but related procedures in the physical therapy process and should not be considered independently. The process as a whole is supported by the therapeutic relationship.

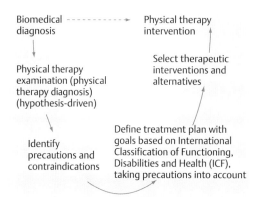

**Fig. 1.2** The biomedical diagnosis alone is not sufficient to perform individualized physical therapy treatment. The physical therapy process begins with the examination, which then forms the basis for a comprehensive treatment plan in accordance with the International Classification of Functioning, Disabilities and Health (ICF) (Hengeveld 1994; WHO 2001).

The process of formulating hypotheses has been described as a cyclical process in which hypotheses are formulated, confirmed, modified, and rejected throughout the entire physical therapy process. The process begins during the first encounter and continues throughout all the sessions with a patient (Jones 1989, 1992; Higgs et al 2008). It is essential that physical therapists use different forms of assessment, and these will be described at a later stage in this chapter (see pp. 21–33) (Hengeveld and Banks 2005). From one session to the next, therapists need to evaluate treatment results in disciplined reassessment procedures and must reflect on the hypotheses they have formulated to guide the treatment process (**Fig. 1.3**).

## 1.1.2   Paradigms in Physical Therapy

As a result of scientific developments in the physical therapy profession, various authors questioned to which body of knowledge the research outcomes should contribute (Hislop 1975; Cott et al 1995; Higgs and Jones 1995; NPI 1997). Hence, for some time now numerous authors have also been reflecting on the paradigms that form the basis of the clinical practice and research of physical therapists and what specific contributions physical therapists make to a society's health (Kuhn 1962; Engel 1977; Antonowsky 1987; Waddell 1987; Krebs and Harris 1988; Pratt 1989; Tyni-Lenné 1989; Hullegie 1995; APTA 1998; Hengeveld 1998 b; WCPT 1999).

For historical reasons, physical therapists seem mainly to follow the dominant biomedical model of reasoning (Hengeveld 2003 b, c), even though there is growing recognition that this model is inadequate when it comes to planning and executing physical therapy interventions. There is increasing support for the notion that physical therapists are following paradigms that are specific to the profession and different from the models used in other areas of medicine (Hislop 1975; Tyni-Lenné 1989; Roberts 1994; APTA 1998).

## Movement as the Common Denominator

In the discussion on different paradigms it has been recognized that the common denominator of all physical therapy concepts can be found in different aspects of movement functions. Hence, the WCPT defines physical therapy within a biopsychosocial movement paradigm (WCPT 1999):

---

**The Nature of Physical Therapy**
Physical therapy is about working with people and populations to maintain and restore maximum movement and functional ability throughout their lives. Physical therapy is particularly important in circumstances where movement and function are threatened by the process of aging or by injury or disease. It places full and functional movement at the heart of what it means to be healthy.

It is concerned with identifying and maximizing movement potential, within the spheres of promotion, prevention, treatment, and rehabilitation. This is achieved through interaction between physical therapist, patients or clients and caregivers, in a process of assessing movement potential and in working towards agreed objectives using knowledge and skills unique to physical therapy.

Assumptions underlying the knowledge and practice of physical therapy include the following:
- Movement: The capacity to move is an essential element of health and well-being. Movement is dependent upon the integrated, coordinated function of the human body at a number of different levels of a movement continuum (Cott et al 1995).
- Movement is purposeful and is affected by internal and external factors.
- Physical therapy is directed towards the movement needs and potential of the individual. (WCPT 1999)

---

Although the biopsychosocial movement paradigm seems to be the leading paradigm of physical therapists, they will often need to incorporate other models in their decision-making processes (see **Fig. 1.4**):

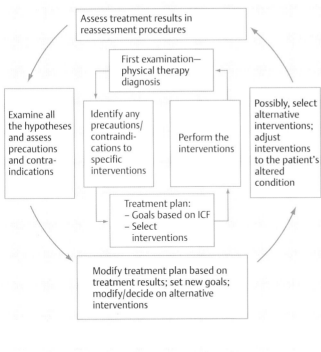

**Fig. 1.3** The physical therapy process is a cyclical process in which, from one session to the next, the therapist assesses whether the treatment goals have been achieved and whether the treatment plan and hypotheses the treatment was based on need to be modified (Hengeveld 2003 b, c).

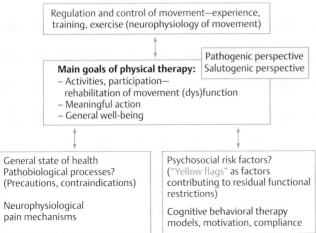

**Fig. 1.4** Different models are used for comprehensive treatment in physical therapy processes (Hengeveld 2004).

- The biomedical paradigm, in order to identify possible precautions and contraindications to examination and treatment. Within this paradigm physical therapists make use of knowledge from pathology, physiology, and other biomedical sciences.
- Cognitive behavioral therapy models, which are relevant for motivating, teaching, and monitoring behavioral changes in patients with regard to patterns of habitual movement and consistently applying self-management strategies in daily life.

- Neurophysiological models, for instance, serve to understand the factors underlying the symptoms and pain, as well as to teach patients about the benefits of movement, relaxation, and other modalities in the treatment of pain.
- The rehabilitation model with the ICF (WHO 2001). Most movement (dys-)functions should be analyzed based on levels of function (impairment), activity, and participation. Furthermore, it is recommended that treatment goals are defined on the basis of this classification.

• The dominant movement paradigm can also be interpreted in various ways:
  – From a pathogenic perspective, where abnormal movement patterns, control processes, and biomechanical deviations are analyzed.
  – From a salutogenic perspective, where approaches are established that are important to enable the patient to engage in meaningful activities in daily life. Salutogenic aspects, such as a sense of coherence, a sense of control over well-being, and understanding treatment objectives, play an important role (Antonowsky 1987; Schüffel et al 1998).

In order to play a successful part in interdisciplinary teams physical therapists should be aware of their identity in the medical field and the unique role they play in treating patients. Therefore, an awareness of the different paradigms underlying decision-making processes is essential (Parry 1991; Rothstein 1994; Bélanger 1998; Beeston 1999). Conflicts may arise when members of multidisciplinary teams are unaware of the various paradigms and behavior of the different team members, and instead strictly adhere to the biomedical model (Hengeveld 2000). For instance, a physical therapist may succeed, after much effort, in motivating a patient to regularly perform specific exercises and relaxation techniques for pain control and to improve their sense of well-being, rather than relying on a structural-biomedical diagnosis in which a "quick fix" can be expected. As a result, the patient starts to become aware of a movement paradigm for treating his or her disorder. The pain may indeed already have decreased, but it may not yet have completely disappeared.

However, when a patient says during a consultation with his or her physician that he or she is still in pain, the physician may not have clarified the actual degree of pain. Based on this statement the physician may decide, without consulting the other team members, to refer the patient to another medical specialist. The patient, by being returned to the biomedical model, may then assume that "something must be wrong," which can only be remedied by injections or surgery. This in turn may reduce their motivation to follow the self-management strategies offered by physical therapy.

## 1.1.3    Physical Therapy Diagnosis

As part of the above-mentioned emancipation process, which involves reflecting on various paradigms and on professional identity, a number of authors have argued that a profession-specific diagnosis should play a central role in the overall therapeutic process (Sahrmann 1988; Rose 1989; Guccione 1991). Generally speaking, the physical therapy diagnosis is expressed in terms of an analysis of movement and function. It has also been argued in physical therapy research processes that criteria should be defined that correspond to the physical therapy diagnosis. Such inclusion criteria should describe movement dysfunction, such as motor control patterns (Maluf et al 2000; O'Sullivan 2005), or symptom behavior during repeated active movements (McKenzie 1981; Maluf et al 2000), and others.

Physical therapy diagnosis has been described by the WCPT as follows:

---

**Diagnosis**
Diagnosis represent[s] the outcome of the process of clinical reasoning [and] ... may be expressed in terms of movement dysfunction or may encompass categories of impairments, activity limitations, participatory restrictions, environmental influences or abilities/disabilities. (WCPT 1999)

---

## Is Biomedical Thinking Outdated?

Despite the increasing focus on specific physical therapy diagnostics, biomedical thinking continues to be of great importance in the physical therapy decision-making process. On the one hand, biomedical information helps to determine the course and prognosis of a given disorder, while on the other it also helps to assess any precautions and/or contraindications related to certain physical therapy interventions.

In fact, both methods of diagnosis can be reciprocally beneficial: just as a physical therapy diagnosis may point to a biomedical diagnosis, a biomedical diagnosis may also provide clues to the physical therapy diagnosis. Nevertheless, it is recommended that physical therapists do not skip the specific physical therapy process of examination and evaluation when planning and implementing treatment.

**Specific characteristics of the physical therapy process**
· It includes examination and assessment, diagnosis, planning, interventions, and reassessment.
· It involves analysis and synthesis within a clinical reasoning process.
· The diagnosis represents the outcome of the clinical reasoning process.
· Planning includes determining the need for interventions and developing a treatment plan,
  including measurable, observable, and achievable treatment goals.
· The interventions are implemented and modified in order to achieve the agreed goals.
  This can include the following:
  – Manual handling
  – Movement enhancement
  – Physical, electrotherapeutic, and mechanical applications
  – Aids and orthotics
  – Patient instruction and education
  – Documentation, coordination
  – Communication
· The interventions are aimed at treating and preventing restrictions of function and movement, impairments,
  and injuries, as well as supporting the promotion of health, quality of life, and fitness at every stage of life
  and in every population group.
· Reassessment serves to evaluate the treatment outcomes.

**Fig. 1.5**  Specific characteristics of the physical therapy process (WCPT 1999).

## 1.2    Clinical Reasoning as Part of the Physical Therapy Process

The WCPT has described the process of physical therapy in detail and clinical reasoning plays a central role (**Fig. 1.5**).

Clinical reasoning is often mentioned in connection with decision-making processes and problem-solving strategies. This has its origins in the early history of research on the clinical reasoning process.

The term "clinical reasoning" originated in learning psychology. Since the 1950s, research has been undertaken in many areas, such as chess, physics, computer science, and medicine, on how experts and novices differ in their decision-making and problem-solving processes.

Several phases in this research can be identified (Patel and Arocha 1995):
- During the first phase, the precognitive era, studies focused on behavioral differences between experts and novices. It was found that experts employed more efficient and better problem-solving processes (Elstein et al 1978). During this phase, various instruments were developed for studying clinical reasoning, for instance simulation methods that imitate actual patient situations. Written case studies, actors re-enacting actual clinical situations, and, somewhat later, computer simulations, are examples of simulation methods used to observe differences in behavior between experts and novices.
- Later, cognitive research came more to the fore. In this phase it was discovered that experts have a better organized, more in-depth, and broader knowledge base. It was recognized that many

decisions are based on hypotheses and pattern recognition (Elstein et al 1978; Norman and Patel 1987). As far as medical practitioners are concerned, it has been established that many of their decisions are based on their direct experiences with other patients, stored in the practitioner's memory. These stories are directly accessible. Over time, theoretical knowledge gained during initial training becomes increasingly embedded in clinical experiences with patients and recedes into the background ("encapsulation of knowledge") (Schmidt and Boshuizen 1993; Robertson 1996 a, b).
- In the fields of medicine, occupational therapy, and physical therapy, research has in recent years increasingly focused on interpretative, cognitive functions. This type of clinical reasoning research has shown that, along with hypothesis-guided clinical reasoning, other forms of reasoning are being used that are of particular relevance in interactions with people. Indeed, it has been observed that experts often employ various forms of clinical reasoning simultaneously (Fleming 1991; Mattingly and Fleming 1994; Edwards et al 1998; Hengeveld 1998 a; Higgs et al 2008), that they have different interactions with patients (Jensen et al 1990, 1992), and often take a person's individual story and illness experience into more consideration when planning treatment (Mattingly and Fleming 1994). The expert's personal knowledge base, feelings, and aspects of intuition are starting to play an increasing role in clinical

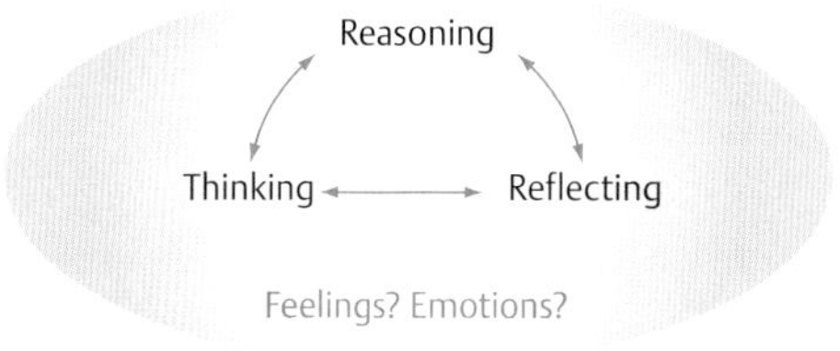

Fig. 1.6 Clinical reasoning is a mixture of thinking, feeling, and reflecting. Reflection is an essential aspect of developing experiential knowledge and expertise.

reasoning processes (Carroll 1988; Higgs and Titchen 1995). Research has increasingly focused on this kind of implicit clinical reasoning. There is growing recognition that, along with a theoretical knowledge base, people working in professions that require practical skills (e.g., carpenters, physical therapists, surgeons) also draw on another knowledge base that differs from the cognitive, theoretical one, and that has long been neglected in the scientific world. This knowledge derived from practical experience has been called the *experiential knowledge base* (Schön 1983).

## Reasoning, Thinking, and Reflecting

A mixture of *thinking* (as a more automatic process) and *reflection* (as a conscious process) play an important role in clinical reasoning (**Fig. 1.6**). It has been recognized that people who are true experts in their profession have reflective skills (Schön 1983), Therefore, in order to develop their expertise, it is recommended that physical therapists regularly reflect on their own way of thinking, their decisions, their feelings, the chosen examination and treatment procedures, the therapeutic results, and any interactions between the client and therapist. This process of regular, disciplined reflection allows one to learn from each encounter with a patient, which in itself will then contribute to further developing one's *experiential knowledge base*. Especially in professions such as physical therapy, which are frequently considered "an art as well as a science" (Peat 1981; Grant 1995), experiential knowledge plays a key role in clinical decision-making processes (Nonaka and Takeuchi 1995).

## Definitions of Clinical Reasoning

There are several views of clinical reasoning as well as of its training and research, all of which are equally valuable (Ryan 1995). This has resulted in a number of definitions, each of which reflects the philosophical and historical background of its authors:

- In their original definition, the physical therapists Higgs and Jones tended toward a cognitive perspective. They interpreted clinical reasoning as the "thought processes and decision-making processes which underpin clinical practice" (Higgs 1992 a, b; Higgs and Jones 2000).
- The anthropologist Mattingly and the occupational therapist Fleming (1994) adopt a more phenomenological perspective. They consider clinical reasoning as primarily a tacit, implicit, complex problem-solving process. The focus is not only on the biomedical diagnosis, but also on the person with his or her individual experience of the disorder. It is more than applied science, and rather like "applied phenomenology." During a treatment session the therapist will normally not only assess the possible causes and potential treatments of the disorder, but also how to actively integrate the patient into the rehabilitation process. Often therapists may themselves not be fully aware of all of the subtle decisions they are taking during this process (Mattingly and Fleming 1994).
- The occupational therapist Ryan regards clinical reasoning as a continuous process that also takes place outside of the therapeutic setting. She postulated that clinical reasoning is a process that occurs before, during, and after treatment sessions. It occurs in both therapeutic and in private situations. Many steps in this process are implicit, unconscious, and automatic. These processes must be made explicit in comprehensive clinical practice. They may include cognitions and emotions (Ryan 1995, 1996; Alsop and Ryan 1996).
- Over the course of many years of research and exchange with like-minded researchers, Higgs and Jones (2008, p. 4) expanded the definition of clinical reasoning as follows:

*Clinical reasoning (or practice decision making) is a context-dependent way of thinking and decision making in professional practice to guide practice actions. It involves the construction of narratives to make sense of the multiple factors and interests pertaining to the current reasoning task. It occurs within a set of problem spaces informed by the practitioner's unique frames of reference, workplace context and practice models, as well as by the patient's or client's contexts. It utilizes core dimensions of practice knowledge, reasoning and metacognition and draws on these capacities in others. Decision-making within clinical reasoning occurs in micro, macro and meta levels and may*

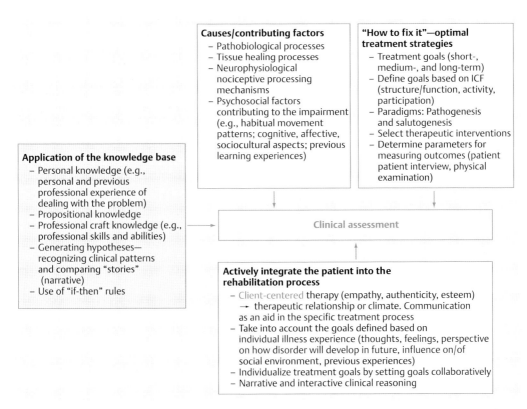

**Causes/contributing factors**
- Pathobiological processes
- Tissue healing processes
- Neurophysiological nociceptive processing mechanisms
- Psychosocial factors contributing to the impairment (e.g., habitual movement patterns; cognitive, affective, sociocultural aspects; previous learning experiences)

**"How to fix it"—optimal treatment strategies**
- Treatment goals (short-, medium-, and long-term)
- Define goals based on ICF (structure/function, activity, participation)
- Paradigms: Pathogenesis and salutogenesis
- Select therapeutic interventions
- Determine parameters for measuring outcomes (patient patient interview, physical examination)

**Application of the knowledge base**
- Personal knowledge (e.g., personal and previous professional experience of dealing with the problem)
- Propositional knowledge
- Professional craft knowledge (e.g., professional skills and abilities)
- Generating hypotheses— recognizing clinical patterns and comparing "stories" (narrative)
- Use of "if-then" rules

Clinical assessment

**Actively integrate the patient into the rehabilitation process**
- Client-centered therapy (empathy, authenticity, esteem) → therapeutic relationship or climate. Communication as an aid in the specific treatment process
- Take into account the goals defined based on individual illness experience (thoughts, feelings, perspective on how disorder will develop in future, influence on/of social environment, previous experiences)
- Individualize treatment goals by setting goals collaboratively
- Narrative and interactive clinical reasoning

**Fig. 1.7** The clinical reasoning processes of the physical therapist are complex. Decisions must be made about the possible causes of the problem, optimal treatment strategies, and actively integrating the patient into the process. A broad, in-depth knowledge base significantly influences the process (Mattingly 1991; Higgs and Titchen 1995; Hengeveld 1998 a; Edwards et al 1998).

*be individually or collaboratively conducted. It involves metaskills of critical conversations, knowledge generation, practice model authenticity and reflexivity.*

- In contemporary physical therapy, where the focus is on evidence-based practice, clinical reasoning has also been referred to as "wise action," in which a balanced approach to scientific and clinical information guides the decision-making processes. It is recommended that physical therapists base their decisions on the "best of science," the "best of therapies," and the "best of the patient and therapist" (Linton 1998; Higgs and Jones 2000; Higgs et al 2008).

To conclude, the processes of clinical reasoning in physical therapy are complex. The physical therapist must simultaneously make many decisions on various levels to adequately address the patient's overall clinical situation.

In order to allow for individualized treatment, a clinical judgment must be made with regard to:

- The possible causes of and factors contributing to the problem
- Treatment strategies
- Actively integrating the patient into the treatment process

The physical therapist's knowledge base and the use of various paradigms, as described on pages 16–18 and 4–6 respectively, have an important role to play in this process.

These decision-making processes are largely tacit, implicit processes. They should be made explicit, however, to help novices become experts in the course of their training, to promote the development of the profession as a whole, and to instigate meaningful clinical research to be performed (**Fig. 1.7**).

## Basic Models

As described above, the treatment process is a cyclical process in which assessment, treatment, and reassessment procedures guide the overall therapy.

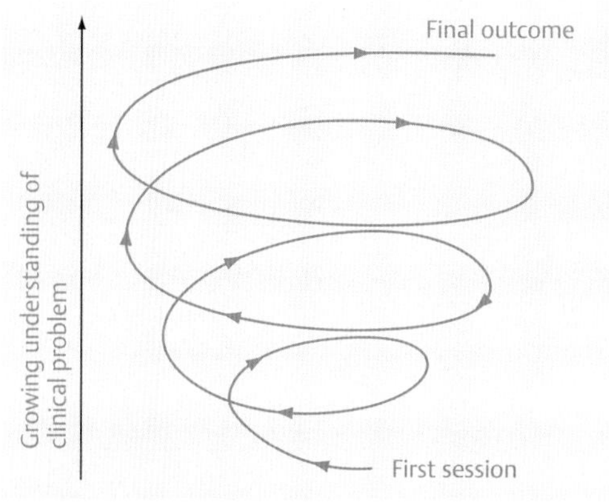

Fig. 1.8 Clinical reasoning as a cyclical process (Higgs and Jones 1995).

Within this context two basic, complementary models of clinical reasoning have been proposed:

- A cyclical model (Higgs and Jones 1995)
- Multiple forms or the "three-track mind" model (Fleming 1991; Mattingly and Fleming 1994)

Higgs and Jones (1995) describe clinical reasoning as a developing process that resembles a spiral and that occurs during all the sessions with the patient (**Fig. 1.8**). It is essential that physical therapists recognize and acknowledge the patient's unique situation at all times and understand that the therapeutic process often, if not always, allows for different interpretations and solutions (Higgs and Jones 1995).

The central elements of this process are:

- The therapist's personal and profession-specific knowledge base
- Cognition (thought processes, insights)
- Metacognition (reflecting on one's own thinking and decision-making processes)

### Generating and Testing Hypotheses

Over the course of the therapeutic process, different hypotheses are generated that support the conceptualization of the problem. Various hypotheses are generated while interviewing the patient during the subjective examination and while performing the physical examination, as well as during all subsequent treatment. These hypotheses may be confirmed, refined, or rejected over the course of the treatment process, provided the therapeutic process is guided by a consistent, disciplined process of reassessment to monitor the effects of the therapeutic interventions (Hengeveld and Banks 2005). Hypothesis development will be influenced by the theoretical and experiential knowledge base that therapists

have developed over the course of their training and clinical experience. Well-developed patient interviewing and physical examination skills are required in order to obtain the relevant and comprehensive information on which multiple hypotheses need to be based. The reassessment procedures are an essential part of confirming, refining, and/or rejecting hypotheses (Jones 1992; Hengeveld and Banks 2014a, b) (**Fig. 1.9a**).

Throughout the entire therapeutic process therapists refine their understanding of the patient's disorder, the cause, contributing factors, and optimum treatment interventions. However, patients themselves can go through a similar, cyclical process of refining and deepening their understanding of their problem and the therapeutic possibilities, particularly if therapists attend carefully to their roles as advisor, provider of information, and teacher (Edwards et al 1998) (**Fig. 1.9b**).

### Multiple Forms of Clinical Reasoning: The Therapist with the "Three-track Mind"

It has been recognized that various forms of clinical reasoning are employed in physical therapy (Edwards et al 1998; Hengeveld 1998a). This has been further researched in the various specialties in physical therapy, such as manual therapy, neurological rehabilitation, and community physical therapy (Edwards et al 2004).

While the physical therapists Higgs and Jones initially concentrated on clinical reasoning with hypothesis-guided thinking,[*] including pattern recognition, the anthropologist Mattingly and the occu-

---

[*] Hypothesis-guided clinical decision-making processes have been referred to as a hypothetico-deductive process. In fact, however, they are an aspect of both inductive and deductive reasoning processes. As inductive processes, hypotheses are generated on the basis of cues gathered mainly during subjective and physical examination procedures, as well as when monitoring reactions when applying treatment. In a sense the deductive process can be observed in the reassessment of therapeutic interventions in which, depending on the outcome, hypotheses may be confirmed, modified, refined, or rejected. Furthermore, experienced therapists can take future decisions with new clients deductively based on the clinical experience they have gained in earlier, similar clinical presentations with other patients. Also, if a therapist applies recommendations from evidence-based guidelines, a more deductive reasoning process takes place in which generalized observations from scientific studies are applied to the individual patient's situation. However, in any kind of induction and deduction, therapists need to give clinical proof of whether the induced hypotheses or deduced generalizations are indeed of benefit to individual clients. Critical thinking and observation as well as in-depth reflective skills are essential to this process.

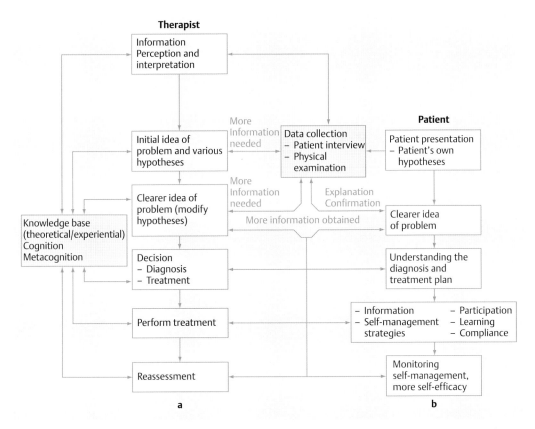

**Fig. 1.9a, b** During the treatment process, hypotheses may be modified or confirmed by the therapist (a), as well as by the patient (b) (Jones 1992; Edwards et al 1998).

pational therapist Fleming have focused on multiple forms of clinical reasoning employed in practice (Fleming 1991; Mattingly and Fleming 1994). They found that, regardless of individual personality and preferences, therapists frequently use various forms of clinical reasoning simultaneously. They call this the "therapist with the three-track mind." This occurs with various intentions and is guided by the specific features of the clinical problem. It appears that, with increasing years of professional experience, therapists seem to switch more easily between various forms of clinical reasoning without even being aware of doing so (Fleming 1991; Mattingly and Fleming 1994).

### Forms of Clinical Reasoning

Various forms of clinical reasoning have been described over the years. Depending on the clinical context and the problem, these can be used in combination. **Table 1.1** sets out these different types of clinical reasoning (see also **Table 1.2**—Exercise 1: Case study).

### Factors Influencing Clinical Reasoning

Various factors have been described that influence a physical therapist's clinical reasoning:
- Cognition, metacognition, reflective skills, professional knowledge, and experiential knowledge (Higgs and Jones 1995)
- The therapist's values and views
- The patient's values and views
- The therapist's life experience and personal knowledge base
- Emotions
- The patient's knowledge base
- The patient's and therapist's previous experiences
- Cultural factors (which contribute to values)
- The patient's social environment, occupation, economic status
- The clinic's biomedical or biopsychosocial focus
- The clinic's management structure
- The collaborative structure (authoritarian, multidisciplinary, interdisciplinary, or transdisciplinary)

**Table 1.1** Forms of clinical reasoning

| Form | Description |
| --- | --- |
| Diagnostic reasoning | This is used to determine possible underlying pathobiological processes. Evaluating the impairment of structures, local functions, activity limitations, resources, and restrictions on participation based on the ICF (WHO 2001) can also be considered an aspect of this type of clinical reasoning. It generally uses predetermined examination procedures (procedural reasoning) |
| Theoretical reasoning | Theories are used as a guide, providing a system-oriented approach to the planning and organization of therapeutic interventions<br>For instance, in manual therapy, the convex–concave rule of biomechanics can help in deciding how passive mobilization techniques need to be applied (Williams and Warwick 1980). In restricted knee bending, for example, dorsal gliding and internal rotation may be used. However, the appropriateness of the decision must be proven clinically. Regular reassessment procedures are essential for evaluating the treatment outcome (Maitland 1986) |
| Practical reasoning | Practical reasoning is distinct from theoretical reasoning. The result is clinical action. The context and the patient play an important role (Mattingly 1991). This type of clinical reasoning is largely done unconsciously and decisions are more likely determined by experiential (often intuitive) knowledge (Schön 1983):<br>• The result of the above-mentioned convex–concave rule can be the following: If dorsal gliding applied to the tibia fails to achieve the desired outcome (improved knee bending) ventral gliding, lateral gliding, or rotational accessory movements could perhaps be attempted instead, particularly if these movement directions seem more restricted than on the unaffected side (Maitland 1987)<br>• For instance, if according to an evidence-based program a stressed mother of three children is told to practice for 45 minutes a day, practical reasoning would suggest tailoring this program to her individual situation to avoid increasing her burden |
| Procedural reasoning | This follows predetermined procedures in the examination and treatment planning, usually along with hypothesis-guided thinking, which is increasingly based on pattern recognition as one gains professional experience over the years |
| Interactive reasoning | This is involved in shaping the therapeutic relationship. It also involves the complex interpretation of subtle interactive clues that are perceived during a treatment encounter, such as the therapist's and patient's choice of words and intonation, and verbal and nonverbal behavior |
| Conditional reasoning | This occurs regularly throughout treatment. The therapist reflects on how the current interventions might affect the patient's future functioning and actions |
| Narrative reasoning | This may be expressed in various ways:<br>• Using stories experienced with other patients to underline recommendations or instructions<br>• Actively listening to patients' personal stories to gain a deeper understanding of their individual illness experience<br>• Therapy as a story between the patient and therapist, which unfolds from one session to the next.<br>• The therapist enters the patient's personal life story and can take on a minor or major role in that life story<br>• Therapists tell each other stories to increase their understanding of the illness experience<br>The purpose of narrative reasoning is to design a truly meaningful treatment with the patient and establish a therapeutic relationship based on understanding and trust |
| Ethical reasoning | The patient's values, needs, and individual goals are taken into account when choosing a treatment method |
| Pragmatic reasoning | This is oriented to feasibility within a given framework (e.g., setting priorities when defining treatment objectives if the number and/or time of treatment sessions is reduced due to sociopolitical or other restrictions) |
| Collaborative reasoning | This is related to the process of joint decision-making by the patient and therapist about treatment goals and the choice of interventions (and may also be seen as a component of interactive reasoning) |
| Education/teaching as reasoning | This form of clinical reasoning is used when counseling, advising, instructing, and guiding patients in order to improve their understanding of the effects of their own (movement) behavior (and also includes aspects of narrative, procedural, and interactive clinical reasoning) |
| Intuitive, implicit, silent ("tacit") reasoning | This is a very common form of reasoning and increases over the years of professional experience. Intuitive reasoning is often "tacit" reasoning, and decisions based on this type of reasoning cannot be discussed with colleagues. As intuitive reasoning is mostly an unconscious process, clinicians need to develop their reflective skills to be able to share reasons for their clinical decisions with colleagues and students, to enhance further personal and professional development, and thus to contribute to the overall development of the profession |

Sources: Mattingly (1991); Mattingly and Fleming (1994); Munroe (1996); Higgs and Jones (2000).

**Table 1.2** Clinical reasoning processes occur immediately in the early phase of the encounter with a patient (

| | | |
|---|---|---|
| *Exercise 1: Case study—analysis of the various types of clinical reasoning and application of knowledge in the greeting phase of treatment* | | |

- An older gentleman, about 70 years old, is sitting in the waiting room. He greets you with a smile. You smile back and greet him. You know that he has been referred to you with shoulder symptoms. He shakes your hand while still seated. He winces and can barely raise his arm
- **Take a moment to write down your thoughts about this encounter—before reading the next paragraph**
- You introduce yourself too, stating your name and function. You also explain that you would like to perform a physical therapy examination before proceeding with treatment. The man agrees to this and smiles again. Then he says: "I'm glad I could come. My arm has been bothering me for ages. I can't lift it at all, and I'm right-handed. I can barely do anything I need to"
- As you walk toward the treatment room you ask him: "Did something happen to cause the problem?"
- He says: "I slipped on ice about six months ago. It hurt so badly I could hardly lift my arm. The pain has gone, but I still can't lift my arm"
- **Now write down your thoughts, taking this new information into consideration—have your thoughts and hypotheses changed?**

*Analysis*

| | Perhaps your thoughts went along the following lines | Now evaluate which types of clinical reasoning were used in the encounter and thought processes: |
|---|---|---|
| **First part**<br>An older gentleman, about 70 years old, is sitting in the waiting room. He greets you with a smile. You smile back and greet him. You know that he has been referred to you with a shoulder symptom. He shakes your hand while still seated. He winces and can barely raise his arm | **First part**<br>"Ah, this is a friendly man. I can probably work well with him; he's smiling at me and seems open-minded. But I'm not happy about the way he winced when he tried to raise his arm and greet me—does it hurt that much? If so, then I'll have to examine his shoulders and neck. They might be sources of the nociceptive process. Of course, other sources might be responsible for the pain as well. But in older people these are often the first things to consider. Of course, I should ask him first, because there can be many reasons why a person winces and cannot lift their arm" | Interactive<br>Procedural<br>Conditional<br>Narrative<br>Diagnostic |
| **Second part**<br>Next, you introduce yourself, stating your name and function. You also explain that you would like to perform a physical therapy examination before proceeding with treatment. The man agrees to this and smiles again. Then he says: "I'm glad I could come. My arm has been bothering me for ages. I can't lift it at all, and I'm right-handed. I can barely do anything I need to"<br>As you walk toward the treatment room, you ask him: "Did something happen to cause the problem?" He says: "I slipped on ice about six months ago. It hurt so badly I could hardly lift my arm. The pain has gone, but I still can't lift my arm" | **Second part**<br>So he is glad to be here, and he appears very motivated. But he seems to be severely restricted in everyday life. Does he have the resources to look for alternatives to certain things he can't do with his right hand? Hmm, he had a fall...I don't like hearing that from an elderly person, since several structures may be damaged—the neck, the shoulder joint itself, neurodynamics, and the musculature. In any case, I will have to examine him closely for possible structural and functional impairments. He says it no longer hurts, but then I would expect him to be able to lift his arm again. Why is it causing such a problem? This could be due to a "frozen shoulder." If so, I'll have to mobilize the structures as best as possible. But it could also be a partial or even a complete muscle lesion. I want to find out for certain from his history which physicians have already examined him and what they thought about treatment within their own discipline. If it is a large muscular tear, then I wonder why surgery was not considered... anyway, I'll have to ask him first. If we're lucky, then it's not half as bad as I think | |

Continued ▷

**Table 1.2** Clinical reasoning processes occur immediately in the early phase of the encounter with a patient (continued)

Although only a small amount of information is available at this point, the clinical reasoning process begins immediately. It involves many thoughts as well as emotions: the therapist is pleased, for instance, that the older gentlemen smiles and she is concerned that her hypothesis about a possible complete muscle lesion will be confirmed

An analysis of the therapist's **knowledge base** shows the following:

- She has an understanding of the **procedural knowledge** applied in her profession; she knows which questions she would like to ask during the patient interview and which areas she would like to assess during the functional evaluation
- She has **experiential knowledge**—she seems to have treated many patients with such problems. (*First part: … Of course, other sources might be responsible for the pain as well. But in older people these are often the first things to consider. … Second part: … Hmm, he had a fall… I don't like hearing that from an elderly person, since several structures may be damaged… He says it no longer hurts, but then I would expect him to be able to lift his arm again. Why is it causing such a problem? This could be due to a "frozen shoulder." If so, I will have to mobilize the structures as best as possible. But it could also be a partial or even a complete muscle lesion…*)
- She has a **theoretical knowledge** of potential sources of arm pain (first and second parts), of the pathology of a "frozen shoulder," and muscle lesions. She is also familiar with ICF terms (WHO 2001) and uses them in analyzing the problem. She also uses medical knowledge, because she says she would expect a larger muscle lesion to be managed surgically rather than conservatively

**Cognitive**: She is able to formulate her thoughts in an orderly fashion, although her thinking may not necessarily be linear during the actual process

**Metacognition—reflection**: During the first and second parts, one aspect of metacognition can be identified:

(*First part: … Of course,* I should ask him first, *because there can be many reasons why* a person winces *and cannot lift their arm. Second part: … If we are lucky, then it's not half as bad as I think*)

We can also observe the cyclical process of clinical reasoning: in the second part the therapist obtains more information and her thinking goes deeper—she develops more hypotheses and she already rejects one ("the primary problem is pain"). Categorizing the hypotheses generated during the reflective phases of the therapeutic process can enhance the efficiency of clinical reasoning (see **Table 1.5**)

- Number of staff
- The clinic management's legal structure
- Policy decisions regarding health care and decisions by professional associations
- Professional paradigms (Alsop and Ryan 1996)

These contextual factors often play a crucial role in clinical situations. The following examples give an indication of how these contextual factors influence clinical reasoning processes:

- Given a sociopolitical situation in which therapists are forced to reduce treatment time and the number of therapeutic sessions, therapists should avoid feeling pressured into fulfilling all of the treatment goals that could be achieved in an ideal setting. Thus, pragmatic and interactive reasoning are needed to help set priorities collaboratively with the patient.
- Personal values, such as the therapist's dominant biomedical perspective, probably lead to a more object-oriented approach to clinical practice, with more procedural reasoning processes being applied and less interactive or narrative reasoning.
- If a patient does not appear to understand that specific movements or meaningful activities can also help to relieve pain and enhance overall well-being, information strategies will often have to be applied that emphasize cognitive behavioral therapeutic approaches using interactive, educational, and narrative clinical reasoning strategies.

## Differences between Experts and Novices

Over the years, research on clinical reasoning in various professional domains has identified several differences between experts and novices. Insights gained serve the teaching of physical therapists on undergraduate and postgraduate programs, to establish profession-specific declarative knowledge, and domain-specific research on the profession.

Various stages have been described that novices pass through on their way to gaining expertise (Dreyfus and Dreyfus 1985):

- Novice
- Advanced beginner
- Competent
- Proficient
- Expert

Experts in a given domain generally have at least 10 years of professional experience, although it is possible that not everyone develops into an expert in their field after 10 years of work experience.

Based on various studies, the various features that distinguish an expert from a novice in a given profession can be summarized as follows:

- Experts develop reflective qualities. They take the time to reflect on unusual or difficult situations in a practice setting or to seek others' advice.
- Experts appear to more efficiently and completely analyze a problem and to have more effective

treatment results. They can demonstrate superior clinical treatment outcomes with more rapid and in-depth problem-solving. Their interpretations and conclusions are more often correct, more thorough, and more self-critical than those of novices.

- Experts have well-organized, active access to their knowledge base and continue to develop their reflective (metacognitive) characteristics.
- Due to their experience with patients, experts appear to have more patient stories in their clinical memory that influence their decision-making processes (encapsulated illness scripts).
- Experts have a larger number of clinical patterns stored in their clinical memory.
- Experts know and apply more "if-then" rules and use them in forward reasoning processes. This reflects their enhanced knowledge organization.
- Given the many patient stories in their clinical memory, experts are more likely to have the greater potential for "reflection-in-action," while novices often require more time for "reflection-on-action."
- Experts may take more time for qualitative problem analysis, that is, they can better take the patient's individual illness experience into account in their treatment planning.
- Experts appear to differ from novices and advanced beginners regarding their time management. While there do not appear to be any great differences with regard to the content of their reasoning, they differ with regard to the quality and quantity of the time they take. Beginners seem to need more time and often repeat themselves without noticing it, while experts can move on more quickly to the next step in clinical reasoning and action.
- Experts are more likely to develop creative—and sometimes unusual—solutions (creative thinking, lateral thinking, thinking "outside the box").
- Experts are aware of their weaknesses as regards clinical reasoning and also understand their preferred pathways in decision-making processes.
- Experts change more smoothly between various forms of clinical reasoning.
- Experts demonstrate conscious, interactive reasoning and actively shape the patient–therapist relationship. They appear to be more empathetic in their communication.
- Experts make more frequent use of nonverbal clues such as a patient's facial expression, intonation, and choice of words in their decision-making processes.

- Experts are not as easily distracted by telephone calls, for instance. After being distracted during a treatment, they tend to be better at picking up where they left off (both interactively as well as procedurally).
- Experts' actions are often less focused on physical processes alone, and they praise their patients more often.

(Jensen et al 1990, 1992; Schmidt and Boshuizen 1993; Mattingly and Fleming 1994; Higgs and Jones 1995; Jones 1995; Ryan 1995; Thomson et al 1997; King and Bithell 1998; Jensen et al 1999.)

In the course of developing their expertise, professionals will increasingly demonstrate the characteristics mentioned above. In order to assist in this process, it is important to give newly qualified physical therapists sufficient time to reflect on their own actions and decisions (reflection-on-action). Experienced professionals are also advised to take the time needed to reflect when confronted with unusual or difficult clinical situations (Alsop and Ryan 1996).

## Reflection-in-action and Reflection-on-action

The terms *reflection-in-action* and *reflection-on-action* were coined by Schön (1983), who found that many experienced practitioners were able to reflect on their actions while performing them (reflection-in-action). Novices, on the other hand, first have to perform the actions and reflect on them afterward (reflection-on-action). Consequently, experienced professionals are better able to perform *forward reasoning* and can, therefore, be more efficient and thorough in their treatments.

Experienced professionals will have no difficulty imagining, before performing an examination, how a patient with a torn rotator cuff muscle that is healing without post-operative complications will present clinically (forward reasoning), because they will often have encountered this problem in clinical practice. They can, therefore, also more quickly recognize when the clinical presentation differs from what they normally see. In addition, they can often already formulate a complete treatment plan, including a prognosis, during the examination and then discuss it with the patient at the end of the session (reflection-in-action = thinking during the action). If, however, they are confronted with a new problem that they have not previously treated, or a highly complex one, such as chronic pain syndrome, then they will probably need to apply reflection-on-action. In such circumstances professionals

**Table 1.3**  Common errors in clinical reasoning processes

| Error | Example |
|---|---|
| Giving preference to certain hypotheses | For instance, aiming treatment only at the glenohumeral joint (GHJ) during the rehabilitation of movement functions after a rotator cuff operation |
| Categorically neglecting other hypotheses | In the same example: forgetting that the cervical spine, the acromioclavicular joint (ACJ), scapulothoracic junction, neurodynamics, and soft tissues can also contribute to the movement limitations |
| A hypothesis is just that and not yet the truth | This misconception can occur in everyday clinical practice, for instance, when early on, pain is explained by a movement dysfunction of the GHJ and thus other options are not considered. The hypothesis must first be confirmed by clinical evidence, based on assessment and reassessment procedures |
| Acting automatically without reflection | In clinical practice, particularly given the tight schedules and long working days, it is possible that no time is available for conscious reflection on new and/or unusual clinical presentations. Errors can easily occur. Also, therapists may not look for unusual or creative solutions to the patient's presentation |
| Insufficient lateral thinking | Nearly always choosing the same treatment interventions for similar clinical presentations |
| Knowledge gaps | What someone does not know, they cannot apply in clinical reasoning |

should not put themselves under any pressure to provide a complete treatment proposal at the end of the first session. Often, it is wise for therapists to explain to the patient that they wish to organize all the information they have gathered during the first session and collect their thoughts (reflection-on-action) and that they would like to clear up any remaining questions at the beginning of the next session and then suggest a treatment plan. Novices and students in particular should be given the necessary time to reflect, in order to guide them in developing their clinical expertise (Alsop and Ryan 1996).

## Advantages of and Common Errors in Clinical Reasoning

It is generally believed that conscious clinical reasoning processes lead to greater efficiency and thoroughness in clinical practice. If therapists recognize certain patterns in a clinical presentation based on past experience, they may take short cuts in various examination procedures.

At this point readers may be feeling uncomfortable with the term "clinical reasoning" and may be wondering whether working with clinical reasoning and using short cuts could lead to superficial actions and mistakes. This is justified and something every experienced professional should consider. It appears to show the difference between an expert and a therapist with many years of professional experience. Experts know where their strengths and weaknesses are in clinical reasoning; they know what their preferred decisions are and where their "blind spot" in clinical reasoning is.

The most common mistakes in clinical reasoning processes are set out in **Table 1.3**.

## Knowledge Base: Development and Role

It has been said that an effective clinician must have developed both a good knowledge base and comprehensive clinical reasoning processes. In this context it has been postulated that knowledge is more likely continuously (re)constructed rather than discovered (Higgs 1992 b). Knowledge is dynamic and personal. It is created by human consciousness in order to understand the world with its related events and personal experiences. It is built upon changing and subjective experience, the interpretation and the understanding of one or more people (Higgs 1992 b).

The knowledge base can be divided into different areas (Higgs and Titchen 1995):
- Personal knowledge
- Propositional knowledge
- Professional craft knowledge

### Personal Knowledge

Personal knowledge is the sum of personal experiences and insights gained over a lifetime. It is shaped by personal experiences as well as by experiences of people in one's immediate environment. Personal interests, values, previous learning experiences, beliefs, and worldview influence the development of one's personal knowledge base. Personal knowledge encompasses affective, conative, spiritual, and esthetic awareness, interpersonal knowledge, and knowledge of being (Higgs and Titchen 1995; Hooper 1997).

> *What learners bring to the situation has an important influence on what is experienced and how it is experienced. Learners possess a personal foundation of experience, a way of being present in the world, which profoundly influences the way in which that world is experienced and which particularly influences the intellectual and emotional content of the experience and the meanings that are attributed to it. (Boud and Walker 1994.)*

However, many therapists seem unaware of their personal viewpoints and motives, although these can unconsciously influence their clinical reasoning.

### Propositional Knowledge

This type of knowledge is determined by theoretical learning processes, schools of thought, research, and the declarative knowledge of the profession. It can contain discursive knowledge, research knowledge, and declarative knowledge (Higgs and Titchen 1995).

Although propositional knowledge forms the basis for clinical reasoning, it must still be applied in practice. In an actual encounter with a patient, therapists must always determine whether propositional knowledge is applicable to the specific, individual case (theory-in-use), as propositional knowledge has its limitations, despite evidence-based practice.

### Professional Craft Knowledge

Professional craft knowledge encompasses practical knowledge, procedural knowledge, and theory-in-use (Higgs and Titchen 1995). It concerns the examination and treatment procedures taught in undergraduate and postgraduate training. It is also related to the use of theoretical models as applied in physical therapy. An essential aspect is *experiential knowledge*, which is acquired in the course of professional experience and has a considerable influence on clinical reasoning processes (Schön 1983; Jensen et al 1990; Higgs 1992 a, b; Nonaka and Takeuchi 1995).

### Knowledge is Constructed, Not Discovered

In clinical reasoning, the knowledge base is constructed rather than discovered. The knowledge base thus continuously develops and is constantly being reorganized (Higgs 1992 a).

Developing a knowledge base is not a passive fact-collecting process. The notion that teachers have all the relevant knowledge and that students are merely passive recipients ("funnel effect") is outdated. This would mean learning from an authority figure who may never be questioned. Such an educational approach would not be conducive to developing an independent and well-founded attitude to learning.

Various forms of knowledge generation have been described (DePoy and Gitlin 2010):
- Following an authority.
- Hearsay (unverified information).
- Trial and error—knowledge developed through specific use, verification, and modification until a desired result is achieved. Trial and error has negative overtones, but it is an important problem-solving process (*heuristic search*). This can be crucial for developing experiential knowledge and recognizing clinical patterns.
- History—knowledge from collective experience.
- Spiritual understanding (knowledge through belief in a higher power).
- Intuition.
- Research—systematic inquiry.

### Reorganization of the Knowledge Base—Encapsulation

On the path toward gaining professional expertise, the knowledge base is continuously reorganized over the course of years of clinical experience (Case et al 2000). Direct experience with patients plays an important role in this process.

Schmidt and Boshuizen (1993) have studied the influence and development of clinical memory in the clinical reasoning processes of medical practitioners. Physicians were given patient case studies and asked for their diagnosis and treatment proposal. The authors found that more experienced physicians linked their biomedical knowledge to direct experiences with patients. This *encapsulation* of knowledge means that their basic theoretical knowledge can no longer be called up in as much detail as just after medical school. In making diagnoses they were strongly guided by past experiences with patients ("patient stories") and the diagnosis was often more efficient and comprehensive. When they are confronted with patients who do not remind them of previous encounters, they try to recognize a pattern. If they are not able to recognize an apparent pattern, they resort to basic examination procedures using hypothesis-guided thinking and directly applying basic theoretical knowledge and consult a book or colleague (Schmidt and Boshuizen 1993) (**Fig. 1.10**).

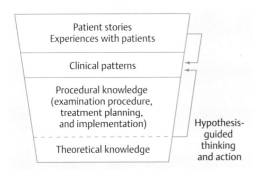

**Fig. 1.10** Memory structure. Adapted from Schmidt and Boshuizen (1993). The clinical memory seems to consist of various layers. Clinical patterns take shape in the therapist's mind as a result of direct experiences with patient stories (narrative reasoning) and hypothesis-guided thinking. Novices can only become experts in their field through lived experiences with patients and by consciously generating and testing hypotheses (Hengeveld, 2001).

Experienced physical therapists presumably use similar decision-making processes. However, many therapists may be unaware of the value of their lived experiences with previous patients for problem-solving in new patients. Therefore, it is essential during undergraduate physical therapy training to develop basic theoretical knowledge along with sound, specific examination and treatment procedures, including clinical reasoning processes with hypothesis-guided thinking and structured reflection. Together, these form the foundation of the therapist's future general knowledge base: lived experiences with patients will lead to the formation of more clinical patterns while more patient stories are recorded in clinical memory. Furthermore, these stories will increasingly influence subsequent clinical decision-making processes.

## Hypothesis Generation, Hypothesis Categories, and the Development of Clinical Patterns

In physical therapy, the notions of procedural reasoning and hypothesis-guided thinking have become widely known as a result of in-depth research by Higgs, Jones, and Payton. It appears that most adults use problem-solving approaches based on hypothesis generation and testing in many different situations in life (Payton 1985).

In therapeutic encounters with patients, therapists are alert to various cues to base their hypotheses on. Therapists usually form several hypotheses early on in the encounter. These are then further developed and modified during all the phases of the treatment process. This is an automatic process and numerous clinical reasoning studies suggest making this a conscious procedure. In general, it is strongly recommended that therapists become consciously aware of these hypotheses following the end of the patient interview, at the end of the functional examination, and after every treatment session.

### Categorizing Hypotheses

In comparative studies of experienced therapists versus novices, it was found that experienced therapists were more thorough in their assessments and gathered more specific information and asked more clarifying questions. Both experienced and novice therapists employed similar procedures during the patient interview and physical examination. The experienced therapists also seemed to be able to summarize the information more completely after the examination and appeared to be less liable to forget important things than novices. In addition, they were better able to distinguish between the relevant main issues and incidental information (Thomas-Edding 1987). It was concluded that the main difference between the two groups regarding clinical reasoning was how they organized the information they were given. While novices tended to absorb information indiscriminately and wanted to organize the information later, after the session with the patient, experienced therapists already did this to a certain degree during the examination. According to Larkin et al (1980), experienced therapists are already *categorizing* the information ("chunking" information). **Table 1.4** summarizes various hypothesis categories that have been described in (neuromusculoskeletal-oriented) physical therapy.

It appears that hypothesis-guided thinking plays a role in all areas of physical therapy (Case et al 2000; Edwards et al 2004). Yet, the hypothesis categories originate from a predominantly orthopedically focused area of physical therapy (Payton 1985; Thomas-Edding 1987; Jones 1989). For instance, for neurological rehabilitation, all categories except for "sources of (local) movement dysfunctions" may be useful in clinical reasoning. However, if a patient with hemiplegia presents with restricted mobility of the hip joint (impairment on a bodily or local functional level) that is making it difficult for them to get up out of a chair, the hypothesis category "sources of stiffness in the hip" could be used, as local hip mobilization and neurodynamic mobilization (impairment treatments) may facilitate the activity.

**Table 1.4** Hypothesis categories

| | |
|---|---|
| Pathobiological mechanisms | Hypotheses on possible tissue pathology ("end organ dysfunction"; Apkarian and Robinson 2010), as well as stages of tissue healing; neurophysiological pain mechanisms, such as peripheral nociceptive, peripheral neurogenic, central nervous system (CNS), and autonomic nervous system mechanisms |
| Sources of movement dysfunctions and nociception | These sources of movement dysfunction may be related to sources of the pain as well as to sources of restricted mobility. This affects hypotheses on the movement dysfunction of joints (local or referred symptoms), muscles, neurodynamic functions, soft tissues, and other vascular and visceral structures that may be contributing to the patient's problem (e.g., check whether pain in the gluteal area originates more in the hip, sacroiliac joint [SIJ], lumbar spine, or from another movement dysfunction) |
| Precautions and contraindications | These are determined by the intensity of the perceived pain, pathobiological processes, as well as stages of tissue regeneration after trauma or operations. Also, contraindications for certain interventions need to be considered in this category. This category influences the "dosage" of examination procedures, the decision as to whether treatment is indicated, and the choice and "dosage" of treatment interventions |
| Prognosis | The prognosis can be made during the initial sessions, as a result of an entire treatment series, or as a long-term prognosis after completing treatment. Various factors determine the prognosis. Sufficient experiential knowledge is needed to provide a differentiated prognosis:<br>• Mechanical versus inflammatory presentation<br>• Irritability of the disorder<br>• Degree of trauma/disability<br>• Length of history and progression of the disorder<br>• Prior dysfunctions<br>• Unicomponential/multicomponential problem<br>• Unidimensional/multidimensional approach to treatment<br>• Patient's expectations<br>• Patient's personality and lifestyle<br>• Cognitive, affective, sociocultural aspects, learning processes<br>• Patient's movement behavior |
| Contributing factors | Any predisposing or additional factor that could be responsible for the movement problem developing or continuing:<br>• Physical<br>• Biomechanical<br>• Social/environmental<br>• Behavioral<br>• Emotional<br>(Examples: Posture, muscular imbalance, motor control patterns movement habits in everyday life, understanding the usefulness of movement when in pain, affective factors such as fear of moving etc.) |
| Degree of disability | This is determined by the limitations and resources with regard to local function and structures, activities, and participation (ICF—WHO 2001) |
| Management | Determine therapeutic goals and treatment interventions while respecting precautions and contraindications<br>These include short- and long-term goals and are related to movement paradigms |
| Individual illness experience | This refers to the patient's individual experience of the disorder. It can be influenced by thoughts, feelings, previous experiences, beliefs, and knowledge about how the disorder will develop in the future, environmental factors, coping possibilities, knowledge, and behavior and other factors |

Sources: Jones (1992, 1995); Hengeveld (1998 a–c, 1999); Higgs and Jones (2000); Hengeveld and Banks (2005); Higgs et al (2008).

Note: Hypothesis categories can be determined individually. In orthopedic musculoskeletal-oriented treatments, the above categories can be applied universally; however, additional categories may be defined depending on the therapist's preferences and paradigms.

**Table 1.5**  Case study and hypothesis development (see **Table 1.2**)

| *Exercise 2: Case study—underline relevant sentences in the text and write the hypothesis category in the right-hand column* | |
|---|---|
| The following information was gathered in the patient interview (subjective examination): | |
| Sometime in the middle of February (it is now the middle of May) the man slipped on an icy street. He turned quickly and grabbed onto a railing, but in doing so twisted his right arm and hit his head. He had severe pain in his upper arm and had difficulty raising his arm. About a week later, on the advice of his wife, he went to see his physician because house-hold remedies, such as ointments, had not been helping much. The physician examined him and ruled out the presence of a fracture. He prescribed a new ointment and asked the patient to return in two weeks if the pain persisted. Three weeks later he went back to his physician, who then gave him an injection in the joint. The pain subsided and he found it somewhat easier to lift his arm and use it for everyday activities (e.g., carrying plates). Yet the pain still made it impossible for him to perform activities that involved lifting his arm above his head. Two weeks later the man went back to see his physician and was given another injection in the joint. The pain practically disappeared after that and he was able to lift his arm more easily, but only up to a certain height. Now he was compensating more with his left arm, but that was very inconvenient for his hobbies, as he spends a great deal of time doing crafts and renovating antique furniture. Also, his grandson, who has Down syndrome, visits him and his wife regularly. He likes to play with the boy and they both enjoy walking along the river. Walking is not a problem, but if they play ball he has diffi-culty throwing the ball with his right arm. It still hurts a little, but he says it is "not worth mentioning." Also, the pain always disappears immediately. It does not disturb his sleep. That only happened during the first 3 to 4 weeks. | |
| He had never had any problems with his arm before. When he was still working as a book-keeper, he occasionally had a little neck pain, but that disappeared after applying ointment or if his wife massaged the area. He has hardly had any problems since retiring, only occa-sionally if he falls asleep watching television and wakes up with his head in a funny posi-tion. Then he does some stretching exercises and "everything is all right again". | |
| He says he feels healthy and does not take any medication. His heart is normal. He is not diabetic. His physician diagnosed an enlarged prostate, but he is now taking pumpkin seed tablets for that. He does not smoke and only occasionally drinks wine or beer. He has no history of serious disease. He is content with his health. | |

## Exercise 3: Example Case Study and Hypothesis Generation

Re-read the case study in **Table 1.2** and then read the information in **Table 1.5**, which is taken from the patient interview (subjective examination). Which hypotheses have you developed based on this information? Underline relevant sentences in the text and write down the corresponding hypoth-esis categories:

Perhaps your thoughts and hypotheses, including the reason (clinical signs), went along the following lines:

- Pathobiological mechanisms, neurophysiologi-cal pain mechanisms, stage of tissue healing:
  - Did he develop a "frozen shoulder" following traumatic capsulitis? If so, then it must have already healed quite well because he says he is in hardly any pain.
  - However, it is possible that he really does have a muscle lesion, because I'm not sure whether the physician performed an ultrasound or a functional radiography examination.
  - But if he is in pain, it is of a stimulus–response nature, which suggests a predominantly noci-ceptive pain mechanism. Also, right now there are no indications of any specific precautions

regarding the "dosage" of physical examina-tion tests due to major pathobiological pro-cesses that should be taken into account.

- Based on the data available at this point, there are no real contraindications to treatment. I am a little bit more cautious given the possibility of a muscle lesion. On the other hand, if his shoulder girdle is stiff (which is quite probable) and there is a muscle lesion, an attempt should still be made to mobilize the structures in order to opti-mize range of motion. I see no particular medical precautions against passive and active joint mobilization. The (minimal) pain tends to come and go, indicating a more simple nociceptive neurophysiological pain mechanism. Further-more, there is no evidence of bone disease or similar problems. He feels healthy and seems always to have been in good health.
- I do not see any significant factors contributing to the impairment experienced by Mr. M. He is not afraid to move his arm. He wants to use his arm and seems to have a high pain tolerance, considering that it was his wife who initially sent him to see his physician. Although he says it still hurts, it is "not worth mentioning." He may have a very stiff thorax. He has already had this prob-

lem for 3 months. If joint stiffness really is the main problem, then I hope that it is not too severe.

- *Sources of the dysfunctions:* If pain and stiffness are the problem, this will become clear during the physical examination with active testing. Then, during the first three sessions I will definitely have to examine the following sources of pain and movement limitation and, if indicated, perform the relevant probationary treatments: glenohumeral joint, acromioclavicular joint, cervical spine, thoracic spine and first four ribs, neurodynamic movements of the upper extremity.
- At a later stage I should examine the muscle length, but—assuming that joint stiffness is the problem—this is not yet relevant to treatment. If my hypothesis about a muscle lesion is right, then I will notice it during the active and passive tests. If there is a large discrepancy between active and passive mobility, then my hypothesis will be confirmed. If so, I will focus more on examining the muscles of the rotator cuff and perform a few instability tests. If a muscle lesion is not confirmed, due to only a slight discrepancy between active and passive mobility, then I will focus fully on the above hypothesis of pain combined with stiffness.
- **Management (goals and interventions):**
  - *Impairments:* These will depend on the functional examination. If the patient has pain and stiffness in the above-mentioned areas, then I will use passive, manual techniques to treat all the affected areas. I should focus on the glenohumeral joint; however, I should not neglect the other areas that may be contributing to the movement disorder. The patient will also be given an accompanying self-management program.
  - If the hypothesis of a muscle lesion is confirmed, or if it is only a partial lesion, then I will try to recruit the musculature using local exercises, which in the medium term should become part of the patient's everyday activities. If this does not work, I should consult his physician to discuss further medical investigation and possible alternative medical (surgical?) treatment.
  - *Activities:* Based on the information I currently have (there are still some pieces missing, e.g., body care, dressing on his own), I think it will be important for him to be able to play (ball) with his grandson again and to pursue his hobbies.
- *Individual illness experience:* The patient appears to have a high pain threshold. It seems that he is not suffering too much as long as he can perform those everyday activities that are important to him. That is why it is important to me that he quickly realizes that he will be able to do so again.

I think he has a rather more internalized locus of control regarding his own sense of well-being. However, in the current situation he does not know what he himself can do about his problem or to improve his sense of well-being. If the hypothesis on joint stiffness proves correct, then I am considering teaching him simple automobilization exercises, which he will definitely also do at home—especially if he starts to feel that his condition is improving. In order to keep him motivated to carry on with the treatment: in the event of stiffness, he could draw marks on the wall so he can occasionally measure his success.

- **Prognosis (short-term, medium-term, long-term):**
  - He has a history of neck pain, although he does not appear to have consulted a physician or therapist for treatment. The pain could also be influencing his shoulder problem, however. Also, he is 72 years old and so his collagen certainly has less elastin than 30 years ago. Still, he seems to be very motivated and open to therapy. If we can cooperate well (and I do not doubt that we will), we will definitely make progress.

    I expect he will regain his full level of activity. If the stiffness is extreme, he may not regain 100% of his mobility, although we will try to achieve his maximum movement potential. If the muscle lesion is small, then the problem is more one of stiffness. If the muscle problem is bigger than expected, then I wonder whether a surgeon should not examine him. I will first do the functional examination. Then I will see which of these hypotheses apply and which do not and whether we are in for any surprises.

---

Thus, it can be said that physical therapists generate numerous, often competing, hypotheses in the examination and treatment process. They need to *deliberately* decide which of these to follow up first during the examination and treatment. There may be an element of trial and error in this where newly qualified physical therapists are concerned, although the process is basically heuristic: decisions need to be based on the therapist's theoretical and clinical knowledge base. When it comes to developing clinical expertise it is important to become aware of all the decisions that need to be taken. A *decision tree* (Watts 1985, 2000) can contribute to an analysis of all the available options (**Fig. 1.11**).

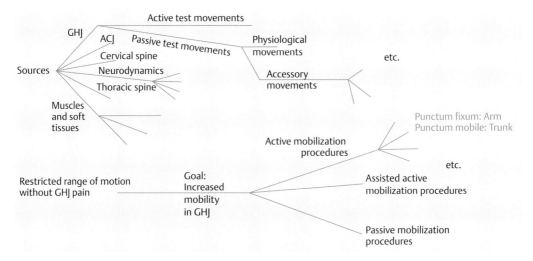

**Fig. 1.11** A "decision tree" helps in determining hypotheses about the sources of the movement dysfunction or treatment options.

## Developing Clinical Patterns

Previous clinical reasoning studies have shown that, compared to novices, experts have developed a wider array of clinical patterns, use more "if-then" rules, and have more possibilities for forward reasoning at their disposal.

Clinical patterns cannot be developed by theoretical learning alone, since this requires lived clinical experiences. A sound theoretical knowledge base will certainly support the process of developing clinical patterns. However, without direct contact with patients and regular, disciplined reassessment procedures, only limited clinical patterns will develop.

### What are Clinical Patterns?

Various studies in different medical areas have shown that, compared with novices, experts are often able to assess a situation almost at a glance. They seem to know, almost immediately, what the problem is and how it should be treated. An important element in this process is clinical pattern recognition (Elstein et al 1978; Tanner 1987; Jones 1989; Jensen et al 1990, 1992; Robertson 1996a,b).

> Clinical patterns can be defined as follows: the recognition of identical relationships in symptoms and signs in different patients that help to identify diagnostic titles, precautions and contraindications, examination and treatment strategies, and the therapeutic climate.

Clinical patterns are often expressed in terms of a biomedical diagnosis. However, it is essential to consider the consequences for clinical actions and to ask how examination procedures or therapeutic interventions need to be adapted to the defined clinical pattern.

For example, during the patient interview, the therapist might recognize a pattern in the clinical presentation that makes him or her think that the underlying cause of the movement problem may be a cervical radicular syndrome. In such cases, the physical examination should include neurological conduction tests that should be re-evaluated regularly in reassessment procedures to check whether the condition is worsening.

As well as helping to recognize pathobiological processes, clinical patterns may also be related to specific examination and treatment procedures; hence, the recognition if a patient may be presenting with a unicomponent or a multicomponent movement disorder. This is illustrated by the following example:

---

**Case Study**
A 24-year-old physical therapist with one year of clinical experience is working in an outpatient unit at a medium-sized hospital in Switzerland. A rheumatologist who has trained in manual medicine routinely refers patients to her for treatment. One day, the physical therapist ends an initial session by performing a subjective and physical examination, probationary treatment, and reassessment. Later she discusses the session with a colleague. The physical therapist is quite frustrated. Dr. S. referred the patient to her with a diagnosis of lumbovertebral syndrome (LVS). She had thought the woman would be similar to any number of patients who had previously been referred to her with the same medical diagnosis: she had expected

---

the patient to present with local pain in the lower back and buttocks, she had expected to reproduce the pain with lumbar bending and sidebending, and had thought that local treatment with passive L4–L5 mobilization, ultrasound, and piriformis muscle stretches might be effective. When asked by her colleague why she was so frustrated, she replied that the patient had not presented with those symptoms at all and that she could not recognize anything of what she had anticipated.

What the physical therapist had failed to recognize was that a clinical pattern had already automatically formed in her memory, as she had treated patients with the same diagnosis in the past and had noticed that the therapies chosen often led to satisfying outcomes in reassessment procedures. Under normal circumstances, this would allow her to take certain short cuts during the examination and treatment planning for a new patient. However, now she was working with a patient with a different clinical presentation. Hence, she needed to return to basic examination procedures without taking any short cuts and applying reflection-on-action, as she could not recognize a pattern that she already had some clinical experience of. It was important for her to recognize that she had already started to develop an experiential knowledge base and to become aware of the value of this development for clinical decision-making processes.

> Clinical patterns are dynamic and continue to develop throughout one's entire professional career. They involve more than the mere recognition of pathobiological processes.

Clinical pattern recognition enables therapists to take short cuts and achieve greater efficiency in their work. There is a risk of superficial reasoning, however: clinical patterns are merely hypotheses that need to be tested and proved in everyday practice using specific reassessment procedures. If therapy fails to achieve the anticipated result, the clinician may need to reconsider the hypotheses or clinical patterns that provided the basis for his or her therapeutic decisions. **Table 1.6** presents various clinical patterns.

### *"If-then" Rules and Forward Reasoning*

Another essential part in the development of professional experience and pattern recognition are "if-then" rules. Experts seem to have numerous such rules at their disposal and make specific use of them in their evaluation procedures. They form part of stored patterns in a practitioner's clinical memory. The "if-then" rules are an element of forward reasoning in which clinicians speculate about potential clinical presentations and the actions they may take in a specific case.

For example, *if* the patient has radiating pain with pins and needles, *then* he or she might have radicu-

**Table 1.6** Clinical patterns

| | |
|---|---|
| Unistructural versus multi-structural problem | As in the case study on pp. 13–14 and 20–21, is the cause of the problem in a 72-year-old man only a dysfunction affecting a single joint complex or might several dysfunctions in other joint complexes play a role? (E.g., as well as the glenohumeral dysfunction, acromioclavicular, cervical, thoracic, and neurodynamic dysfunction may be contributing to the disorder and may need to be addressed during treatment) |
| Unidimensional or multi-dimensional approach to treatment | Can treatment focus only on the movement dysfunctions or should one also consciously take cognitive, affective, sociocultural, and experiential factors into account? In the latter case, the quality of the therapeutic relationship and communication is essential |
| Pathobiological processes with consequences for examination and treatment | If pathobiological processes ("end organ dysfunction") are considered, precautions often need to be taken in examination and treatment until these processes have stabilized. On the other hand, the patterns may indicate a first treatment choice. For example, movement dysfunctions in the lumbar spine due to discogenic causes can often successfully be treated with gentle passive rotation mobilization until just before the onset of pain during movement (Maitland et al 2005) |
| Prognosis (short-, medium-, and long-term) | A differentiated prognosis is dependent on clinical experience |
| Choice and implementation of treatment | This depends on the pathobiology, neurophysiological pain mechanisms, patient behavior, coping strategies, and individual illness experience and behavior |
| Active integration into the therapeutic relationship | Actively integrate the patient into the rehabilitation process. This pattern deals with aspects of patient motivation, explanations, and behavioral changes |

lar syndrome. *Then* it is essential to perform neurological conduction tests. *If* the conduction is altered, *then* I should proceed more carefully with treatment and regularly reassess conduction and see whether it is stable or at least has not worsened. *If* it is worse, *then* I should contact the patient's physician for further advice.

**Note:** In teaching situations, students can perform exercises using the "if-then" rules before treating a patient. Before treatment they can record their thoughts using a tape recorder or write them down. After transcribing their thoughts they can then analyze the "if-then" rules they have generated. This exercise can help to make clinical reasoning processes explicit and to recognize clinical patterns that are already stored in memory. An exchange with fellow students enhances mutual learning and the expansion of clinical patterns.

## Clinical Reasoning and Evidence-based Practice

In recent decades, physical therapy, like all medical professions, has been faced with the challenge of scientific scrutiny and defining the knowledge base that underpins clinical practice.

As described on pages 16–17, different types of knowledge are key to making decisions in daily clinical practice (Higgs and Titchen 1995). If, in evidence-based practice, only the theoretical knowledge base (propositional knowledge) were to be of any value and no account taken of the professional craft and personal knowledge bases, the latter's influence on clinical decisions and clinical outcomes may be neglected in research.

*Evidence-based practice (EBP)* has become a widespread term in research and many professions have acknowledged it as an important component of clinical practice.

EBP has been defined as follows: "The conscientious, explicit and judicious use of current best evidence in making decisions about the care of individual patients" (Sackett et al 1996).

EBP means integrating individual clinical expertise with the best available evidence from systematic research (Sackett et al 1998).

Some clinicians are concerned that EBP may lead some therapists to simply follow a "recipe" without deliberate decision-making, reflection, and reassessment in clinical reasoning processes. This has been refuted by Sackett et al (1998). However, the definition of EBP implies that it should go hand in hand with conscious clinical reasoning processes.

Nevertheless, clinicians may face a dilemma when applying knowledge from research processes to actual clinical practice. Schön (1983) voiced concern about the increasing gap between knowledge derived from research versus a knowledge base developed from professional experience. In everyday practice, clinicians often have to use incomplete or ambiguous information for clinical decision-making processes, for which no backup by scientific research is available.

Furthermore, the "best evidence" is not yet available for all the problems that professionals are confronted with in actual practice. Sackett et al (1998) therefore described various levels of evidence that were refined in 2008 (Sackett et al 2008). It should be noted that the levels of evidence as defined by van Tulder et al (1999) stand in contrast to those of Sackett et al (**Table 1.7**).

Looking at the various levels of evidence, particularly the classification by van Tulder et al, can present clinicians with a dilemma. In everyday practice, physical therapists are routinely required to make decisions about patients' problems for which no published randomized controlled trials (RCTs) or systematic reviews are available. Furthermore, clinicians may sometimes learn more with regard to their decision-making processes for *individual* patients from a clinical case study or expert opinion than from an RCT that deals with homogeneous groups of people. Hence, van Tulder et al's classification can leave a clinician feeling uncomfortable, particularly as the classification has been included in some practice guidelines (KNGF 2001). Although systematic reviews have been considered as the highest level of evidence, it should be noted that they may not always be free of bias and error (Linton 1998; Jones and Higgs 2000).

Another central issue with regard to research processes is whether all the relevant clinical questions have been asked and systematically investigated. An important aspect in the therapeutic process—be it undertaken by a physician, physical therapist, or occupational therapist—is the direct encounter with the patient, in other words the therapeutic relationship. The clinician's decision-making processes are often influenced by subtle, hardly quantifiable clues: the pitch of the patient's voice, the patient's choice of words, intonation, and body language may all have a significant influence on how the clinical information is interpreted (Linton 1998; Hengeveld 2000). The question is whether the effects of a good therapeutic relationship, as the basis of clinical practice, have already been sufficiently studied, not to

**Table 1.7** Levels of "best evidence" described by various research groups

| Level[a] | | Level[b] | | Level[c] | | |
|---|---|---|---|---|---|---|
| I | Systematic review | 1A | Systematic review/RCTs[d] | 1 Strong/high | Consistent results in several high-quality RCTs | |
| | | 1B | RCTs with narrow confidence interval | | | |
| | | 1C | All or none case series | | | |
| II | RCT | 2A | Systematic review, cohort studies | 2 Moderate | Consistent results in several high-quality RCTs | |
| | | 2B | Cohort study/low-quality RCTs | | | |
| | | 2C | Outcomes research | | | |
| III | Quasi-experimental studies | 3A | Systematic review/case-controlled studies | 3 Limited/contradictory | One RCT or inconsistent results in various RCTs | |
| | | 3B | Case-controlled study | | | |
| IV | Pre-experimental studies | 4 | Case series, poor cohort case-controlled | 4 None | No RCTs | |
| V | Expert opinions | 5 | Expert opinion | | | |
| VI | "I once heard that…" | | | | | |

Notes:
[a] Described by Sackett et al (1998).
[b] Described by Sackett et al (2008).
[c] Described by van Tulder et al (1999) in KNGF (2001).
[d] Randomized controlled trials.

mention whether an RCT or meta-analysis would be possible at this point (Linton 1998).

The inclusion and exclusion criteria used in studies may not correspond to their relevance to physical therapy. Inclusion criteria are often based on pathobiological, biomedical diagnoses. Some authors have suggested defining inclusion criteria for specific physical therapy research on movement dysfunction and motor control patterns (Maluf et al 2000; O'Sullivan 2005) or symptom localization and reactions to repeated movements (McKenzie 1981). Other authors have suggested using outcome instruments that are clinically relevant to physical therapy practice (Jones and Higgs 2000). Physical therapists are increasingly expected to use clinimetric instruments in everyday practice to detect more quantifiable, measurable changes. This would certainly be a very welcome development. Nevertheless, there is a risk of therapists focusing too much on their own measurements rather than assisting and guiding their patients in *experiencing for themselves* any positive changes and thus enhancing their confidence in their own potential for influencing their well-being.

In everyday practice, clinicians are faced with questions for which no RCTs or meta-analyses are yet available. The question arises of whether this means that the best evidence has not yet been provided or whether "it has not been proven and would therefore be ineffective." However, it seems that there are some power issues at play in these arguments. On occasion, insurance companies appear to exploit this situation by arguing that no treatment will be reimbursed until satisfactory evidence has been provided for its efficacy. The following question was posed by Margareta Nordin, a physical therapist and the first nonphysician to serve as president of the North American Spine Society at her inaugural lecture: "When is evidence sufficient?" She noted the benefits of activity in the treatment of low back pain—a fact that was confirmed in 1997 by 16 well-designed RCTs, but did not seem to have been taken into account by many medical professionals (Nordin 1998).

It is certainly desirable for the best results from research to be incorporated into decisions made in clinical practice, and clinicians are advised to understand research processes and to stay abreast of current developments. Nevertheless, clinicians must also maintain a critical, but open-minded attitude to information from EBP in order to be able to make the best decisions for individualized patient care.

In every newly formed scientific community similar discussions seem to be sparked that do not seem to be free of a certain degree of polemics. For example, for several decades, in different scientific communities all over the world, the issues of validity, reliability, sensitivity, and specificity of examination and treatment methods have been investigated in studies on inter-tester and intra-tester reliability. Several, often related examination techniques, such as palpation methods in medicine and manual therapy, have demonstrated low inter-tester and intra-tester reliability. This has led some researchers to advise against using them in everyday practice. It is worth noting that the values increase if information is collected in clusters, that is, if they are placed in relation to other test procedures (DePoy and Gitlin 2010). They also change when reference standards other than a comparison between therapists are used (Jull and Bogduk 1988; Phillips and Twomey 1996). Although it is sometimes crucial to throw outmoded methods overboard, important examination procedures on which relevant clinical decisions are based should not be discarded before viable alternatives are available.

Another aspect of a dilemma in EBP is that many everyday problems that physical therapists are faced with are multicomponential and multifactorial, while most studies often need to focus on problems arising from a single cause and a single approach to treatment.

In sum, as Linton (1998, p. 49) stated: "In the field of pain, the way the treatment is applied, the communication between the caregiver and patient, the setting, the level of anxiety, and so forth, may all influence the results of techniques designed to relieve pain."

Everyday clinical practice that is supported by rigorous reassessment procedures corresponds to level 4 evidence according to Sackett et al. This applies in particular if the therapist not only focuses on the subjective and functional parameter of examination, but also endeavors to implement test procedures that have an acceptable reliability and validity. Adopting a strict quantitative science approach, performing treatment and reassessment procedures based on conscious clinical reasoning may already be considered a single clinical case study that has the potential to contribute to the body of knowledge underpinning the science and practice of physical therapy.

It is therefore essential for therapists to be well aware of their own clinical reasoning processes, including certain decision-making habits they may have; then the results from EBP will support, rather than limit, their clinical decision-making processes. The process of delivering the clinical proof for the hypotheses generated, and regular planning and reflecting during the critical phases of the treatment process allow physical therapists to develop in-depth expertise while incorporating insights from relevant research.

## 1.3   Critical Phases in the Physical Therapy Process—Reflection Phases

As described on page 8, clinical reasoning involves a mixture of thinking (a more automatic process) and reflecting (a conscious process). It has been recognized that people with a high level of professional expertise also have good reflective abilities (Schön 1983). In other words, they have developed the habit of reflecting (during and after treatment sessions) on their own ways of thinking, their decisions, their emotions, the chosen examination and treatment procedure, the therapeutic outcomes, and the interactions between the client and therapist.

The physical therapy process consists of various critical phases (Hengeveld and Banks 2005), and these should be deliberately planned and implemented. A few of these phases are illustrated in this section:

- Greeting and information phase (may extend over one to three sessions)
- Patient interview (subjective examination)
- Planning the physical examination
- Physical examination, with probationary treatment and reassessment
- Analysis of initial findings, treatment planning
- Planning the second, third, and subsequent sessions
- Reassessment procedures
- Retrospective assessments
- Final phase of treatment

**Table 1.8** Goals of physical therapy examination procedures

| Goals/Objectives | |
|---|---|
| Physical therapy diagnosis | To analyze movement dysfunctions, which may best be described using terms such as impairment, activities, and participation. Movement dysfunctions (and resources) may include all bodily functions related to movement, such as cardiac and pulmonary functions. In manual therapy, an analysis of the movement impairments of joints, muscles, neurodynamics, and soft tissues has a key role to play (component concept) (Hengeveld and Banks 2005) |
| Precautions and contra-indications | To identify precautions and potential contraindications to certain therapeutic interventions |
| Screening questions and tests | Physical therapists must use screening questions and tests based on parts of bodily systems used in medicine to identify any contraindications (Goodman and Snyder 2007; Boissonnault 2011). This is especially important in countries where patients have direct access to physical therapy |
| Parameters for measuring the outcome of treatment | These refer to information gained from the patient interview (subjective examination), as well as from the physical examination |
| Parameters from patient interviews/subjective examination | Patient interview information may include: symptom localization, quality, intensity, frequency, and duration; activity levels; confidence in moving; use of medication; the use of coping strategies to influence overall well-being |
| Physical examination parameters | The parameters of the physical examination usually involve those test movements that reproduce the symptoms. For pulmonary treatment, however, they may include stethoscopic or other findings. Each specialized area within physical therapy should define these parameters |
| Determine treatment goals | Once the short- and long-term goals of treatment have been defined collaboratively with the patient, meaningful treatment interventions are selected, taking into account any precautions |
| Develop hypotheses | The therapist is encouraged to develop several hypotheses as already described on pp. 18–21 |

## 1.3.1 Goals of Physical Therapy Examination Procedures

The physical therapy examination has various objectives and may take two to three sessions, assuming that the examination process includes probationary treatments and re-examination procedures. Every question and every test in the examination process should be aimed at achieving these goals (Hengeveld and Banks 2005). These objectives are listed in **Table 1.8**.

## 1.3.2 Assessment

Various types of assessment have been described that should be used specifically in the context of the overall physical therapy process (Maitland 1987; Hengeveld and Banks 2005; Maitland et al 2005):
- Initial assessment with patient interview, planning, and physical examination
- Reassessment procedures
- Assessment during the therapeutic intervention
- Reflection after two to three sessions
- Retrospective assessment
- Final analytical assessment

The various types of assessment are described in the following.

## 1.3.3 Initial Assessment

### Greeting and Information Phase

The greeting is an essential part of the treatment process, and one that is often performed hastily (Brioschi 1998). However, in this phase of treatment, if planned carefully, therapists can obtain invaluable information about the patient's beliefs and expectations. Furthermore, it provides therapists with the opportunity to communicate information about the specific goals of physical therapy, that is, optimizing movement potential and restoring functional capacity. Also, this phase can lay the foundation for developing a good therapeutic relationship based on trust and mutual understanding. Patients and therapists often have different expectations about the treatment in general, the setting, and the roles of both patient and therapist within the overall process. If possible, these factors need to be clarified in an early phase of treatment, otherwise the chances of a successful therapeutic outcome may be limited due to persistent misunderstandings.

The greeting should include the following elements (Brioschi 1998):
- Introduction, including name and function.

- Joining, bonding (e.g., "ice-breakers," usually friendly remarks intended to establish a personal relationship with the patient.
- Preliminary information on the specific (movement) paradigms of physical therapy and a comparison with the patient's expectations (see the example below).
- Clarification of the setting: In some cases it may be important to determine before starting the therapy whether the patient would rather be treated by a man or a woman, and whether the door should be left open or closed (Schachter et al 1999). This is considered sensitive practice (Rothstein 1994).
- Course of the first session and the patient's role during this session.
- During this phase therapists may become aware of some of the patient's boundaries if they pay careful attention and respond sensitively to non-verbal signals and verbal clues.

---

**Example Preliminary Communication**
"I would like to briefly explain what modern physical therapy does. We physical therapists focus on movement. I am aware that your physician diagnosed your condition as a 'herniated disk.' We physical therapists keep that diagnosis at the back of our minds. But in physical therapy we must carefully examine your movement functions. You may have certain movement habits in your daily life, perhaps some joints are stiff or your muscles may not react quickly enough. This is something I have to first ask you about and take a look at before I can treat your problem specifically adapted to your situation and life. Is that what you were expecting?"

---

## Patient Interview and Planning

### Patient Interview/Subjective Examination
The main goal of the patient interview is to understand the disorder from the patient's perspective. In general it is important to know which everyday activities may be restricted and which resources are available to help the patient overcome them. This forms the basis for determining the most important treatment outcomes.

Various factors can restrict everyday activities, including:
- Pain and other symptoms
- Regulation and control, for example in neurological rehabilitation
- Cardiovascular factors
- Neuropsychological aspects, for instance spatial orientation or apraxia

If pain is the primary problem, it is best to record the affected sites on a body chart (Maitland 1986; McCombe et al 1989). This increases the reliability of the information and, most importantly, helps in developing clinical patterns.

Often it is helpful to divide the patient interview into the following main areas (Maitland 1986; Hengeveld and Banks, 2014a,b):
- Personal information, such as name, address, profession, hobbies.
- Main problem: It is important to understand how the disorder is affecting the patient in his or her daily life (irrespective of whether the main problem is described as pain, shortness of breath, or other problems). The patient may describe being very restricted, moderately restricted, or perhaps not restricted at all.
- Body chart, precisely sketching in the symptoms, symptom-free areas, qualification of symptoms, and the relationship between the symptom areas.
- Twenty-four-hour symptom behavior and activities: This includes various aspects:
  - Symptom behavior in certain positions and during certain activities.
  - Behavior of the main problem throughout the course of the day.
  - Activity levels during the day or week.
  - Coping possibilities: Which interventions has the patient learned to maintain control over his or her main problem or well-being?
- History of the problem: This may be divided into a short- and long-term history (of recurrent problems). The following factors should be included in the short-term history:
  - When was the onset of symptoms?
  - Which contributed to their development?
  - Course of the symptoms and disability: How has the problem developed since the onset of symptoms?
  - How is the patient doing now, regarding symptoms and everyday activities, compared to the beginning?

Symptoms may develop spontaneously or after trauma. In the case of a traumatic onset, the therapist should determine the mechanism of trauma. If symptoms seem to have occurred spontaneously, the therapist should distinguish how the structures were used before they developed and if the structures' overall ability to withstand stress may have been restricted. In both instances, the therapist should ask detailed questions about when and where the patient noticed the initial symptoms:

- Specific questions:
  - This phase focuses on various aspects of the patient's social history, dietary influences and so on. This category also includes screening questions according to biomedical bodily systems (Boissonnault 1995; Goodman and Snyder 2000).
- Eliciting the patient history is an important part of the examination. It provides an opportunity to set the course for determining the treatment goals collaboratively (clarify tasks), to determine any precautions regarding the subsequent functional examination, and to set subjective parameters to measure success with in subsequent sessions.
- Good communication plays a vital role in the overall examination and therapeutic process. It will enhance the patient's learning process from the very beginning of the interview.

### Questionnaire or Interview

Various questionnaires have been developed for use in scientific research to better understand the patient's perspective. These can be very useful when performing the patient interview. Yet, physical therapists should understand which problems the questionnaire was developed for, as it may be restricted to a specific kind of research question. Furthermore, a questionnaire should not become a substitute for direct contact with the patient during the subjective examination, as this phase is therapeutic in itself and lays the foundation for the therapeutic relationship.

### Psychosocial Assessment

It has been postulated that physical therapists should also perform a psychosocial assessment if indicated (Kendall et al 1997; Watson 1999). The purpose of this is to determine the psychosocial factors that might hinder or restrict progress toward the full restoration of functioning (Main 2004). If there are any indications of psychosocial factors ("yellow flags"), they often need to be addressed in treatment or they may influence the way in which therapy is delivered. Psychosocial factors and those that are relevant to physical therapy have been described elsewhere in the literature (Hengeveld 2003 b; Hengeveld and Banks 2014a,b).
A few questionnaires have been developed for this purpose. Nevertheless, if a physical therapist listens carefully and pays attention from the greeting phase onward, and reacts to keywords or gestures, then the psychosocial assessment can become an integral part of the routine examination and can be considered an example of "good patient handling skills" in which the therapist can gain a deeper insight into the patient's individual illness experience.

*Planning*

Planning of the functional examination should include the following:

- Reflecting on the patient interview ("subjective examination") based on the following questions:
  - Are there enough parameters to evaluate outcomes in the second session?
  - Have all those questions been asked that could provide clues about potential precautions or contraindications?
- The following hypotheses should be made explicit:
  - Sources of the nociceptive processes and movement impairment (for patients with predominantly painful movement problems who require an orthopedic manipulative physical therapy examination).
  - Contributing factors that are sustaining the movement problem (cognitive, affective factors; muscular imbalance; in neurological patients, e.g., joint status). In many hemiplegic patients, a stiff hip after joint replacement prevents them from practicing leaning forward when getting up out of a chair.
  - Pathobiological processes: Consideration of potential pathobiological tissue processes ("end organ dysfunction"), stage of tissue regeneration, and neurophysiological symptom mechanisms.
  - Contraindications and precautions: Whether extra care should be taken during the functional examination will depend on the pain that is experienced during everyday activities (concept of severity and irritability (Maitland et al 2005; Hengeveld and Banks 2014a,b) and other factors such as pathobiological processes, additional diagnoses, stages of healing, stability of the disorder, and psychosocial factors such as confidence when moving (Maitland et al 2005; Hengeveld and Banks 2014a,b).
- "Dosage" and exact order of steps in the physical examination, including reassessments.

## Physical Examination

The physical examination includes various actions and test movements, with the following goals:

- To reproduce the patient's main problem: This may be pain or restricted movement due to pain. In the case of neurological disorders the movements that are restricted as well as the resources for achieving movement goals are assessed. Pulmonary and cardiovascular physical therapy evaluates the functioning as well as any limitation of the lungs and heart.

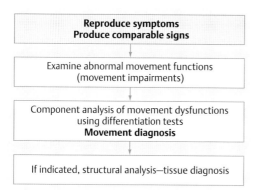

**Fig. 1.12** Component concept—specific taxonomy in the orthopedic manipulative physical therapy analysis of painful movement dysfunction.

Joint functions
- Local
- Referred symptoms

Neurodynamic functions
- Local
- Referred

Soft tissues
- Skin
- Fasciae
- Connective tissue

**Mechanosensitivity—movement dysfunction**

Muscle functions
- Contractile functions
- Trigger points

Other
- Blood vessels
- Viscera

**Reproduce symptoms**
**Produce comparable signs**

Examine abnormal movement functions
(movement impairments)

Component analysis of movement dysfunctions
using differentiation tests
**Movement diagnosis**

If indicated, structural analysis—tissue diagnosis

**Fig. 1.13** Algorithm showing the goals of the physical examination in physical therapy, specifically in orthopedic manipulative physical therapy.

- To evaluate any impairments of movement functions in the case of pain: The components that may be contributing to the impairment can be analyzed using different kinds of differentiation tests (Pfund and Zahnd 2001; Maitland et al 2005) or probationary treatments with succesive reassessments (Maitland et al 2005; Hengeveld and Banks 2014a) (**Fig. 1.12**).

The physical therapy diagnosis is usually expressed in terms of movement dysfunctions. There are clinical situations, however, in which a structural analysis may be important. A structural analysis is especially important for the precise treatment of soft tissues (e.g., deep frictions, trigger point treatment) or if the patient has acute symptoms due to trauma that may need to be evaluated by a physician.

Some schools of thought propose that treatment should be based on structural diagnosis and suggest following a standardized protocol of examination procedures (Cyriax 1982; Winkel et al 2003). However, a primary structural analysis creates a dilemma

for the clinician, because one or two movement tests are not usually enough to assess which structures could be activating the nociceptive processes. Furthermore, it may be possible that the patient's symptoms and movement disorder may not be explained by any pathobiological, structural changes (Waddell, 2004).

Therefore, it is essential when pursuing the objective of the physical examination, to follow an algorithm when assessing painful movement dysfunctions. The primary goal will be to reproduce the patient's symptoms. The test movements that reproduce the symptoms will be the impairments that lay the foundation for defining the treatment objective and serve as a parameter for reassessment procedures. The process of analysis and probationary treatment of the components that are contributing to the impairments may provide a sufficient basis for drawing up a comprehensive treatment plan even if no structural analysis has been done (Hengeveld and Banks 2014a, b) (**Fig. 1.13**):
- Along with analyzing the restriction in movement functions, the resources for different activities also often need to be evaluated. This is especially important if it does not appear possible to achieve complete functional restoration of certain activities.
- When analyzing movement dysfunction with pain, the physical examination includes observation, active and passive test movements, neurological tests, muscular testing procedures, and palpation. Comparable examinations are often used in pulmonary, cardiovascular, or neurological physical therapy. In such cases the examination procedures are adapted to the specific clinical problem. A detailed description of examination procedures can be found in the relevant literature (Maitland et al 2005; Hengeveld and Banks 2014a,b).

- The examination procedures should ideally be performed in such a manner that they can be consistently repeated during subsequent reassessment processes. If possible, the tests should correspond to a "gold standard" in terms of validity and reliability. However, therapists should nevertheless be able to adapt all the test procedures to the patient's specific condition and should be prepared to depart from the "gold standard" if this seems clinically justified. Some therapists prefer to use only test movements that have demonstrated acceptable inter-tester and intra-tester reliability. Yet, a certain degree of skepticism is called for with regard to suggestions that tests with a high inter-tester reliability coefficient are also immediately ready for use in clinical practice (Keating and Matyas 1998; Bruton et al 2000) or the reverse, namely that tests with low reliability are of absolutely no use to the clinician. Often it is the combination of test parameters, both in the subjective examination and in the functional examination, that provides clinicians with meaningful parameters for reassessment procedures (MacDermid et al 1999).
- Routine reassessment procedures should also be performed during the initial physical examination. In cases of severe or irritable symptoms (Hengeveld and Banks 2014 a, b), the level of pain should be monitored regularly to record any increase or decrease. If the therapist suspects an inflammatory process, then temperature, swelling, and any redness should be checked regularly.

Those test procedures that may also be used as a treatment technique should be monitored regularly during the examination process for their possible therapeutic effect. For example, neurodynamic tests, tests of muscle length, and passive joint mobilizations such as accessory movements or joint play techniques can be used as an examination as well as a treatment technique. Hence, the examination and treatment processes merge. As a result, a brief examination procedure can already have a therapeutic effect that needs to be carefully monitored in reassessment procedures even if the initial physical examination has not yet been completed.

### Analysis of Initial Findings

As described in the above, it may take as many as three sessions to perform an initial analysis of a movement dysfunction and to decide on optimal treatment strategies. However, this process should also include initial probationary treatments, which

may be considered as an aspect of "differentiation by treatment" (Maitland et al 2005). Initial treatment planning and initial probationary treatment are often done during the first session. Further treatment planning depends on the outcome of the probationary treatments and supplementary physical therapy examinations. Thus, it is often crucial for the future physical therapy process to analyze the first and second sessions. This analysis should include the following:

- Reflection: Summary of the main features of the patient interview and physical examination (movement diagnoses).
- Hypotheses formulation: All hypothesis categories should be made explicit during this phase. If the therapist identifies any clinical patterns, these should be described. It is also essential to describe the consequences for further management.
- Planning the second session and anticipating the course of the third session, based on the following questions:
  - Which subjective parameters and functional parameters will be evaluated in the reassessment processes?
  - Which supplementary procedures are needed in addition to the subjective examination and physical examination undertaken during the first session?
  - Which movement components require further analysis?
  - Which therapeutic interventions, including self-management strategies, are useful?
- Precise planning as to when the reassessments will be performed: Anticipation of possible responses to the interventions supports the development of forward reasoning and "if-then" rules (see pp. 23–24).

### 1.3.4 Reassessment

As previously mentioned, reassessment processes are an essential part of all physical therapy procedures. However, the basis for in-depth monitoring of treatment outcomes is laid in the initial assessment. Without a thorough evaluation of the patient's disorder at the start of the therapeutic process, the evaluation of treatment outcomes in subsequent sessions will be severely limited.

Reassessments should be performed regularly and can cover various aspects. As an exception, in cases involving severe pain, this can involve merely asking about the patient's overall well-being. Also, during educational sessions reassessment needs to be performed after determining whether the patient has understood the information given and can actually apply it to everyday life (cognitive reassessment; Hengeveld and Banks, 2014 a, b). Usually, however, reassessment consists of a routine evaluation of any changes in the most relevant test movements performed in the physical examination.

Reassessments should ideally include the following:

- At the beginning of a session: Checking subjective parameters and parameters of the physical examination. The effects of any self-management strategies should also be evaluated.
- At the end of each session: Checking the parameters of the physical examination. This should also include information about the patient's overall well-being, and reflecting on the session during which the patient perhaps reports what they may have learned from the session.
- After each individual treatment intervention: Evaluating the aspects described in the above.

Reassessment processes are essential to the treatment process and they fulfill various purposes:

- They are an evaluation of therapeutic outcomes. Treatment results are compared before and after the application of an intervention, on the basis of which the value of the selected intervention can be assessed.
- Reassessment procedures aid differential diagnosis. Not only the examination tests, but also the results from (probationary) treatments contribute to an understanding of which movement dysfunctions are contributing to the disorder ("component analysis"). This applies in particular to treatments involving passive mobilization and joint manipulation.
- Reassessments are almost ideal phases for reflection. They provide a good opportunity to confirm, modify, or discard hypotheses about the sources of the dysfunction, contributing factors, and optimal treatment strategies. By consistently using reassessment procedures, physical therapists start to develop and deepen the patterns of clinical presentations that may be stored in their clinical memory. These patterns may be accessible in later encounters with patients with similar clinical presentations. Not only the patient, but also the therapist may directly experience which interventions seem more or less beneficial. Thus, consistent reassessment processes contribute to developing a therapist's personal, experiential knowledge base.
- Routine reassessment processes support the patient's learning process. From a cognitive behav-

ioral therapy perspective, reassessment procedures can help patients train their perception and show them that positive changes are occurring even if the pain stills seems to persist. During reassessments patients can understand for the first time that positive changes are occurring, even if they feel that no improvement is possible given their condition.

> Reassessment processes, along with conscious communication strategies and a thorough understanding of the possible changes in subjective and physical examination parameters, are key moments in the treatment process.

## 1.3.5    Assessment During the Application of Treatment

It is essential that therapists conduct an assessment while performing treatment. The following questions should be taken into consideration in order to optimize treatment:

- Are the treatment goals being achieved?
- Are there any undesired side-effects? For example, increased pain in the case of increased severity or irritability of pain, increased general muscle tone, autonomic responses, signs of inflammation, changes in soft tissues or fracture pain during the early phase of healing, increased fear of moving/being moved, reduction of self-efficacy/externalization of the locus of control, development of passive coping strategies, confusion caused by too much information.

## 1.3.6    Reflection after Two to Three Sessions

As repeatedly stated in this chapter, a comprehensive clinical assessment and the confirmation of hypotheses can often only take place based on a reassessment following (probationary) treatments. It is therefore suggested that therapists spread out their analysis of the impairments involved in a movement problem over several sessions. If too many sources are evaluated using probationary treatments in the first session, this may confuse the analysis in subsequent sessions. It may be difficult to judge which kind of treatment may have actually contributed to the patient's condition improving.

Therefore, after two to three sessions, it is usually necessary to reflect on the overall therapeutic process up until that point. The therapist should also determine whether additional sources should be examined. However, generally speaking, it can be expected that after three sessions the therapist will have an in-depth understanding of which components are contributing to the problem and which appear not to be involved, and a comprehensive treatment plan should then be defined.

Also, after two to three sessions the therapist should assess whether the treatment goals need refining. In defining a comprehensive treatment plan it is suggested that therapists work backward from the desired final state, and evaluate which factors of this optimum final state are already present and which still need treating if possible.

### 1.3.7    Retrospective Assessment

Retrospective assessments are performed at regular intervals throughout the therapeutic process. The goals of a retrospective assessment are to analyze the treatment process so far, to reformulate the treatment goals if necessary, and to adjust the parameters for measuring treatment success if necessary.

The following aspects should be taken into account:

- An evaluation of the patient's overall well-being—current well-being compared to the start of treatment.
- Which parameters are showing what level of improvement (subjective parameters and physical examination parameters)—now compared to the start of treatment?
- Will the treatment goals be achieved? Which goals have been achieved and which need more attention?
- Check the effect of various interventions, including the patient's learning process.
- Set (new) goals for the next interval of treatment collaboratively with the patient.
- Set (new) parameters for assessing the goals discussed with the patient.

### 1.3.8    Final Analytical Assessment

The final phase of treatment should be well prepared. It is recommended that therapists prepare the completion of therapy during the third-to-last or second-to-last session so that treatment can be adjusted if necessary.

The final analysis includes an analysis of the learning process between the physical therapist and the patient. Together they should check whether and how the treatment goals have been achieved. This phase is characterized by reflection as well as anticipation. The patient reflects on which interventions were helpful, which self-management strategies were most useful, and what he or she learned during the treatment sessions. The physical therapist also reflects on which interventions were helpful by reviewing his or her treatment notes. This contributes to developing clinical pattern recognition. In addition, the physical therapist makes a prognosis about possible recurrences and potential residual disabilities and considers whether further medical interventions are necessary.

Together, the therapist and patient anticipate which difficulties may arise in the future and which self-management interventions the patient could then use. If a collaborative style of communication has been chosen, this kind of discussion enhances long-term compliance with instructions, exercises, and suggestions that have been given throughout the treatment period long after treatment is completed (Hengeveld 2003a, Hengeveld and Banks 2014a).

**Summary**

The physical therapy process is a complex process in which the therapist uses various clinical reasoning strategies and develops a treatment plan with the patient based on a wealth of often ambiguous information. Thorough examination procedures and careful planning play a central role. If physical therapists are trained in these processes early on, apply them in a targeted fashion, and reflect on their clinical decisions, they will be making optimal use of all the possibilities available for developing true expertise in their field of practice.

## References

Alsop A, Ryan P. Making the Most of Fieldwork Education—A Practical Approach. London: Chapman & Hall; 1996

Antonowsky A. The salutogenic perspective: towards a new view of health and illness. Advances 1987;4(1):47–55

Apkarian AV, Robinson JP. Low back pain. IASP, Pain Clinical Updates 2010;VXIII(6):August

American Physical Therapy Association (APTA). Definitions of house of delegates. In: Bélanger G. Confused identity hurts the image of physical therapy. Physiother Can. 1998;50:245–247

Beeston P. Movement as Central Component in WCPT Description of Physical Therapy. E. Hengeveld. London: University of East London; 1999

Bélanger A. Confused identity hurts the image of physical therapy. Physiother Can. 1998;50:245–247

Boissonnault W. Primary Care for the Physical Therapist. Examination and Triage. 2nd ed. Amsterdam: Elsevier-Saunders; 2011

Boud D, Walker D. Experience and Learning: Reflection at Work. Geeling, Victoria: Deakin University Press; 1994

Brioschi R. Kurs: die therapeutische Beziehung. Leitung: Brioschi R, Hengeveld E. Zurzach: Fortbildungszentrum; Mai 1998

Bruton A, Conway JH, et al. Reliability: what is it, and how is it measured? Physiother. 2000;86(2):94–99

Carroll E. The role of tacit knowledge in problem solving in the clinical setting. Nurse Educ Today 1988;8(3):140–147

Case K, Harrison K, et al. Differences in the clinical reasoning process of expert and novice cardiorespiratory physical therapists. Physiother. 2000;86:14–21

Cott CA, Finch E, et al. The movement continuum theory for physical therapy. Physiother Can 1995;47:87–95

Cyriax J. Textbook of Orthopaedic Medicine Vol 1, Diagnosis of Soft Tissue Lesions. London: Baillière Tindall; 1982

DePoy E, Gitlin LN. Introduction to Research: Multiple Strategies to Health and Human Services. 4th ed. St. Louis: Mosby; 2010

Dreyfus H, Dreyfus P. Mind Over Machine: The Power of Human Intuition and Expertise in the Era of the Computer. New York: Free Press; 1985

Edwards I, Jones M, et al. Clinical reasoning in three different fields of physical therapy—a qualitative study. Fifth International Congress. Melbourne: Australian Physical Therapy Association; 1998

Edwards I, Jones M, et al. Clinical reasoning strategies in physical therapy. Phys Ther 2004;84(4):312–330

Elstein A, Shulman LS, et al. Medical Problem Solving: An Analysis of Clinical Reasoning. Cambridge, MA: Harvard University Press; 1978

Engel GL. The need for a new medical model: a challenge for biomedicine. Science 1977;196(4286):129–136

Fleming MH. The therapist with the three-track mind. Am J Occup Ther 1991;45(11):1007–1014

Goodman CC, Snyder TEK. Differential Diagnosis for Physical Therapists: Screening for Referral. 4th ed. Amsterdam: Elsevier-Saunders; 2007

Grant R. The pursuit of excellence in the face of constant change. Physiother 1995;81:338–344

Grant R, Jones M, et al. Clinical Decision Making in Upper Quadrant Dysfunction. Physical Therapy of the Cervical and Thoracic Spine. New York: Churchill Livingstone; 1988

Guccione AA. Physical therapy diagnosis and the relationship between impairments and function. Phys Ther 1991;71(7):499–503

Hengeveld E. Der Entscheidungsfindungsprozess in der Physiotherapie zwischen Überweisung und Behandlung—eine Standortbestimmung. Physiotherapie (Schweiz) 1994;1:4–16

Hengeveld E. Clinical reasoning in Manueller Therapie—eine klinische Fallstudie. Manuelle Therapie 1998a;2:42–49

Hengeveld E. Theorie der Physiotherapie: Plädoyer für einen Paradigmenwechsel. Teil 1 und Teil 2. Physiotherapie (Schweiz) 1998b;11:18–28, 12:13–20

Hengeveld E. Gedanken zum Indikationsbereich der Manuellen Therapie Teil 1. Manuelle Therapie 1998c;2:176–181

Hengeveld E. Gedanken zum Indikationsbereich der Manuellen Therapie. Teil 2. Manuelle Therapie 1999;3:2–7

Hengeveld E. Psychosocial issues in physical therapy: manual therapists' perspectives and observations. MSc thesis. Dept. of Health Sciences. London: University of East London; 2000

Hengeveld E. Clinical reasoning als Weg zu einer bewussten Beziehungsgestaltung. Ergotherapie (Schweiz) 2001; l:14–18

Hengeveld E. Compliance und Verhaltensänderung in Manueller Therapie. Manuelle Therapie 2003a;7(3):122–132

Hengeveld E. Das biopsychosoziale Modell. In: van den Berg F. Angewandte Physiologie. Band 4: Schmerzen verstehen und beeinflussen. Stuttgart: Thieme; 2003b

Hengeveld E. Theorie der Physiotherapie. Osnabrück: Fachhochschule; 2003c

Hengeveld E. In: Hüter-Becker A, Dölken M. Theoriemodelle und ihre Bedeutung für die Physiotherapie. In: Beruf, Recht und wissenschaftliches Arbeiten. Stuttgart, Thieme; 2004

Hengeveld E, Banks K. Maitland's Peripheral Manipulation. 4th ed. Edinburgh: Elsevier-Butterworth; 2005

Hengeveld E, Banks K. Maitland's Vertebral Manipulation. Management of Neuromusculoskeletal Disorders. Vol 1. 8th ed. Edinburgh: Elsevier-Butterworth; 2014a

Hengeveld E, Banks K. Maitland's Peripheral Manipulation. Management of Neuromusculoskeletal Disorders. Vol 2. 5th ed. Edinburgh: Elsevier-Butterworth; 2014b

Higgs J. Developing clinical reasoning competencies. Physiother 1992a;78:575–581

Higgs J. Developing knowledge: a process of construction, mapping and review. NZ J Physiother 1992b;20(2):23–30

Higgs J, Jones M, eds. Clinical Reasoning in the Health Professions. Oxford: Butterworth-Heinemann; 1995

Higgs J, Jones M, eds. Clinical Reasoning in the Health Professions. 2nd ed. Oxford: Butterworth-Heinemann; 2000

Higgs J, Jones M, et al. Clinical Reasoning in the Health Professions. 3rd ed. Amsterdam: Butterworth-Heinemann/Elsevier; 2008

Higgs J, Titchen A. The nature, generation and verification of knowledge. Physiother 1995;81:521–530

Hislop HJ. Tenth Mary McMillan lecture. The not-so-impossible dream. Phys Ther 1975;55(10):1069–1080

Hooper B. The relationship between pretheoretical assumptions and clinical reasoning. Am J Occup Ther 1997;51(5):328–338

Hullegie W. Fysiotherapie, een wetenschapstheoretische en vakfilosofische analyse. Utrecht: De Tijdstroom; 1995

Jensen GM, Gwyer J, et al. Expertise in Physical Therapy Practice. Boston, MA: Butterworth-Heinemann; 1999

Jensen GM, Shepard KF, et al. The novice versus the experienced clinician: insights into the work of the physical therapist. Phys Ther 1990;70(5):314–323

Jensen GM, Shepard KF, et al. Attribute dimensions that distinguish master and novice physical therapy clinicians in orthopedic settings. Phys Ther 1992;72(10):711–722

Jones M. Clinical reasoning in manipulative therapy. Aust J Physiother 1989;35:122

Jones M. Clinical reasoning in manual therapy. Phys Ther 1992;72(12):875–884

Jones M. Clinical reasoning and pain. Man Ther 1995;1(1):17–24

Jones M, Higgs J. Will evidence-based practice take the reasoning out of practice? In: Clinical Reasoning in the Health Professions. 2nd ed. Oxford: Butterworth-Heinemann; 2000

Jull G, Bogduk N, et al. The accuracy of manual diagnosis for cervical zygapophyseal joint pain syndromes. Med J Aust 1988;148:233–236

Keating J, Matyas T. Unreliable inferences from reliable measurements. Aust J Physiother 1998;44(1):5–10

Kendall NAS, Linton SJ, et al. Guide to Assessing Psychosocial Yellow Flags in Acute Low Back Pain: Risk Factors for Long-term Disability and Work Loss. Wellington: Accident Rehabilitation & Compensation Insurance Corporation of New Zealand and the National Health Committee; 1997

King C, Bithell C. Expertise in clinical reasoning: a comparative study. Br J Ther Rehabil 1998;5(2):78–87

Koninklijk Nederlands Genootschap voor Fysiotherapie (KNFG). KNGF Richtlijn Lage-rugpijn. Amersfoort: KNGF, 2001

Krebs DE, Harris SR. Elements of theory presentations in physical therapy. Phys Ther 1988;68(5):690–693

Kuhn T. The Structure of Scientific Revolutions. Chicago: University of Chicago Press; 1962

Larkin J, McDermott J, et al. Expert and novice performance in solving physics problems. Science 1980;208(4450): 1335–1342

Linton P. In defense of reason. Meta-analysis and beyond in evidence-based practice. Pain Forum 1995;7(1):46–54

MacDermid JC, Chesworth BM, et al. Validity of pain and motion indicators recorded on a movement diagram of shoulder lateral rotation. Aust J Physiother 1999;45(4): 269–277

Main CJ. Communicating about pain to patients. Schmerzen, alles klar? Zurzach; 2004

Maitland GD. Vertebral Manipulation. Oxford: Butterworth-Heinemann; 1968

Maitland GD. Vertebral Manipulation. Oxford: 5th ed. Butterworth-Heinemann; 1986

Maitland GD. The Maitland Concept: Assessment, examination and treatment by passive movement. In: Twomey LT, Taylor JR, eds. Physical Therapy of the Low Back. New York: Churchill Livingstone; 1987

Maitland GD, Hengeveld E, et al. Maitland's Vertebral Manipulation. Oxford: Butterworth-Heinemann; 2005

Maluf KS, Sahrmann SA, et al. Use of a classification system to guide nonsurgical management of a patient with chronic low back pain. Phys Ther 2000;80(11):1097–1111

Mattingly C. The narrative nature of clinical reasoning. Am J Occup Ther 1991;45(11):998–1005

Mattingly C, Fleming M. Clinical Reasoning: Forms of Inquiry in a Therapeutic Practice. Philadelphia: F.A. Davis Company; 1994

McCombe PF, Fairbank JC, et al. 1989 Volvo Award in Clinical Sciences. Reproducibility of physical signs in low-back pain. Spine 1989;14(9):908–918

McKenzie R. The Lumbar Spine: Mechanical Diagnosis and Therapy. Waikanae: Spinal Publications; 1981

Munroe II. Clinical reasoning in occupational therapy. Br J Occup Ther 1996;5(59):196–202

Nederlands Paramedisch Instituut (NPI). Evidence-based paramedische zorg. Een balans tussen "consensus based evidence" en "research based evidence." 1997;4:44

Nonaka I, Takeuchi H. The Knowledge-creating Company. New York, Oxford: Oxford University Press; 1995

Norman G, Patel V. Current models of clinical reasoning: implications for medical teaching. Symposium; 1987

O'Sullivan P. Diagnosis and classification of chronic low back pain disorders: maladaptive movement and motor control impairments as underlying mechanism. Man Ther 2005;10(4):242–255

Parry A. Physical therapy and methods of inquiry: conflict and reconciliation. Physiother 1991;77:435–439

Patel V, Arocha J. Methods in the study of clinical reasoning. In Higgs J, Jones M, eds. Clinical Reasoning in the Health Professions. Oxford: Butterworth-Heinemann; 1995

Payton OD. Clinical reasoning process in physical therapy. Phys Ther 1985;65(6):924–928

Peat M. Physiotherapy: art or science? Physiother Can 1981;33(3):170–176

Pfund R, Zahnd F. Leitsymptom Schmerz, Band I. Stuttgart: Thieme; 2001

Pfund R, Zahnd F. Leitsymptom Schmerz, Band II. Stuttgart: Thieme; 2003

Phillips DR, Twomey LT. A comparison of manual diagnosis with a diagnosis established by a uni-level lumbar spinal block procedure. Man Ther 1996;1(2):82–87

Pratt JW. Towards a philosophy of physical therapy. Physiother 1989;75:114–120

Roberts P. Theoretical models of physical therapy. Physiother 1994;80:361–366

Robertson L. Clinical reasoning. Part 1: the nature of problem solving, a literature review. Br J Occup Ther 1996a;59(4):178–182

Robertson L. Clinical reasoning. Part 2: Novice/expert differences. Br J Occup Ther 1996b;59(5):212–216

Rose SJ. Physical therapy diagnosis: role and function. Phys Ther 1989;69(7):535–537

Rothstein JM. Disability and our identity. Phys Ther 1994;74(5):375–378

Ryan P. The study and application of clinical reasoning research. Br J Ther Rehabil 1995;2:265–271

Ryan P. Developing reasoning skills. In: Alsop A, Ryan P. Making the Most of Fieldwork Education—A Practical Approach. London: Chapman & Hall; 1996

Sackett D, Richardson W, et al. Evidence-based medicine—how to practice and teach EBM. Edinburgh: Churchill Livingstone; 1998

Sackett D. Richardson W, et al. Evidence-based medicine—how to practice and teach EBM. 3rd ed. Edinburgh: Churchill Livingstone; 2008

Sackett D, Rosenberg W, et al. Evidence based medicine: what it is and what it isn't. BMJ 1996;312:71–72

Sahrmann SA. Diagnosis by the physical therapist—a prerequisite for treatment. A special communication. Phys Ther 1988;68(11):1703–1706

Schachter CL, Stalker CA, et al. Toward sensitive practice: issues for physical therapists working with survivors of childhood sexual abuse. Phys Ther 1999;79(3):248–261, discussion 262–269

Schmidt H, Boshuizen H. On acquiring expertise in medicine. Educ Psychol Rev 1993;5(3):205–221

Schön DA. The Reflective Practitioner. How Professionals Think in Action. New York: Basic Books; 1983

Schüffel W, Brucks U, et al, eds. Handbuch der Salutogenese—Theorie und Praxis. Wiesbaden: Ullstein Medical; 1998

Tanner C. Teaching Clinical Judgement. Annu Rev Nurs Res 1987;5:153–173

Thomas-Edding D. Clinical problem solving in physical therapy and its implications for curriculum development. Proceedings of the 10th International Congress of the World Confederation of Physical Therapy, Sydney; 1987

Thomson D, Hassenkamp AM, et al. The measurement of empathy in a clinical and non-clinical setting. Does empathy increase with clinical experience? Physiother 1997;83:173–180

Tyni-Lenné R. To identify the physiotherapy paradigm: a challenge for the future. Physiother Theory Pract 1989;5:169–170

van Tulder M, Koes BW, Assendelft WJJ, Bouter IM. The effectiveness of conservative treatment of acute and chronic low back pain. Amsterdam: EMGO Institute; 1999

Waddell G. 1987 Volvo Award in Clinical Sciences. A new clinical model for the treatment of low-back pain. Spine 1987;12(7):632–644

Waddell G. The Back Pain Revolution. 2nd ed. Edinburgh: Churchill Livingstone; 2004

Watson P. Psychosocial Assessment. Zurzach: IMTA Educational Days; 1999

Watts N. Decision analysis: a tool for improving physical therapy practice and education. In: Wolf S, ed. Clinical Decision Making in Physical Therapy. Philadelphia: F. A. Davis; 1985:7–23

Watts N. Teaching clinical decision analysis in physical therapy. In: Higgs J, Jones M, eds. Clinical Reasoning in the Health Professions: Oxford: Butterworth-Heinemann; 2000:236–241

Williams PL, Warwick R. Gray's Anatomy. Edinburgh: Churchill Livingstone; 1980

Winkel D, Vleeming A, et al. Diagnosis and Treatment of the Spine: Nonoperative Orthopaedic Medicine and Manual Therapy. Texas: Pro-Ed; 2003

World Confederation of Physical Therapy (WCPT). Description of Physical Therapy. London: World Confederation of Physical Therapy; 1999

World Health Organization (WHO). ICF—International Classification of Functioning, Disability and Health. Geneva: World Health Organization; 2001

# 2 Examination of Structures and Functions of the Locomotor System

# 2 Examination of Structures and Functions of the Locomotor System

## 2.1 Testing Structures

### 2.1.1 Joint Measurement According to the Neutral Zero Method
*Barbara Trinkle*

The range of motion of a given joint may be measured using a goniometer.

> Synonyms found in the literature for the extent of movement include "range of motion" (ROM) and "joint range of motion" (JROM).

The "neutral zero measuring method" is a standardized method. Establishing the neutral (0°) position of a joint allows for a comparison of results. This point is defined as the neutral or zero position and it corresponds to the position in the upright standing person (**Fig. 2.1**). The arms are hanging next to the body, and the thumbs, feet, knees, and gaze are directed forward. The longitudinal axes of the feet and lower legs form a right angle and the feet are placed hip-width apart. In this starting position, the joints are in a *neutral position* from which various possible ranges of motion may be measured.

The neutral position may be applied to other starting positions (e.g., supine, lateral recumbent, or prone). The distal joint component is moved in one of the three defined planes of the body (sagittal, frontal, and transverse) while the proximal joint component remains stationary.

#### Placement of the Goniometer
The fulcrum of the goniometer is placed over the axis of motion of the joint, and its two extending arms are aligned with the virtual (imagined) longitudinal axes of the bone.

It is important to carefully palpate the reference points and to mark them to limit the variability of measurement results (Cabri 2001):

#### Examples:
- *Measurement of knee joint bending/extension:*
  - Place the fulcrum of the goniometer laterally over the center of the knee joint.
  - Align the proximal arm with the longitudinal axis of the femur using the trochanter major as the reference point.
  - Align the distal arm with the longitudinal axis of the lower leg using the lateral malleolus as the reference point.
- *Measurement of hip joint abduction/adduction:*
  - Place the fulcrum of the goniometer from ventral over the center of the hip joint.
  - Align the proximal arm with a connecting line between the anterior superior iliac spines.
  - Align the distal arm with the longitudinal axis of the femur using the center of the knee joint as the reference point.

> The goniometer must be accurately positioned, applying active or passive support to prevent any change to the patient's position.

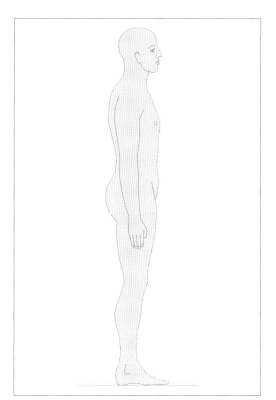

**Fig. 2.1** The neutral or zero position.

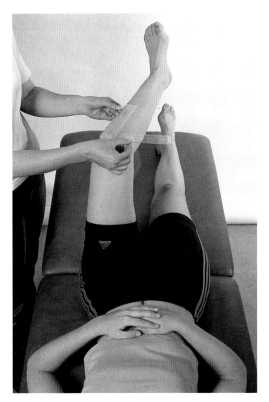

**Fig. 2.2** Measuring rotation of the hip joint with 90° hip and knee joint bending (rotation in the frontal plane). The fulcrum of the goniometer is placed ventrally over the hip joint and moved parallel to it.

If the goniometer cannot be placed over the center of the joint, the fulcrum may be placed over a parallel position (**Fig. 2.2**).

### Obtaining Measurements

The available active and/or passive range of motion of a joint may be measured. To do so, the distal joint component is moved away from the proximal joint component as far as possible.

If the patient is able to actively perform the movement without any pain, this is preferable to a passive measurement because they use their own muscles for the fully available range of motion. When taking passive measurements, the therapist measures not only the angular position, but also the quality of the end-feel or the stopping point of the motion (e.g., muscular, capsular, bony) of the joint being examined (Cabri 2001).

> For the analysis and interpretation of painful or non-painful movement limitation, and in patients with paralysis, the differentiation between passive and active ranges of motion is essential.

For the purpose of comparison (e.g., for repeated measurements or in the event that the patient sees another therapist), and to prevent measurement errors, readily identifiable reference points (landmarks) or connecting lines between two points on the body should be chosen. The measurement results should be recorded and compared with *normal values* (see **Tables 2.1–2.7**).

### Documentation of Measurement Results

The notation (documentation) of the measurement results must be easily understood by relevant third parties. In order to facilitate assessment and follow-up, measurements should always be performed in the same order.

### Procedure

- Name the joint (e.g., knee joint).
- State the directions of joint movement in a single plane and around an axis of motion (e.g., bending/extension).
- The measurement value is understood to be in degrees; a degree sign is not used.
- Record the measured ranges of motion in the order cited.
- If the neutral position can be reached, the 0 is *between* the two measured values.
- If the neutral position cannot be reached, the 0 is entered for the movement direction in which there is *no* available range of motion.
- Each value is separated from the next by a forward slash.

> A comparison of sides is essential when measuring extremity joints.

*Examples:*
- *Freely moving knee joint: Bending/extension on the right 130/0/0, left 130/0/0:*
  - The neutral position is reached.
  - End-range movements are possible in the knee joints.
- *Bending contracture of the right knee joint: Bending/extension right 130/20/0, left 130/0/0:*
  - An extension deficit of 20° is noted in the 0° space.
  - This indicates that the neutral position of the joint cannot be reached.
- *Contracture of the right knee joint: Bending/extension right 30/30/0, left 130/0/0:*
  - If there is a joint contracture, the joint position is noted twice.

***Normal Values and Measurement Procedures***
The following tables list normal values (Hepp and Debrunner 2004), describe goniometer placement, and provide additional details. On the following pages are photographs showing the procedure for taking measurements.

**Table 2.1** Normal values for movements of the **hip joint** based on the neutral zero method

| Movement | Normal values | Starting position | Placement of the goniometer and additional details (Fig. 2.3a–e) |
|---|---|---|---|
| Bending/extension | 130/0/12 | • Supine<br>• Lateral recumbent | • Normal mobility in the lumbar spine:<br>  – F: Projecting at the level of the trochanter major<br>  – PA: Longitudinal axis of the body with bending of the lumbar spine using the Thomas grip<br>  – DA: Longitudinal femoral axis/center of the knee joint<br>Due to the lumbar lordosis, the functional neutral position of the hip joint is about 12° bending<br>The Thomas grip (end-range bending with slight external rotation of the opposite leg) moves the pelvis further in the hip joint by ca. 12° extension → bending of lumbar spine<br>If the thigh of the hip joint being measured remains in contact with the examining table, hip joint extension of 12° is possible<br>• Immobile lumbar spine:<br>  – F: See above<br>  – PA: Longitudinal axis of the pelvis (highest point of the iliac crest to the ischial tuberosity)<br>  – DA: Longitudinal femoral axis/center of the knee joint |
| Abduction/adduction | 40/0/30 | • Supine | • F: Center of hip joint<br>• PA: Connecting line between the iliac spines<br>• DA: Longitudinal femoral axis/center of the knee joint |
| Transverse abduction/adduction | 80/0/20 | • Supine | • F: Center of hip joint projects to the connecting line of the iliac spines<br>• PA: Connecting line between the iliac spines<br>• DA: Longitudinal femoral axis/center of the knee joint |
| Internal rotation/external rotation from the neutral position of the hip joint | 40/0/30 | • Supine | • F: Center of hip joint projects to sole of foot, center of heel<br>• PA: Connecting line between the iliac spines<br>• DA:<br>  – Bending/extension axis of the knee joint, or<br>  – Along the anatomical longitudinal axis of the foot (with stabilized dorsal extension of the upper ankle joint) |
| Internal rotation/external rotation with 90° bending of the knee | 40/0/30 | • Prone | • F: Center of hip joint projects to center of knee joint<br>• PA: Connecting line between the iliac spines<br>• DA: Longitudinal axis of the lower leg/center of ankle |
| Internal rotation/external rotation with 90° hip and knee bending | 30/0/50 | • Supine<br>• Sitting | • F: Center of hip joint projects to center of knee joint<br>• PA: Connecting line between the iliac spines<br>• DA: Longitudinal axis of the lower leg/center of ankle joint |

Note: F = fulcrum; PA = proximal arm; DA = distal arm.

**Table 2.2** Normal values for movements of the **knee joint** based on the neutral zero method

| Movement | Normal values | Starting position | Placement of the goniometer and additional details (Fig. 2.4) |
|---|---|---|---|
| Bending/extension | 150/0/5 | • Supine | • F: Middle of the lateral joint space of the knee<br>• PA: Longitudinal femoral axis/trochanter major<br>• DA: Longitudinal axis of lower leg/middle of lateral malleolus |
| Internal rotation/external rotation with 90° bending of the knee joint | Comparing sides | • Supine<br>• Sitting | • Assess (estimate) without goniometer, with 90° knee bending<br>• DA: Anatomical longitudinal axis of the foot (with stabilized dorsal extension [DE] in upper ankle joint) |

Note: F = fulcrum; PA = proximal arm; DA = distal arm.

**Table 2.3** Normal values of movements of the **ankle joints**, the **metatarsus** and the **joints of the toes** based on the neutral zero method

| Movement | Normal values | Starting position | Placement of the goniometer and additional details (Fig. 2.5a, b; Fig. 2.6) |
|---|---|---|---|
| Dorsal extension/plantar bending of the upper ankle joint | 20/0/50 | • Supine | • F: Lateral malleolus<br>• PA: Longitudinal axis of lower leg<br>• DA: Longitudinal axis of the foot/fifth metatarsal |
| Inversion/eversion of the lower ankle joint | • 60/0/30<br>• Comparing sides | • Supine | • F: Bases of fifth/first metatarsals<br>• PA: Horizontal<br>• DA: Connecting line between the bases of metatarsals I–V/V–I<br>The range of motion is usually estimated; precise measurement in degrees is only possible with special devices |
| Supination/pronation of the metatarsus | • 30/0/15<br>• Comparing sides | • Supine | • F: Points toward first metatarsal (pronation); points toward fifth metatarsal (supination)<br>• PA: Transverse axis of the heel<br>• DA: Transverse axis of the metatarsal heads |
| Bending/extension of the toe joints | Comparing sides | • Supine | • F: Metatarsophalangeal joint/interphalangeal and distal interphalangeal joints<br>• PA: Metatarsal/proximal and middle phalanges<br>• DA: Proximal/middle/distal phalanx |

Note: F = fulcrum; PA = proximal arm; DA = distal arm.

**Table 2.4** Normal values for **shoulder girdle** movements based on the neutral zero method

| Movement | Normal values | Starting position | Placement of the goniometer and additional details |
|---|---|---|---|
| Elevation/depression | Comparing sides | • Sitting | • F: Points toward the superior angle of the scapula<br>• PA: Spine<br>• DA: Medial border of the scapula |
| Abduction/adduction of the scapula | Comparing sides | • Sitting | • F: Crown (of the head)<br>• PA: Horizontal<br>• DA: Spine of the scapula |
| Ventral/dorsal rotation of clavicle | Comparing sides | • Sitting | Inferior angle of the scapula moves along the thorax 8–10 cm cranially during ventral rotation, and it moves back during dorsal rotation |

Note: F = fulcrum; PA = proximal arm; DA = distal arm.

**Table 2.5** Normal values for movements of the **shoulder joint** based on the neutral zero method

| Movement | Normal values | Starting position | Placement of the goniometer and additional details (Fig. 2.7a–e) |
|---|---|---|---|
| Bending/extension | 170/0/40 | ▪ Supine<br>▪ Sitting | ▪ F: Middle of shoulder joint from lateral<br>▪ PA: Longitudinal axis of body<br>▪ DA: Longitudinal axis of humerus/lateral epicondyle |
| Abduction/adduction | 180/0/40 | ▪ Supine<br>▪ Sitting | ▪ F: Middle of shoulder joint from ventral<br>▪ PA: Parallel to longitudinal axis of body<br>▪ DA: Longitudinal axis of humerus |
| Transverse bending/extension | 130/0/40 | ▪ Sitting | ▪ F: Points toward acromion<br>▪ PA: Horizontal<br>▪ DA: Longitudinal axis of humerus/middle of wrist |
| Internal/external rotation from the neutral position with 90° elbow bending | 100/0/40 | ▪ Supine<br>▪ Sitting | ▪ F: Points toward acromion/olecranon<br>▪ PA: Horizontal<br>▪ DA: Longitudinal axis of lower arm/middle of wrist |
| Internal/external rotation with 90° abduction of shoulder joint and 90° bending of elbow joint | 70/0/70 | ▪ Supine<br>▪ Sitting | ▪ F: Points toward olecranon<br>▪ PA: Longitudinal axis of body<br>▪ DA: Longitudinal axis of lower arm/ middle of wrist |
| Internal/external rotation with 90° bending of the shoulder and 90° bending of the elbow joint | 70/0/80 | ▪ Sitting | ▪ F: Points toward acromion/olecranon<br>▪ PA: Horizontal<br>▪ DA: Longitudinal axis of lower arm/middle of wrist |

Note: F = fulcrum; PA = proximal arm; DA = distal arm.

**Table 2.6** Normal values for movements of the **elbow and radioulnar joints** based on the neutral zero method

| Movement | Normal values | Starting position | Placement of the goniometer and additional details |
|---|---|---|---|
| Bending/extension | 150/0/5 | ▪ Sitting | ▪ F: Olecranon<br>▪ PA: Longitudinal axis of upper arm/middle of shoulder joint<br>▪ DA: Longitudinal axis of lower arm/middle of wrist |
| Supination/pronation of lower arm (Fig. 2.8) | 90/0/90 | ▪ Sitting with 90° elbow bending and closed fist | ▪ F: Points toward metacarpophalangeal joint of the middle finger<br>▪ PA: Longitudinal axis of upper arm<br>▪ DA: Transverse axis through metacarpophalangeal joints |

Note: F = fulcrum; PA = proximal arm; DA = distal arm.

**Table 2.7** Normal values for movements of the **wrist joint,** the **fingers**, and the **thumb** based on the neutral zero method

| Movement | Normal values | Starting position | Placement of the goniometer and additional details |
|---|---|---|---|
| Dorsal extension/volar bending | 60/0/60 | • Sitting with 90° elbow bending | • F: Points toward the ulnar styloid<br>• PA: Longitudinal axis of lower arm/lateral epicondyle<br>• DA: Fifth metacarpal |
| Ulnar/radial abduction (**Fig. 2.9**) | 40/0/30 | • Sitting | • F: Middle of the wrist<br>• PA: Longitudinal axis of lower arm<br>• DA: Third metacarpal |
| Bending/extension of metacarpophalangeal joints | 90/0/5 | • Supine<br>• Sitting | • F: Metacarpophalangeal joints<br>• PA: Metacarpals II–V<br>• DA: Middle phalanges II–V |
| Abduction/adduction of metacarpophalangeal joints | Distance between fingers | • Sitting | • Evaluate with comparison of sides<br>• Measure distance with ruler (cm) |
| Bending/extension of proximal interphalangeal joints of fingers | 100/0/0 | • Sitting | • F: Proximal interphalangeal joints<br>• PA: Proximal phalanges II–V<br>• DA: Middle phalanges II–V |
| Bending/extension of distal interphalangeal joints of fingers | Distance fingertip to middle phalanx | • Sitting | • F: Distal interphalangeal joints of fingers<br>• PA: Middle phalanges II–V<br>• DA: Distal phalanges II–V |
| Bending/extension of carpometacarpal joint of thumb | 70/0/0 | • Sitting | • F: Carpometacarpal joints of thumb<br>• PA: Longitudinal axis of index finger (fixed)<br>• DA: Longitudinal axis of thumb |
| Abduction/adduction of carpometacarpal joint of thumb (**Fig. 2.10**) | 70/0/0 | • Sitting | • F: Carpometacarpal joints of thumb<br>• PA: Longitudinal axis of index finger (fixed)<br>• DA: Longitudinal axis of thumb |
| Opposition | Tip of thumb reaches proximal interphalangeal joint of fifth metacarpal | • Sitting | • F: Carpometacarpal joint of thumb |
| Bending/extension of carpometacarpal/interphalangeal joints of thumb | Comparing sides | • Sitting | • F: Carpometacarpal/interphalangeal joint of thumb<br>• PA: Metacarpal I/proximal phalanx I<br>• DA: Proximal phalanx I/distal phalanx I |

Note: F = fulcrum; PA = proximal arm; DA = distal arm.

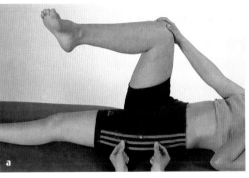

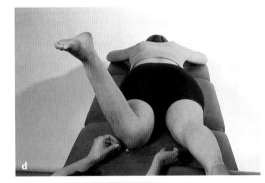

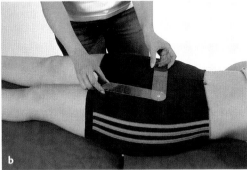

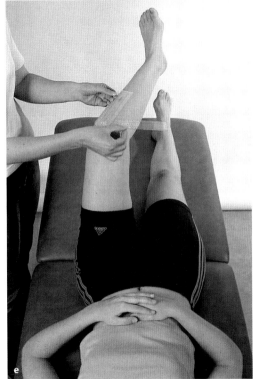

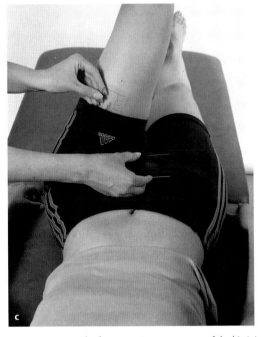

**Fig. 2.3a–e** Examples for measuring movements of the hip joint.
**a** Extension from the pelvis. In the opposite hip joint, the leg moves in the direction of bending with slight external rotation, thereby supporting the continuing movement of the pelvis, with extension in the hip joint.
**b** Adduction of the leg in the hip joint. The fulcrum of the goniometer is resting on the hip joint.
**c** Transverse adduction of the leg in the hip joint.
**d** Internal rotation of the leg in the hip joint in the transverse plane. The lower leg shows the extent of rotation; the pelvis remains in contact with the underlying surface on both sides.
**e** External rotation of the leg in the hip joint in the frontal plane. The lower leg shows the extent of rotation.

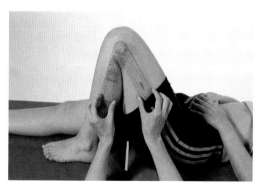

**Fig. 2.4** Measuring knee joint bending.

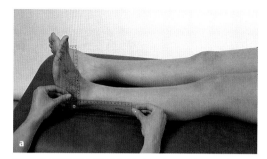

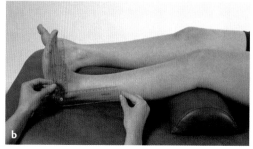

**Fig. 2.5a, b** Measuring dorsal extension of the upper ankle joint.
**a** Multi-joint stretching of the gastrocnemius muscle.
**b** Single-joint stretching of the gastrocnemius muscle.

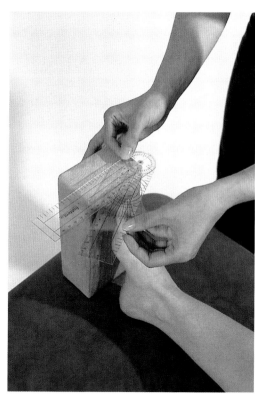

**Fig. 2.6** Example of measurements involving the foot: inversion and supination.

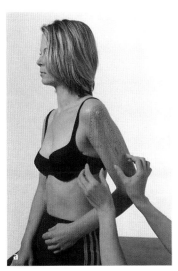

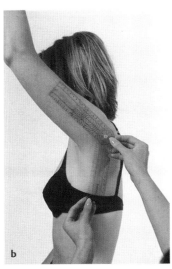

**Fig. 2.7a–e** Examples for measuring shoulder joint movements.
**a** Extension of the arm in the shoulder joint.
**b** Bending of the arm in the shoulder joint.
**c** Abduction of the arm in the shoulder joint.
**d** Transverse bending of the arm in the shoulder joint.
**e** Internal rotation of the arm with 90° abduction in the shoulder joint.

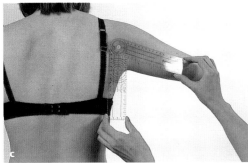

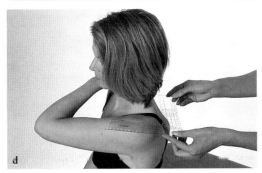

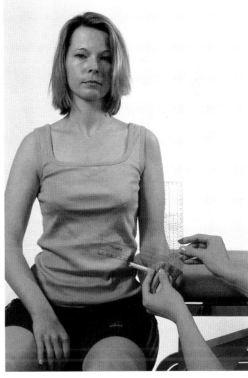

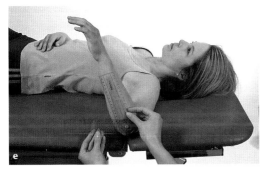

**Fig. 2.8** Measuring pronation. The pen shows the extent of pronation.

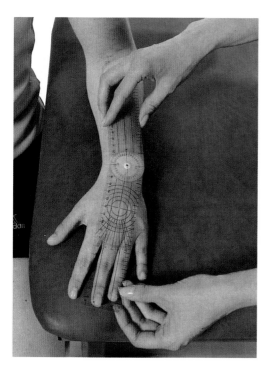

Fig. 2.9 Measuring radial abduction of the hand.

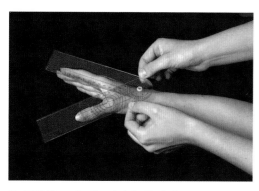

Fig. 2.10 Measuring thumb abduction in the carpometacarpal joint.

## Shapes of Hand Grasps/Grips

There are a variety of grasping shapes of the hand (**Fig. 2.11**), given that slight movements of the fingers produce new shapes. In most of these, the thumb is used in various oppositional positions, which ensures specific or secure grasping of an object. In all grasping shapes, the hand and finger muscles work synergistically.

### Example: Fist closure

Making a fist involves the extensors of the wrist, the flexors, and adductors of the fingers, and the muscles that produce thumb opposition. Along with these, the wrist flexors, the finger extensors and abductors, and the distal interphalangeal joints of the fingers, the carpometacarpal joint of the thumb, and the interphalangeal joint of the thumb may also be simultaneously active in bending.

Kapandji (1985) has described the grasping shapes in detail according to muscle function and the number of fingers used, as well as their position relative to each other. He distinguishes between *static* and *dynamic grasping/gripping shapes.*

### Static Grips

These are used for grasping, gripping, or holding an object:

- Nonprecision or power grips:
  - Handle or hook grip
  - Full fist
  - Flat hand grip
- Precision grips:
  - Pincer grip
  - Key grip
  - Lumbrical grip

### Dynamic Grips

Dynamic grips enable one to hold and simultaneously use (manipulate) an object with the hands.

## Evaluation of Spinal Mobility

The range of motion of the spine is measured by measuring angles, the distance between two points of orientation, or a visual assessment of mobility with a comparison of sides.

> *Palpation and manual therapy test movements may be used as complementary assessments during the examination of mobility, for instance, in patients with partial stiffness or hypermobility and instability of individual spinal segments.*

Before the examination, any difference in leg length must be compensated for, and the pelvis must be positioned so that there is a physiological tilt of 12° in the hip joints. Any deviations from the neutral position should be noted.

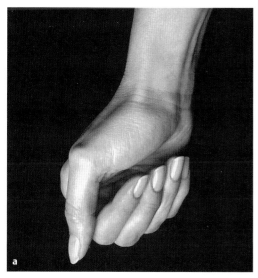

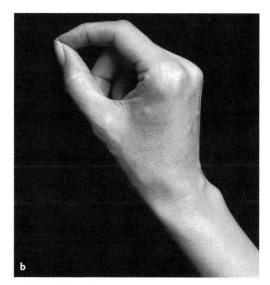

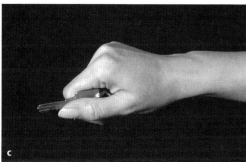

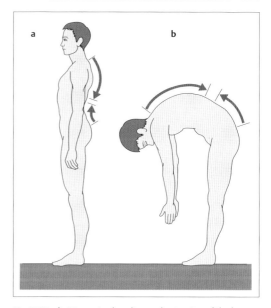

Fig. 2.11a–d  Examples of hand grasping/gripping shapes.
a Handle or hook grip. b Pincer grip. c Key grip.
d Lumbrical grip.

## The Lumbar Spine and the Thoracic Spine

### Bending/Extension (Fig. 2.12a, b)
**Measuring Distance Based on Schober and Ott**
Starting with the patient in the standing position, the following skin markings are placed on the spinal column:

- *Lumbar spine (Schober sign):*
  - The first skin marking is placed over the S1 spinous process and the second marking 10 cm further cranially.
  - When bending the trunk forward, bending should increase the distance between the two markings by about 5 cm.
- *Thoracic spine (Ott sign):*
  - The first marking is placed over the C7 spinous process and the second marking 30 cm caudally from it.
  - When the patient bends forward, the distance increases by about 8 cm.

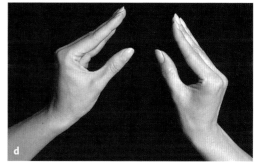

Fig. 2.12a, b  Measuring bending and extension of the lumbar and thoracic spines based on Schober and Ott.
a Starting position. b Final position: Measurement using the Ott method in the thoracic spine region and using the Schober method in the lumbar spine region.

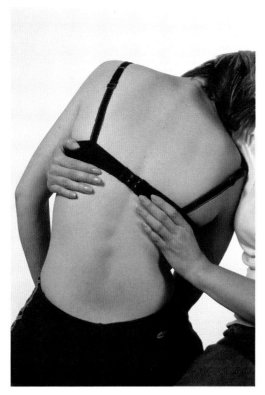

**Fig. 2.13** Evaluating sidebending of the lumbar spine and thoracic spine.

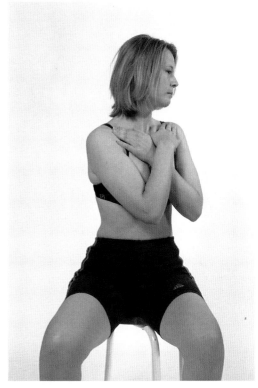

**Fig. 2.14** Evaluating spinal rotation at the thoracolumbar junction. The thorax rotates against the pelvis, which remains in place on the seat.

### Examples: Notation
- Lumbar spine: Bending/extension 15/10/7
- Thoracic spine: Bending/extension 32/30/29

> *The measurements obtained using Schober and Ott's methods do not provide information on the mobility of individual spinal segments.*

### Sidebending (Fig. 2.13)
Normal value: 30°.
- Fulcrum: Thoracolumbar junction
- Stationary arm: Longitudinal axis of the body
- Mobile arm: Straight due to the bent thoracic spine

### Rotation (Fig. 2.14)
Normal value: 30°.
- Fulcrum: Thoracolumbar junction points toward the crown of the head
- Stationary arm: Horizontal
- Mobile arm: Frontotransverse diameter of thorax

## Cervical Spine

### Bending/Extension
Measurements are taken of the degree of bending and the distance between the chin and sternum (in cm).
   Normal values: 35–45/0/35–45.
- Fulcrum: Upper head joints
- Stationary arm: Longitudinal axis of the body
- Mobile arm: Longitudinal axis of the head

### Sidebending
Measurements are obtained in degrees or to assess the distance between the earlobes and shoulders (in cm).
   Normal values: 45/0/45.
- Fulcrum: Middle cervical spine
- Stationary arm: Longitudinal axis of the body
- Mobile arm: Longitudinal axis of the head

### Rotation
Measurements are obtained of the angles in degrees.
   Normal values: 60–80/0/60–80.
- Fulcrum: Crown of the head

- Stationary arm: Sagittotransverse diameter of the thorax
- Mobile arm: Sagittotransverse axis of the head

## Longitudinal and Circumferential Measurements

### Longitudinal Measurements

In regard to longitudinal measurements of the extremities, leg length is especially important, given that any discrepancies will change static stability.

#### Anatomical Leg Length
The following distances are measured:
- Between the trochanter major and lateral knee joint space
- Between the lateral knee joint space and the middle of the lateral malleolus

> *Causes of leg length discrepancies are due to the bones (e.g., after fracture or in patients with growth disorders).*

#### Functional Leg Length
The distance is measured between the anterior superior iliac spine and the middle of the medial malleolus.

> *Reasons for a difference include, for example, improper static alignment of the spine (scoliosis), rotation within the pelvis, or holding the joints in a protective position due to muscle shortening or limited mobility.*

#### Board Test
- By palpating the iliac crests (from dorsal) with the flat of the hand or using a pelvic level device, one can examine whether one hip is higher on one side.
- If so, a small board may be used for support to make the pelvis level.
- The side should be noted and the height of the board (in cm) placed underneath the foot.

> *A difference in leg length may be due to either anatomical or functional causes.*

## Measuring Circumference

Measuring the circumference of the extremities helps to evaluate outcomes, for example, in patients with swelling (**Fig. 2.15, Fig. 2.16**). For documentation, measuring sites are chosen that may be

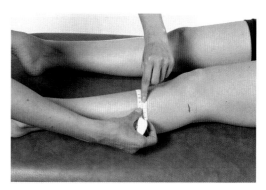

**Fig. 2.15** Before measuring the circumference, the chosen site, for example the joint space of the knee, is marked; when comparing measurements, always choose the same distance (to the knee joint).

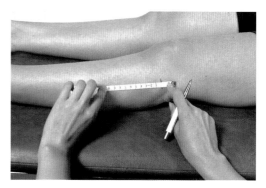

**Fig. 2.16** Measuring the circumference of the lower leg.

changed or added to as needed (**Table 2.8, Table 2.9**). The same ones must be used at each reassessment.

> *Be sure the measuring tape is held taut, without causing any constriction of the tissue.*

### 2.1.2 Tests of Muscle Function
*Barbara Trinkle*

*Manual muscle testing* (MMT), or the *muscle test*, is part of the physical therapy examination. Although only an estimation, this test is well established because it can assess the degree and extent of muscle weakness with minimal technical effort (Wieben and Falkenberg 2012). The test may be performed on any patient with musculoskeletal and neuromuscular disorders.

The test results (muscle values) are expressed in grades from 0 to 6, with each level being precisely defined (**Table 2.10**).

**Table 2.8** Measuring circumferences of the upper extremity

| Measuring site | Date | Right | Left |
|---|---|---|---|
| 10 cm above the lateral humeral epicondyle | | | |
| Lateral humeral epicondyle | | | |
| 10 cm below the lateral humeral epicondyle | | | |
| Wrist at the level of the ulnar styloid process | | | |
| Metacarpophalangeal joints | | | |

**Table 2.9** Measuring circumferences of the lower extremity

| Measuring site | Date | Right | Left |
|---|---|---|---|
| 10 cm above the lateral joint space of the knee | | | |
| Lateral joint space of the knee | | | |
| 10 cm below the lateral joint space of the knee | | | |
| Talar mortise | | | |
| Metatarsophalangeal joint | | | |

**Table 2.10** Muscle grades

| Grade | Definition | Notes |
|---|---|---|
| 0 | No visible or palpable tension of any of the muscles involved in the movement | |
| 1 | Visible or palpable muscle contraction, movement is impossible | Possibly bring the origin and insertion of the muscle closer together during the test |
| 2 | The movement may be done in an antigravity position in the horizontal plane | Friction forces should be eliminated as fully as possible |
| 3 | The movement can be performed fully, without applied resistance, against gravity | |
| 4 | The movement can be performed fully against gravity and moderate resistance | |
| 5 | The movement can be performed fully against gravity and strong resistance | |
| 6 | The movement can be performed 10 times fully against gravity and strong resistance | |

*For grades 3 to 5, if the patient cannot be placed in a starting position that allows for antigravity movement, manual resistance may be used instead.*

### Goals of Muscle Function Tests
- Initial assessment at the patient's first visit
- Evaluate treatment outcomes
- Final evaluation
- Notes for therapy:
  - Change/modification
  - Successes/failures
  - Notes on necessary aids in everyday life
  - Acquisition of compensation strategies for functional deficits
- Optimal design of treatment with exercises increasing in difficulty
- Differential diagnosis
- Prognoses

*Regular evaluations of outcomes can enhance the patient's motivation to perform the exercise treatment.*

### Requirements for Therapists

The therapist should have thorough knowledge of the following:

- Joint mechanics, course, function, and innervation of the muscles, given that imprecise tests can lead to misleading information and erroneous conclusions.
- How the muscles work together: When an agonist muscle produces a movement, the synergist muscles help to perform it. Although the synergists may partially replace an agonist, they cannot perform a movement to the end of its range by themselves. The antagonists of the agonist muscles being tested must have sufficient flexibility.
- Given that the subjective influence of the therapist can often compromise the objectivity of the test result, a certain amount of experience is necessary in order to achieve the most objective status possible.

> *Even the amount of manual resistance applied by the therapist can vary widely (Capri 2001).*

### Performing the Tests

The following criteria should be recalled:

- Correct starting position.
- Optimal positioning.
- Stay in the plane of movement.
- Before determining the amount of force, the passive range of motion should be tested. Any limitations of movement and their causes should be taken into account during the evaluation and documented (e.g., skeletal, ligamentous, capsular, muscular, or pain).
- Joint status based on the neutral zero method should be included.
- The test movement must be precisely explained to the patient.
- The movement is done from the distal joint partner. The therapist or patient actively stabilizes the proximal joint partner. The proximal joint partner should be observed for any movement.
- Objective evaluation: Re-evaluation should be performed by the same person every time. To avoid potential bias, someone other than the therapist should perform the reassessments.
- If there is any uncertainty, both sides should be compared.
- Documentation of the muscle test results.

> *After an injury, tests should only be performed at the level corresponding to the current status of the structure.*

## Testing the Extremity and Trunk Musculature

The following photographs (**Figs. 2.17–2.24**) show examples of test situations.

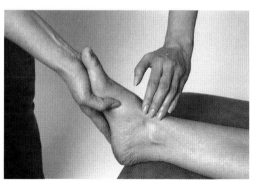

**Fig. 2.17** Test of the tibialis anterior (grade 1): Palpation of the region around the tendon.

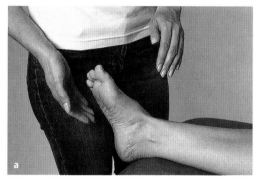

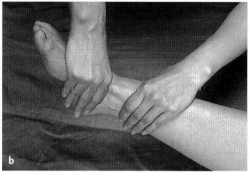

**Fig. 2.18a, b** Supination of the foot.
**a** Grade 2 test result.
**b** Test results of grades 4 and 5.

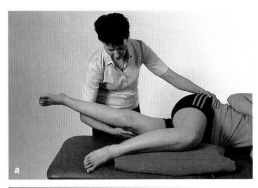

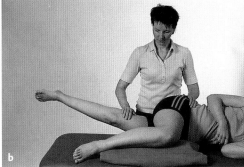

Fig. 2.19a, b Test of the hip joint adductors.
a Grade 3 test result, the leg must be able to be held by itself.
b Test results of grades 4 and 5.

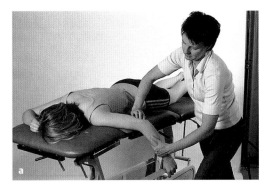

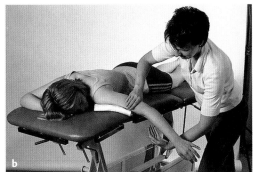

Fig. 2.20a, b Test of the extensors of the elbow joint.
a Grade 1 test result, palpation in the area around the triceps tendon.
b Grade 3 test result.

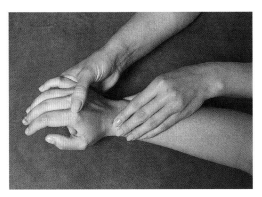

Fig. 2.21 Test of the dorsal extensors of the wrist (grade 1). Shown here: palpation of the region around the tendon of the extensor carpi radialis longus muscle.

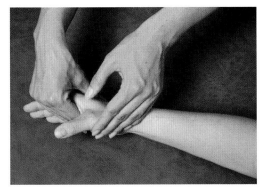

Fig. 2.22 Abductor test of the carpometacarpal joint of thumb (grade 2).

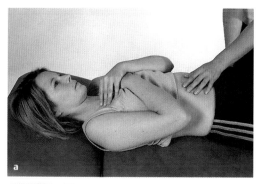

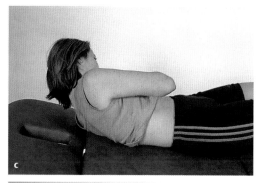

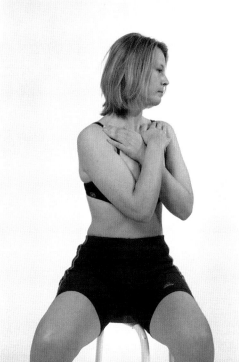

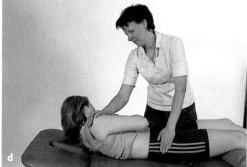

Fig. 2.23a–d  Rotation of the trunk.
a  Test of the oblique muscles of the abdomen (grade 1).
b  Grade 2.
c  Grade 3.
d  Grade 4.

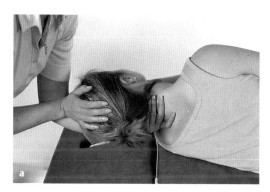

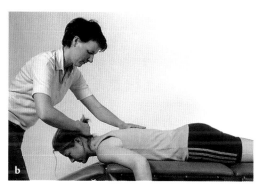

Fig. 2.24a, b  Extension of the cervical spine.
a  Grade 2 test result. b  Test results of grades 4 and 5.

### Documentation

| *The documentation of the test results should be clear and easily understandable.*

The date, patient data, diagnosis/additional diagnosis, and name of evaluator are listed at the top.

For the purposes of documentation, it is useful to list the details in a table containing the movement, the tested muscles, and their segmental innervation. Wieben and Falkenberg (1997) recommend this in the documentation schemes in **Figs. 2.25–2.27**.

Right side — Name of patient: — Date of birth: — Diagnosis: — Name of examiner: — Left side

Date (Right side) / Date (Left side)

T6

**Cervical spine extension**
Cervical portion of autochthonous back muscles, C1–C8, dorsal branches of spinal nerves

**Thoracic spine extension**
Thoracic portion of autochthonous back muscles, T1–T12, dorsal branches of spinal nerves

**Lumbar spine extension**
Lumbar portion of autochthonous back muscles, L1–L5, dorsal branches of spinal nerves

**Cervical spine bending**
Sternocleidomastoid muscle, accessory nerve, and cervical plexus (C1–C2)
Rectus capitis anterior muscle, cervical plexus (C1–C4)
Longus capitis muscle, cervical plexus (C1–C4)
Longus colli muscle, brachial plexus, and cervical plexus (C2–C8)

**Trunk bending**
Rectus abdominis muscle, T5–T12, intercostal nerves
External and internal abdominal oblique muscles, T5–T12, intercostal nerves

**Rotation of the trunk to the right**
External abdominal oblique muscle, T5–T12, intercostal nerves
Internal abdominal oblique muscles T10–T12, intercostal nerves and L1

**Rotation of the trunk to the left**
External abdominal oblique muscle, T5–T12, intercostal nerves
Internal abdominal oblique muscles T10–T12, intercostal nerves and L1

**Sidebending of the trunk**
Erector spinae muscles, C1–S4, dorsal branches of spinal nerves
External abdominal oblique muscle, T5–T12, intercostal nerves
Internal abdominal oblique muscles T10–T12, intercostal nerves and L1
Rectus abdominis muscle, T5–T12, intercostal nerves
Latissimus dorsi muscle, C6–C8, thoracodorsal nerve
Quadratus lumborum muscle, T12, intercostal nerve, L1–L3, lumbar plexus

**Fig. 2.25** Documentation of test results—extremities. (From: Wieben K, Falkenberg B. Muskelfunktion. Stuttgart: Thieme; 2012.)

| Right side (Date) | Name of patient: _____ Date of birth: _____ Diagnosis: _____ Name of examiner: _____ | Left side (Date) |
|---|---|---|
| | **Shoulder blade, cranially** | |
| | Trapezius muscle, ascending part, accessory nerve, and trapezius branch (C2–C4) | |
| | Levator scapulae muscle, C4–C5, dorsal scapular nerve | |
| | **Shoulder blade, caudally** | |
| | Trapezius muscle, ascending part, accessory nerve, and trapezius branch (C2–C4) | |
| | Serratus anterior muscle, C5–C7, long thoracic nerve | |
| | **Shoulder blade, dorsally and medially** | |
| | Trapezius muscle, accessory nerve, and trapezius branch (C2–C4) | |
| | Rhomboid muscles, C4–C5, dorsal scapular nerve | |
| | Latissimus dorsi muscle, C6–C8, thoracodorsal nerve | |
| | **Shoulder blade, ventrally and laterally** | |
| | Serratus anterior muscle, C5–C7, long thoracic nerve | |
| | Pectoralis major and minor muscles, C5–T1, pectoral nerves | |
| | **Shoulder joint, elevation** | |
| | Deltoid muscle, clavicular part, C4–C6, axillary nerve | |
| | Biceps brachii muscle, C5–C6, musculocutaneous nerve | |
| | **Shoulder joint, retroversion** | |
| | Teres major muscle, C6–C7, thoracodorsal nerve | |
| | Latissimus dorsi muscle, C6–C8, thoracodorsal nerve | |
| | Triceps brachii, long head, C6–C8, radial nerve | |
| | Deltoid muscle, spinal part, C4–C6, axillary nerve | |
| | **Shoulder joint abduction** | |
| | Deltoid muscle, C4–C6, axillary nerve | |
| | Supraspinatus muscle, C4–C6, suprascapular nerve | |
| | **Shoulder joint adduction** | |
| | Pectoralis major muscle, C5–T1, pectoral nerves | |
| | Triceps brachii, long head, C6–C8, radial nerve | |
| | Teres major muscle, C6–C7, thoracodorsal nerve | |
| | Latissimus dorsi muscle, C6–C8, thoracodorsal nerve | |
| | **Shoulder joint, external rotation** | |
| | Infraspinatus muscle, C4–C6, suprascapular nerve | |
| | Teres minor muscle, C5–C6, axillary nerve | |
| | **Shoulder joint, internal rotation** | |
| | Subscapularis muscle, C5–C8, subscapular nerve | |
| | Teres major muscle, C6–C7, thoracodorsal nerve | |
| | **Elbow joint, bending** | |
| | Biceps brachii muscle, C5–C6, musculocutaneous nerve | |
| | Brachialis muscle, C5–C6, musculocutaneous nerve | |
| | Brachioradialis muscle, C5–C6, radial nerve | |
| | **Elbow joint, extension** | |
| | Triceps brachii, C6–C8, radial nerve | |
| | **Elbow joint, supination** | |
| | Supinator muscle, C5–C6, radial nerve | |
| | Biceps brachii muscle, C5–C6, musculocutaneous nerve | |
| | **Elbow joint, pronation** | |
| | Pronator quadratus muscle, C8–T1, median nerve | |
| | Pronator teres muscle, C6–C7, median nerve | |
| | **Wrist extension** | |
| | Extensor digitorum communis muscle, C6–C8, radial nerve | |
| | Extensor carpi radialis longus muscle, C5–C7, radial nerve | |
| | Extensor indicis muscle, C6–C8, radial nerve | |
| | Extensor carpi radialis brevis muscle, C5–C7, radial nerve | |
| | **Wrist bending** | |
| | Flexor digitorum superficialis muscle, C7–T1, median nerve | |
| | Flexor digitorum profundus muscle, C7–T1, median nerve, and ulnar nerve | |
| | Flexor carpi ulnaris muscle, C7–C8, ulnar nerve | |
| | Flexor pollicis longus, C7–C8, median nerve | |
| | Flexor carpi radialis muscle, C6–C7, median nerve | |
| | **Wrist joint, ulnar abduction** | |
| | Extensor carpi ulnaris muscle, C7–C8, radial nerve | |
| | Flexor carpi ulnaris muscle, C7–C8, ulnar nerve | |
| | **Finger bending/metacarpophalangeal (MCP)** | |
| | Dorsal and palmar interosseous muscles, C8–T1, ulnar nerve | |
| | Lumbrical muscles, C8–T1, median nerve, and ulnar nerve | |
| | Flexor digitorum superficialis muscle, C7–T1, median nerve | |
| | Flexor digitorum profundus muscle, C7–T1, median nerve, and ulnar nerve | |

**Fig. 2.26** Documentation of test results—extremities. (From: Wieben K, Falkenberg B. Muskelfunktion. Stuttgart: Thieme, 2012.)

Continued ▷

| | | | | | **Finger bending/proximal interphalangeal joint (PIP)** | | | | | | |
|---|---|---|---|---|---|---|---|---|---|---|---|
| | | | | | Flexor digitorum superficialis muscle, C7–T1, median nerve | | | | | | |
| | | | | | Flexor digitorum profundus muscle, C7–T1, median and ulnar nerves | | | | | | |
| | | | | | **Finger bending/distal interphalangeal joint (DIP)** | | | | | | |
| | | | | | Flexor digitorum profundus muscle, C7–T1, median and ulnar nerves | | | | | | |
| | | | | | **Finger extension/MCP** | | | | | | |
| | | | | | Extensor digitorum communis muscle, C6–C8, radial nerve | | | | | | |
| | | | | | Extensor indicis muscle, C6–C8, radial nerve | | | | | | |
| | | | | | Extensor digiti minimi muscle, C6–C8, radial nerve | | | | | | |
| | | | | | **Finger extension/PIP and DIP** | | | | | | |
| | | | | | Extensor digitorum communis muscle, C6–C8, radial nerve | | | | | | |
| | | | | | Extensor indicis muscle, C6–C8, radial nerve | | | | | | |
| | | | | | Extensor digiti minimi muscle, C6–C8, radial nerve | | | | | | |
| | | | | | Dorsal and palmar interosseous muscles, C8–T1, ulnar nerve | | | | | | |
| | | | | | Lumbrical muscles, C8–T1, median and ulnar nerves | | | | | | |
| | | | | | **Finger abduction** | | | | | | |
| | | | | | Dorsal interosseous muscles, C8–T1, ulnar nerve | | | | | | |
| | | | | | Abductor digiti minimi muscle, C8–T1, ulnar nerve | | | | | | |
| | | | | | **Finger adduction** | | | | | | |
| | | | | | Palmar interosseous muscles, C8–T1, ulnar nerve | | | | | | |
| | | | | | **Thumb bending, carpometacarpal joint** | | | | | | |
| | | | | | Flexor pollicis longus muscle, C7–C8, median nerve | | | | | | |
| | | | | | Flexor pollicis brevis muscle, C8–T1, median and ulnar nerves | | | | | | |
| | | | | | Abductor pollicis brevis muscle, C8–T1, median nerve | | | | | | |
| | | | | | Opponens pollicis muscle, C6–C7, median nerve | | | | | | |
| | | | | | **Thumb bending, metacarpophalangeal joint** | | | | | | |
| | | | | | Flexor pollicis longus muscle, C7–C8, median nerve | | | | | | |
| | | | | | Flexor pollicis brevis muscle, C8–T1, median and ulnar nerves | | | | | | |
| | | | | | **Thumb bending, interphalangeal joint** | | | | | | |
| | | | | | Flexor pollicis longus muscle, C7–C8, median nerve | | | | | | |
| | | | | | **Thumb extension, carpometacarpal joint** | | | | | | |
| | | | | | Extensor pollicis longus muscle, C7–C8, radial nerve | | | | | | |
| | | | | | Extensor pollicis brevis muscle, C7–T1, radial nerve | | | | | | |
| | | | | | Adductor pollicis longus muscle, C7–C8, radial nerve | | | | | | |
| | | | | | **Thumb extension, metacarpophalangeal joint** | | | | | | |
| | | | | | Extensor pollicis longus muscle, C7–C8, radial nerve | | | | | | |
| | | | | | Extensor pollicis brevis muscle, C7–T1, radial nerve | | | | | | |
| | | | | | **Thumb extension, interphalangeal joint** | | | | | | |
| | | | | | Extensor pollicis longus muscle, C7–C8, radial nerve | | | | | | |
| | | | | | **Thumb adduction, carpometacarpal joint** | | | | | | |
| | | | | | Adductor pollicis muscle, C8–T1, ulnar nerve | | | | | | |
| | | | | | Flexor pollicis brevis muscle, C8–T1, ulnar nerve | | | | | | |
| | | | | | **Thumb abduction, carpometacarpal joint** | | | | | | |
| | | | | | Abductor pollicis longus muscle, C7–C8, radial nerve | | | | | | |
| | | | | | Abductor pollicis brevis muscle, C8–T1, median nerve | | | | | | |

**Fig. 2.26**  Documentation of test results—extremities (continued). (From: Wieben K, Falkenberg B. Muskelfunktion. Stuttgart: Thieme; 2012.)

| Date | | Right side | | | | Name of patient: ____<br>Date of birth: ____<br>Diagnosis: ____<br>Name of examiner: ____ | Date | | Left side | | | |
|---|---|---|---|---|---|---|---|---|---|---|---|---|
| | | | | | | **Hip joint bending** | | | | | | |
| L2 | | | | | | Iliopsoas muscle, L1–L4, lumbar plexus, and femoral nerve | | | | | | |
| | | | | | | Rectus femoris muscle, L2–L4, femoral nerve | | | | | | |
| | | | | | | Tensor fascia latae muscle, L4–L5, superior gluteal nerve | | | | | | |
| | | | | | | Sartorius muscle, L1–L3, femoral nerve | | | | | | |
| | | | | | | **Hip joint extension** | | | | | | |
| | | | | | | Gluteus maximus muscle, L5–S2, inferior gluteal nerve | | | | | | |
| | | | | | | Semimembranosus and semitendinosus muscles, L5–S2, tibial nerve | | | | | | |
| | | | | | | Gluteus medius and minimus muscles, L4–S1, superior gluteal nerve | | | | | | |
| | | | | | | Adductor magnus muscle, L3–L5, obturator and tibial nerves | | | | | | |
| | | | | | | Biceps femoris muscle, long head, L5–S2, tibial nerve | | | | | | |
| | | | | | | **Hip joint adduction** | | | | | | |
| L1 | | | | | | Adductor muscles, L2–L5, obturator and tibial nerves | | | | | | |
| | | | | | | Gluteus maximus muscle, L5–S2, inferior gluteal nerve | | | | | | |
| | | | | | | Semimembranosus and semitendinosus muscles, L5–S2, tibial nerve | | | | | | |
| | | | | | | **Hip joint abduction** | | | | | | |
| L5 | | | | | | Gluteus medius and minimus muscles, L4–S1, superior gluteal nerve | | | | | | |
| | | | | | | Tensor fascia latae muscle, L4–L5, superior gluteal nerve | | | | | | |
| | | | | | | Gluteus maximus muscle, L5–S2, inferior gluteal nerve | | | | | | |
| | | | | | | **Hip joint, external rotation** | | | | | | |
| | | | | | | Gluteus maximus muscle, L5–S2, inferior gluteal nerve | | | | | | |
| | | | | | | Gluteus medius and minimus muscles, dorsal portion, L4–S1, superior gluteal nerve | | | | | | |
| | | | | | | Short external rotators, L1–S2, obturator nerve, inferior gluteal nerve, sacral plexus | | | | | | |
| | | | | | | **Hip joint, internal rotation** | | | | | | |
| | | | | | | Gluteus medius and minimus muscles, L4–S1, superior gluteal nerve | | | | | | |
| | | | | | | Tensor fascia latae muscle, L4–L5, superior gluteal nerve | | | | | | |
| | | | | | | **Knee joint extension** | | | | | | |
| L3 | | | | | | Quadriceps femoris muscle, L2–L4, femoral nerve | | | | | | |
| | | | | | | **Knee joint bending** | | | | | | |
| | | | | | | Semimembranosus and semitendinosus muscles, L5–S2, tibial nerve | | | | | | |
| | | | | | | Biceps femoris muscle, L5–S2, tibial nerve, and peroneal nerve | | | | | | |
| | | | | | | **Foot, plantar bending** | | | | | | |
| S1 | | | | | | Triceps surae muscle, S1–S2, tibial nerve | | | | | | |
| | | | | | | **Foot, dorsibending** | | | | | | |
| L4 | | | | | | Tibialis anterior muscle, L4–L5, deep peroneal nerve | | | | | | |
| | | | | | | Extensor digitorum longus muscle, L5–S1, deep peroneal nerve | | | | | | |
| | | | | | | Extensor hallucis longus muscle, L4–S1, deep peroneal nerve | | | | | | |
| | | | | | | **Foot pronation** | | | | | | |
| | | | | | | Peroneus longus and brevis muscles, L5–S1, superficial peroneal nerve | | | | | | |
| | | | | | | Extensor digitorum longus muscle, L5–S1, deep peroneal nerve | | | | | | |
| | | | | | | **Foot supination** | | | | | | |
| | | | | | | Triceps surae muscle, S1–S2, tibial nerve | | | | | | |
| | | | | | | Tibialis posterior muscle, L4–L5, deep peroneal nerve | | | | | | |
| | | | | | | Tibialis anterior muscle, L4–L5, deep peroneal nerve | | | | | | |
| | | | | | | **Toe bending** | | | | | | |
| | | | | | | Flexor digitorum longus muscle, S1–S3, tibial nerve | | | | | | |
| | | | | | | Flexor digitorum brevis muscle, L5–S1, medial plantar nerve | | | | | | |
| | | | | | | **Great toe bending** | | | | | | |
| | | | | | | Flexor hallucis longus and brevis muscles, L5–S3, tibial nerve, and medial plantar nerve | | | | | | |
| | | | | | | **Toe extension** | | | | | | |
| | | | | | | Extensor digitorum longus and brevis muscles, L5–S2, deep peroneal nerve | | | | | | |
| | | | | | | **Great toe extension** | | | | | | |
| | | | | | | Extensor hallucis longus and brevis muscles, L4–S2, deep peroneal nerve | | | | | | |

**Fig. 2.27** Documentation of test results—extremities. (From: Wieben K, Falkenberg B. Muskelfunktion. Stuttgart: Thieme; 2012.)

## Testing the Facial Muscles

The facial muscles may be tested by comparing their movements with those on the healthy side (**Table 2.11**).

**Table 2.11** Test grades for the facial muscles

| Grade | Definition | Notes |
|---|---|---|
| 0 | No muscle tension when attempting movement | |
| 1 | When attempting movement, there is a clear palpable contraction | |
| 2 | One-quarter of the range of motion is possible | |
| 3 | Half of the range of motion is possible | |
| 4 | Almost normal | Slight asymmetry |
| 5 | Normal | No apparent asymmetry |

## References

Cabri J. Testverfahren am Bewegungsapparat. In: van den Berg F, ed. Angewandte Physiologie. Band 3: Therapie, Training, Tests. Stuttgart: Thieme; 2001

Daniels L, Worthingham C. Muskelfunktionsprüfung. Stuttgart: G. Fischer; 1982

Kapandji IA. Funktionelle Anatomie der Gelenke, Band 1–3. Stuttgart: Enke; 1985

Kendall FP, Kendall E. Muskeln—Funktionen und Test. Stuttgart: G. Fischer; 1985

Wieben K, Falkenberg B. Muskelfunktion. Stuttgart: Thieme; 2012

## 2.1.3    Body Mass Index (BMI)
### *Jan Cabri*

The body mass index (BMI) is a simple method of determining a person's body composition. The measure is used to estimate obesity. To calculate the BMI, one needs the person's body weight (BW) in kg and his or her body height (BH) in m: $BMI = BW : (BH)^2$

The BMI is widely recognized because extremely large population studies have been used to arrive at normal values. It is also referred to as the *Quetelet index*.

## Procedure and Interpretation of the Results

- Measure the weight (kg) and height (m).
- Calculate the BMI based on the formula.
- Compare the BMI with standard values (**Table 2.12**).

**Table 2.12** Standard values for the BMI

| BMI | Level of obesity |
|---|---|
| 20–25 kg/m² | Desirable range for adult men and women |
| 25–29.9 kg/m² | Grade I overweight |
| 30–40 kg/m² | Grade II overweight |
| > 40 kg/m² | Grade III (obesity) |

> The BMI is a measurement of obesity level. A health risk due to obesity is present at 25 to 30 kg/m².

### *Example: Calculating the BMI*
A man who is 1.80 m tall weighs 95 kg.
$$BMI = 95 \text{ kg} : (1.80 \text{ m})^2$$
$$BMI = 95 \text{ kg} : 3.24 \text{ m}^2$$
$$BMI = 29.32 \text{ kg/m}^2$$

*Result:* With a BMI of 29.32 kg/m² the man is considered overweight (grade I).

## 2.1.4    Measurement of the Skin Folds
### *Jan Cabri*

The measurement of the skin folds is a method for calculating the percentage of body fat that is especially suitable for older persons. The measurements are added to formulas for body density and then for the percentage of body fat.

> Different formulas are used for men and women.

### Formula for Men
% body fat = 0.29288 (sum of four skin folds) – (0.0005 [sum of four skin folds])² + 0.15845 (age) – 5.76377

### Formula for Women
% body fat = 0.29669 (sum of four skin folds) – (0.00043 [sum of four skin folds])² + 0.02963 (age) – 1.4072

The four skin folds are as follows: suprailiac, abdominal, anterior aspect of the thigh, and triceps brachii muscle (see below).

The measurement procedure is based on the assumption that the subcutaneous fatty tissue makes up a consistent proportion of the total available fat mass and that the average thicknesses of the subcutaneous fatty tissue at the selected measuring sites are representative.

## Procedure

The measurement itself is made using a skinfold caliper. These are metal instruments, which may be calibrated or uncalibrated (for more precise results) (**Fig. 2.28**). There are also cheaper and simpler plastic models that are suitable for everyday use (**Fig. 2.29**); these are relatively precise (to 1 mm):

- When taking measurements using a skinfold caliper, the examiner pinches the skin and the subcutaneous fat between his or her thumb and index finger in the direction of the longitudinal muscle fibers.
- Next, the jaws of the caliper are placed on the skin fold so that the surfaces of the jaws, which are perpendicular to the skin fold, exert constant pressure; the caliper jaws should be positioned 1 cm below the examiner's thumb and index finger.
- Then the skin is released slightly and the therapist presses the trigger to apply maximum pressure to the skin fold.
- The measurement may be read after 2 to 3 seconds.

*All measurements should be taken on the right half of the body.*

### Examples:
- *Measuring the area around the triceps brachii muscle (Fig. 2.30):*
  - The examiner pinches the skin fold between his or her thumb and index finger in the middle of the back of the patient's right upper arm.
  - The fold lies parallel to the longitudinal axis of the arm.
- *Measurements in the abdominal region:*
  - The examiner pinches the skin fold with his or her right thumb and index finger 3–5 cm above and to the right of the patient's navel.
  - The skin fold is parallel to the longitudinal axis of the trunk.
  - The jaws of the skin caliper grasp the skin underneath the fingers.

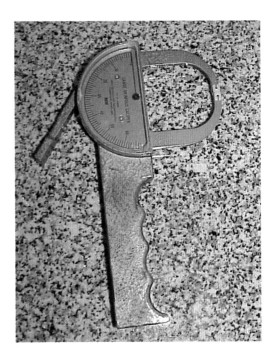

Fig. 2.28 Metal skin caliper.

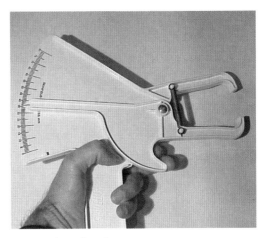

Fig. 2.29 Plastic skin caliper.

### Other Skin Folds that May be Used for Obtaining Measurements
- Biceps brachii muscle
- Subscapular region
- Suprailiac region
- Anterior aspect of the thigh
- Medial aspect of the calf muscle
- Pectoral region

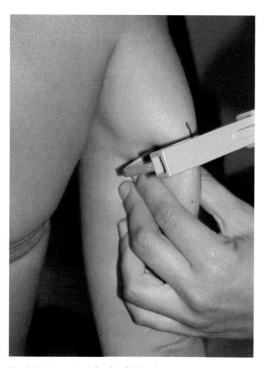

**Fig. 2.30** Measuring the skin fold in the region of the triceps brachii muscle.

### 2.1.5 Examining the Joint and the Surrounding Structures

*Mechthild Doelken*

#### Joint Mobility

Rarely does a patient come in for treatment complaining of limited mobility as the main problem. Usually, pain or irritation, which have developed as a result of altered mobility, is what sends the patient to the doctor and then to a physical therapist. Only when movement limitations interfere with or even impair everyday activities, do patients take them seriously enough to visit a doctor and begin treatment.

The therapist can obtain preliminary signs of the current fitness level of the patient and related functional impairments in everyday life by asking about the patient's individual situation. Questions should focus specifically on the impairment of everyday functions. The patient should explain and/or show which activities are the most difficult at the moment.

Changed movement behavior due to altered mobility is what determines the functional impairment in the patient's everyday life. Movement behavior may be assessed by *observation* and *functional testing*.

Tests may also be used to check the proprioceptive ability of the locomotor system, for example, the muscular stability of the trunk and the leg joints. Deficits influence one's confidence when moving about in everyday life, and severe deficits can affect the patient's freedom and independence.

The examination is not a set procedure. Rather, it is tailored to the individual and determined by his or her history as well as any information already obtained from examination results (findings). In addition to individual data, there are also obligatory elements. Not only mobility, but also the stabilizing ability of the joints are important requirements for being able to move about with confidence.

Patients in good physical condition, who are active at a near-normal everyday level, may be tested to their current limit. Under certain circumstances, reaching the limit may mean it is necessary to perform specific provocations of the patient's typical pain. The therapist should not necessarily avoid this limit for fear of pushing the patient too far. At the same time, care should be taken to gradually increase the difficulty level to avoid injury. Also, adequate safety devices should be available. Determining which provocations are possible and increasing their difficulty level is easier for experienced therapists than for trainees and newly qualified physical therapists. With experience, therapists "store" many clinical patterns. These allow them to better anticipate what may be expected of a given patient.

As the difficulty of the provocation test increases, the patient should be asked whether he or she feels ready for the next step. This helps to determine the patient's own ability to self-assess.

> *Lacking self-assessment ability and inadequate knowledge (e.g., of the current ability of body structures to withstand stress) can negatively influence the healing process.*

#### Active and Passive Examination of Patients with Limited Mobility

> *The goal of the physical therapy examination is to differentiate the body structures that are leading to movement limitation.*

The therapist must identify the cause of limited mobility due to body structures. This "examination of interference fields" is done by tactile perception (palpation) and observation of various behavior strategies. In addition to palpating changes in tension in body structures and specific pain provocation by applying pressure to individual structures, the tactile and visual examination includes perception of resistance to passive movements. If there is resistance to passive movement, the movement quality is compromised. The various defenses may be seen such as counter-tension or changes in facial expression (reaction to pain or fear of pain and movement). The therapist should observe the patient's movement behavior and compare it with normal mobility.

> Three criteria are evaluated when testing joint mobility:
> 1. Range of motion
> 2. Feeling of resistance during movement
> 3. Feeling of resistance at the end of movement (end-feel)

### Principles of Examining Mobility

> Always test movements with a comparison of sides and with active and passive motions.

The following principles should be adhered to whenever possible:
- Test isolated movements of a joint as well as movement combinations.
- The patient should report any change in pain (adapt to the patient's behavior when queried).
- Test the movement with various starting positions and tailor it to the ability and symptoms of the patient (e.g., in weight-bearing and non-weight-bearing positions, especially when testing the weight-bearing joints such as the spinal, hip, knee, or ankle joints).
- Never test joints merely in a single joint; the adjacent joints that are also involved in the movement should also be tested (e.g., when examining the hip joint, examine the lumbar spine as well, because all movements from the proximal lever in the hip joint [pelvis] require motion tolerance in the lumbar spine).

> Even if areas of limited mobility are a causal factor in the patient's symptoms, they may not necessarily be located in the symptomatic region. Often symptoms are produced in areas that compensate with hypermobility to make up for restricted mobility.

- Recognize zones of inhomogeneous use of the locomotor system (e.g., if straightening the spine occurs only in one segment of the lumbothoracic junction).
- Identify functional hypermobile and hypomobile parts of the movement.
- Measuring with the eyes (any deviations and range of motion) and hands (tactile perception of

movement resistance) is equally as important as measuring with a goniometer or tape measure— and in actual practice often even more so. Yet for documentation and verification purposes, standardized measuring methods of mobility are absolutely essential.

- Mobility is measured and documented based on the standardized neutral zero method. See 2.1.1 Joint Measurement According to the Neutral Zero Method.
- The patient's cooperation is essential. They should say whether there is any change in their pain during the movement. It is usually better to ask about any change rather than asking whether the symptoms have improved or worsened; posing an open question is preferable to a suggestive one.

### Testing Active Angular Mobility
The patient should perform angular movements (synonyms: angle altering, rotational movements) while the therapist looks for mechanisms of deviation, range of motion, and notes any reported pain. All of the structures involved in the movement are tested for their range of motion and quality of movement.

> Always perform tests with a comparison of sides.

Active movement testing shows the usefulness of the movement in the patient's everyday life. Along with the active range of motion, it also includes muscle strength and coordination. In patients with acute pain and limited physical capacity, the therapist must assist the active movements by supporting the weight of the body parts being moved.

**Note:** The quality of movement is described and the range of motion is noted based on the neutral zero method. See 2.1.1 Joint Measurement According to the Neutral Zero Method.

### Testing Passive Angular Mobility
The therapist uses one hand to perform the angular movements while the other, which is near the joint, is used for palpation and control. This allows him or her to sense the response of the tissue. In patients with severe arthritis, for example, there may be palpable joint crepitation. Before beginning the movement, the patient should be informed about the planned course of movement so that they can allow the motion to occur along the movement pathway.

> The passive range of motion is normally larger than the active one.

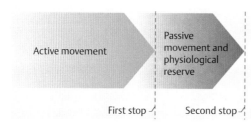

Fig. 2.31 Physiological reserve.

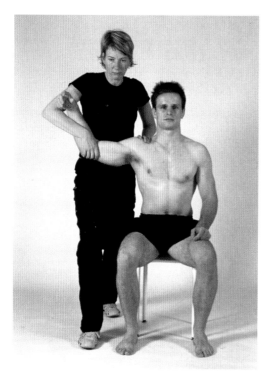

Fig. 2.32 The therapist needs to concentrate during the test movements so that he or she can evaluate the end-feel.

Passive testing also includes the *end-feel* of the movement. Purely passive movements may only be performed in patients with minimal or no pain. Pain triggers muscle guarding and thus limits the range of motion.

Every joint possesses a *physiological reserve*, known as the *elastic zone* (EZ) (Panjabi 1992), which protects the joint structures (**Fig. 2.31**). The elastic zone begins at the end of the active movement pathway and can only be reached passively. This area of the joint is not used during active movements. Otherwise, there would be maximum stretching and compression of passive joint structures with every end-range movement.

Early movement limitations resulting from joint degeneration are initially seen in the physiological reserve. The quality of the end-feel may be altered, or it may occur earlier than normal. During active movements, the joint moves in the neutral zone; the therapist senses the end-feel in the elastic zone (**Fig. 2.32**). It is in the elastic zone that the passive restraint system demonstrates its mechanical effect. The elasticity depends on the connective tissue structure of a joint and is represented by the end-feel.

### Physiological End-feel
Passive movements have different physiological end-feels and are stopped by specific joint structures:
- Firm/springy stop: The capsule and ligaments stop/limit the movement.
- Soft/springy stop: The soft tissues stop/limit the movement.

### Pathological End-feel
- The range of motion is limited and the end-feel occurs prematurely.
- Firm/springy stop due to reflexive shortening of the muscle.
- Firm stop if there is a capsular sign or structural shortening of the muscle.
- Firm/springy stop: Cartilage stops the movement.
- Hard/inelastic stop due to osteophytes.
- If no end-feel is present, the movement is empty (in patients with extreme hypermobility, e.g., instability related to ligamentous injuries).
- The end-feel cannot be tested because the movement is limited by pain.

Mobility of an isolated joint is tested, taking care to avoid tension in multiple joints that would prevent end-range movement of the joint.

**Note:** The therapist should record the range of motion, the end-feel, and the results of movement tests in terms of limiting structures. He or she should always carefully consider which structure may be under tension or compression in the symptom-producing direction of movement.

### Testing Translational Movements of the Joints
The angular movement tests are followed by tests of translational motions. These tests involve an assessment of joint play (or intra-articular) movement.

*Joint play is tested, comparing sides, with traction and compression as well as gliding from the resting and treatment positions of a given joint.*

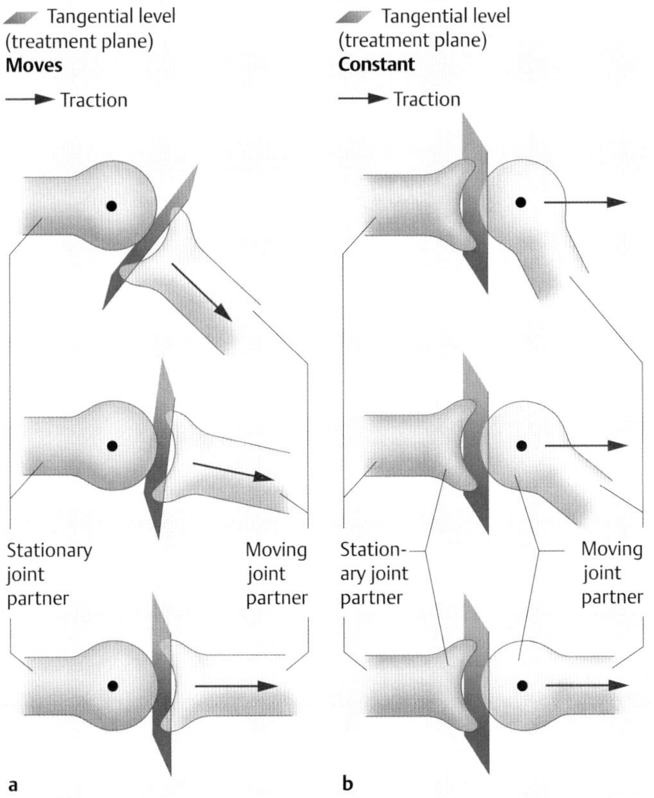

Fig. 2.33a, b Treatment plane.

Joint play can provide the examiner with an overview of changes in joint biomechanics. Joint play involves small movements parallel or perpendicular to the plane of treatment (**Fig. 2.33a, b**). This imaginary plane, which was defined by Kaltenborn (1982), is parallel to the concave joint surface. The directions of movement in the joint techniques are in relation to this plane. Evaluating the quantity and quality of these minimal movements requires a certain amount of experience.

> Joint play is tested in the resting and treatment positions, and always with a comparison of sides.

- Resting position: The capsuloligamentous structure should be completely relaxed to allow for maximum joint play.
- Treatment position: At the pain-free end of active movement, the capsule is already tighter, and thus the amount of mobility is less than in the resting position.

> Every joint has a close-packed position in which the capsuloligamentous unit is under maximum tension with maximum contact pressure between the joint surfaces (**Fig. 2.34**). There is no joint play in this position.

Only in hypermobile joints is movement still detectable in this position. The close-packed position may be used to perform stability tests.

> If joint play is not restricted, the elasticity of the muscles should be tested.

**Note:** The evaluation of joint play is based on the therapist's subjective perception. It is impossible to break down the results into reliable, comparable categories. For the purposes of communication and documentation, the degree of joint play may be divided into minimum (–), significant (– –) and maximum (– – –).

Minimal movements must be tested manually in order to sense differences in tissue resistance. This requires a great deal of experience in tactile perception.

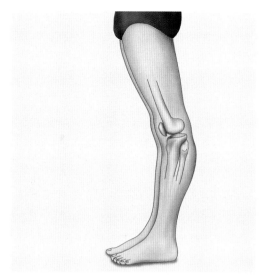

**Fig. 2.34** Close-packed position.

### Measuring Active and Passive Angular Movements of the Extremities

Any deviation from the position of the joints in an upright standing person is noted in degrees. The neutral zero method (see 2.1.1 Joint Measurement According to the Neutral Zero Method) defines the zero position of the joints in the upright standing position. The measurements taken with a goniometer are standardized.

In actual practice, the movement must often be tested in a position other than the starting position in an upright standing person in order to ascertain the entire scope of the functional limitations. Any deviations from using the neutral zero method for taking measurements should be described.

### Examples: Reasons for deviating from the neutral zero method

- Testing adduction of the glenohumeral joint in the transverse plane to identify a ventral labrum defect or acromioclavicular joint involvement.
- If there is severe pain, mobility must often be tested from the actual resting position.
- A patient with acute subacromial pain symptoms can often only tolerate abduction and bending in the scapular plane.
- The rotation of the hip joint is tested from the neutral zero position as well as with 90° hip joint bending:
  - The rotation from the neutral zero position determines the stance phase of the gait cycle. A beginning capsular sign is first seen in the neutral zero position because the weight-bearing part of the femoral head is in contact with the socket of the joint, and ventral capsuloligamentous structures are under maximum tension. This increases the contact pressure of the femoral head in the joint socket and early degeneration becomes apparent.
  - During rotation with hip joint bending, there is also tension on other capsule and muscle components. Changes in the dorsal part of the capsule limit internal rotation, especially in the flexed position.
- Movement tests may be done from both "lever arms" as is necessary in everyday life.
- Rotation of the leg in the hip joint may be possible in a nonweight-bearing starting position without pain or significant limitations. Yet, if rotation is tested on the standing patient, from the proximal lever (pelvis), the patient may report that the same pain is felt when walking. Each step requires rotation tolerance in the load-bearing hip joint. In patients with early degeneration, such movements may be impaired. The result is pain and deviation.

### Measuring Spinal Motion

Spinal movements are always assessed in the following order:

- Active movement is tested without the spine lifting weight against gravity, that is, the axis of motion is vertical.
- Passive movements are tested segmentally.
- Assess the movement in weight-bearing positions as well, for example, standing or sitting. (This is often done at the beginning: omit in patients with acute pain.)

### Measuring Active Movements of the Spine

The neutral zero method is also used to measure the motion of the spinal joints:

### Examples:

- *Schober and Ott signs (see Fig. 2.12a, b):*
  - See 2.1.1 Joint Measurement According to the Neutral Zero Method
- *Finger to floor distance (Fig. 2.35):*
  - This measures the distance between the fingertips and the floor with maximum spinal bending.

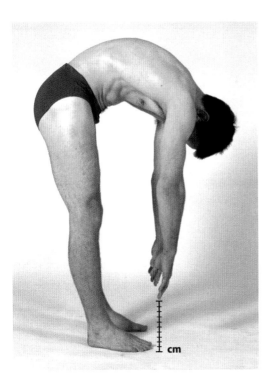

**Fig. 2.35** Finger-to-floor distance.

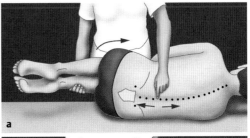

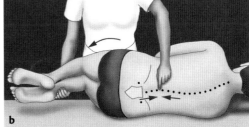

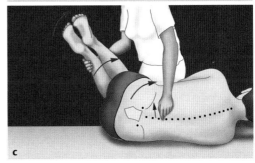

*The measurement methods described here assess only the quantity of motion and not its quality. The number of structures involved prevents any conclusions from being drawn with regard to lack of mobility or hypermobility of spinal segments.*
*In the Schober test of the lumbar spine, shortened hamstring muscles may inhibit the movement prematurely. The entire dorsal musculoskeletal system acts as a brake with the high level of weight-bearing. Patients who have pain may barely tolerate this test.*

**Fig. 2.36a–c** Examining the mobility of the lumbar spinal segments.
**a** Bending.
**b** Extension.
**c** Sidebending.

**Testing Mobility of the Spinal Segments**
Tolerance of segmental motion can only be tested if the therapist relieves the weight of the patient's trunk. The patient must be positioned so that the movement occurs around a vertical axis. The weight of the arms and legs is supported to avoid triggering the braking action of muscles that prevent their falling. **Fig. 2.36a–c** illustrates the examination of segmental mobility of the lumbar spine:

- *Testing extension of the lumbar spine in the side-lying position:*
  - The movement occurs in the sagittal plane around a frontal axis.
  - The frontal axis is vertically oriented when the patient is in the side-lying position.

- A small cushion is placed between the thighs so that the top leg does not trigger a rotational impulse.
- Hip joint bending should not exceed 70°, as the movement will otherwise involve the lumbar spine.
- The upper arm is supported on the table or placed on a cushion.
- *Testing active extension without any weight being lifted against gravity:*
  - The coccyx moves toward the back of the head and folds form in the region of the lumbar spine.
  - The therapist observes whether the sequence of movements is harmonious.
  - Does the movement proceed harmoniously from caudal to cranial or is one vertebral segment pulled along as a block?

- *Passive mobility testing of the spinal segments (Fig. 2.36a–d):*
  - The patient lies near the edge of the bench. The legs are flexed at the hips and the knees rest against the thighs of the therapist.
  - With one hand, the therapist grasps the lower legs of the patient from ventral, guiding them caudally and dorsally and using his or her thighs to press them slightly dorsally.
  - The palpating finger of the other hand is placed interspinously to feel the spinal processes as they approach one another and the relaxing of soft-tissue structures.
  - Extension causes the facets to glide into one another, that is, they converge.
  - Maximum movement tolerance with extension is found at L5–S1. Movement decreases with increasing spinal level.
  - An example of a deviation from the norm would be lacking convergence in the segments L5–S1 and L4–L5.
  - *Note:* L-EXT with diminished extension:
    L5–S1: – – (two minus signs = significantly limited movement)
    L4–L5: – – – (three minus signs = significantly limited movement)

> *Given the minimal amount of movement between individual segments, the therapist must have a certain amount of experience in order to detect any differences.*

**Note:** Distinguishing between ranges of motion is subjective and therefore the differences cannot be reliably divided into categories. For the purpose of communication and documentation, a distinction is made between slight (–), significant (– –), and severe (– – –) restriction. So long as it is impossible to categorize differences with sufficient certainty, the results are of limited use for scientific studies.

**Testing Spinal Motion in Weight-bearing Positions**
In patients who have pain only in weight-bearing positions, for example, in the lumbar spine, movement must also be assessed in pain-triggering positions. If the patient primarily experiences pain when sitting, spinal mobility is tested in the sitting patient using pelvic motion. The aim of this is to reproduce pain symptoms in a weight-bearing position.

*Example: Testing extension of the lumbar spine in the sitting patient*

- The pelvis rolls forward on the supporting surface producing bending of the hip joints and extension of the lumbar spine.

- The therapist observes whether the curvature of the lumbar spine is disrupted, whether the movement occurs smoothly from caudal to cranial, and whether there is any pain associated with movement.

**Analysis of Measurement Results for Various Tests of the Spinal Column**
The results of movement testing are compared with the physician's report. Abnormalities may be caused, for instance, by structural changes to a joint, which may be visible on a radiograph.

**Example:** A patient with osteoarthritis of the lumbar/thoracic/cervical spine has osteophyte formation in the region of the facet joints. Mobility in this segment of the spine is extremely impaired. The patient reports a reduction in pain due to increasing stiffness that leads to less movement of the degenerated vertebral joints.

> *Avoid intense mobilization of the affected spinal segment. Active movements in positions where there is no lifting of weight against gravity can optimize the metabolic situation and thus help nourish the body's structures.*

In addition, any deviations in static posture or patient constitution should be noted when assessing movement tests. The results of testing should be considered with these observations in mind.

---

**Case Study 1**
A patient with a large girth and lumbar symptoms had aberrant static posture in the sagittal and transverse planes with ++ hip joint bending and ++ lumbar lordosis. There was also dorsal translation of the thorax in relation to the pelvis.
Movement testing showed reduced extension tolerance of both hip joints. There was significantly limited bending in the lumbar spine and at the lumbothoracic junction with increased extension.
The patient's constitution is forcing the hip and spinal joints into certain positions. Because he cannot change his constitution overnight, he must be given postures to reduce the weight-bearing of the spine as well as stretching exercises for the hip flexors that he can perform alone. The bending tolerance of the spinal column will improve as the weight is relieved. The patient will also learn to better distinguish between different segments of the body. He is given an individual training plan, which, if performed regularly, will increase ability of the muscles to sustain activity.
The autochthonous muscles are trained in order to improve stability. In addition, the patient is given exercises to perform on his or her own to improve reactive abdominal muscle activity.

---

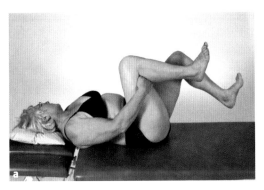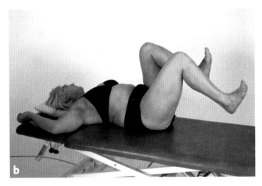

**Fig. 2.37a, b**
**a** Reactive abdominal muscle activation (supine). **b** With more resistance due to greater weight-bearing

**Example:** The patient is in the supine position with both legs in maximum hip bending, with the hands holding the legs to the abdomen (**Fig. 2.37a, b**). One leg is slowly lowered onto the supporting surface without moving the abdomen or allowing the lumbar spine to lose contact with the underlying surface.

This exercise, if performed properly, can strengthen the abdominal muscles as a result of the changing starting position and lever action.

## Examining the Capsule

In patients with structural adhesions and shrinkage (e.g., due to immobility), inadequate capsular elasticity limits joint play. With hypermobile joints in particular, the increased stretching, compressive, and tensile forces resulting from the altered rotational axes can strain the joint capsule and adjacent ligamentous structures.

Due to the increased strain, along with insufficient stability of the joint, strain on the joint structures may irritate the passive system. If there is already irritation, symptoms may develop more rapidly. If there is none, there is a certain level of stress or strain tolerance.

Sufficient strain on the joint can lead to effusion. If the irritation spreads throughout the entire joint, a capsular pattern of movement limitation results. If there is irritation of the joint capsule, the increased tension (e.g., due to traction or passive movements) may lead to an increase in pain.

> Stability problems and diminished mobility may both be present in a single joint.

*Examination Steps*
- Testing active and passive mobility and performing a comparison of any limitations with the capsular patterns:

*Examples: Typical capsular patterns*
- Osteoarthritis of the knee: Bending > Extension
- Osteoarthritis of the hip: Internal rotation > Extension > Abduction > Bending
- Osteoarthritis of the shoulder: External rotation > Abduction > Internal rotation
- Osteoarthritis of the lumbar spine: Extension/Sidebending > Bending
- Osteoarthritis of the thoracic spine: Rotation is limited first and most severely
- Osteoarthritis of the cervical spine: Extension > Rotation/Sidebending > Bending
- Testing joint play:
  – Traction
  – Compression
  – Translational (gliding) movement

> If the rolling/gliding movement is impaired, joint play will be restricted. In patients with restricted joint play due to capsular adhesions, the end-feel is firm and hard.

- Testing of the capsule for *pain with pressure* and of the joint for *effusion*. Both may be present in patients with arthritis or following joint surgery:

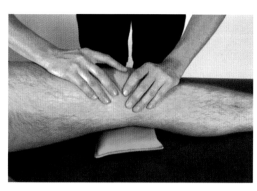

**Fig. 2.38** The dancing patella test.

**Examples:**
- Horseshoe-shaped swelling of the suprapatellar recess
- Dancing patella, which is a sign of effusion in the knee joint capsule:

**Example: Test for a dancing patella (Fig. 2.38)**
- The knee joint is placed in the neutral zero position; if there is an extension deficit a thin cushion should be used for support.
- The suprapatellar recess should be stroked in the direction of the knee joint to force the fluid toward the center of the joint.
- Grasp the medial and lateral borders of the patella and press the index finger (palpating finger) against the center of the patella.

▍ *A dancing patella floats like a saucer on water.*

## Examination of Ligamentous Stability

As already mentioned, around hypermobile joints, if the rotational axes are altered, increased stretching, compressive and tensile forces may strain the ligamentous structures. The ligaments are tender and there may be radiating pain as well. The pain with pressure worsens if the ligament is placed in a position where it is under tension.

▍ *It usually takes time for the ligaments to respond to pressure with pain (20–30 seconds).*

**Examples:**
- Lumbar instability strains the iliolumbar ligaments. These may be palpated between the transverse processes of L4 and L5 and deeper at the pelvic crest. Additional sidebending of the lumbar spine to the opposite side can increase the provocation.

- Between the spinous processes, the supraspinous ligament and interspinous ligament react to pressure with pain. Pain on pressure may be tested with the help of the *coin test*. This involves placing a coin between the spinous processes to exert pressure on the ligamentous structures. Radiating pain from the ligaments occurs after about 30 seconds.

### *Specific Examination of the Ligaments*

**Examining Painful Ligaments**
- *Localization:* Local receptor pain at the insertion sites of the tendons and ligaments often radiating into the muscle.
- *Quality of pain:* The pain is diffuse, dull, pulling, or piercing. Patients commonly say that their "back goes out" after prolonged periods of sitting.
- *Onset of pain:* The pain continually worsens if the patient stays in one position for a longer period of time.
- Pain provocation:
  - Stability tests, consisting of extension stress tests of the ligaments, will cause a response after about 30 seconds, with pain radiating into the corresponding muscles.
  - There is local tenderness on palpation at the insertion site or along the course of the ligament.

▍ *Prolonged pressure can lead to radiating pain (although this is not always the case). It is therefore advisable to evaluate whether there are any changes in the joint position such as those that may occur with axial deviations resulting from ligament damage.*

**Tests of Mobility**
If ligamentous structures are severely damaged, the joint's neutral zone is significantly enlarged (**Fig. 2.39**). There is greater translation between the joint surfaces and the end-feel is empty or limited by the suddenly increased tonus of the musculature as a reactive defense mechanism. The symptom response may also change.

**Example:** After an anterior cruciate ligament tear in the knee joint, anterior translation of the tibia may be greater than in a healthy knee joint. The anterior drawer test with 90° knee bending and the Lachmann test with 25° bending may be used to confirm the increased translation (**Fig. 2.40, Fig. 2.41**).

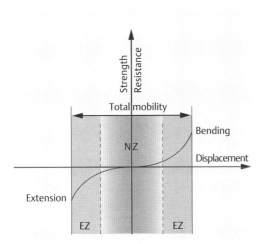

Fig. 2.39 Neutral zone.

There appears to be less firmness at the end of the passive movement in the elastic zone. This is often referred to as an *empty end-feel*.

**Example:** Injury of the anterior cruciate ligament of the knee may lead to passive hyperextension, given the lacking increase in tension with vertical-ization of the cruciate ligament during extension. The quality of the end-feel is different than in a healthy knee joint.

> *The interpretation of the end-feel, as well as of specific instability and translational tests, should be critically considered. The movements are very tiny and the findings are based on the therapist's subjective perceptions.*

Pain and guarding may distort the result. Counter-tension, for instance, may obscure the enlargement of the neutral zone. Correct interpretation of examination findings requires experience. In a therapist with insufficient expertise, there is a risk that he or she may feel what they want to, or rather, what would match their working hypothesis.

> *Despite a normal-sized neutral zone, functional hyper-mobility may be present. Even enlargement of the neutral zone does not necessarily indicate lack of sta-bility. Instability is present if the active system is unable to compensate for deficits of the passive sys-tem during movement. This is why a comparison of active and passive movements is necessary.*

In hypermobile joints, particularly in the treatment position, testing the end-feel and traction may cause discomfort. The ligaments and capsule register an increase in tension and reproduce pain or discom-fort. Pain usually does not occur unless the tension is

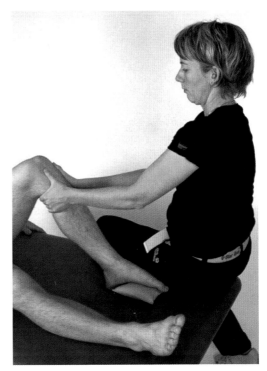

Fig. 2.40 Performing the anterior drawer test.

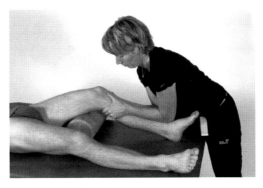

Fig. 2.41 The Lachmann test.

held and sensed by the Golgi tendon organ recep-tors, which is after about 30 seconds.

> *In hypermobile joints, compression is often perceived as pleasant, because bringing the joint surfaces closer together relaxes the capsuloligamentous unit.*

### Stability Tests

The underlying principle of the stability tests is to examine translational movements in joint positions in which the joint capsule or ligaments are under maximum tension. In a stable passive system there is no translation, and there is firm elastic resistance.

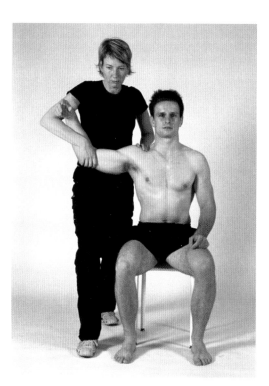

**Fig. 2.42** Anterior apprehension test.

Stability tests are always done with a comparison of sides. Maximum tension of the capsuloligamentous unit will place the joints in the close-packed position.

Specific pain provocation tests of the ligaments and capsule may be performed in these positions. The position of maximum tension is held for about 30 seconds in the position that provoked symptoms. The therapist observes whether the pain is reproduced.

**Specific Stability Tests on Selected Joints**

*Shoulder Joint*

The shoulder joint is often affected by *ventral instability*. The very common ventral decentering of the humeral head involves prolonged laxity of the ventral capsule. If there is inadequate motion tolerance of the thoracic spine, increased mobility of the glenohumeral joint is needed, especially for overhead movements. The ventral shoulder joint structures are thus repeatedly placed under stress.

Anterior apprehension test to examine ventral instability (**Fig. 2.42**):

- Starting position of the patient: Sitting with abduction and maximum external rotation of the shoulder.

- Starting position of the therapist: Standing behind the patient.
- Performing the test:
  - Using one hand, the therapist guides the patient's arm in 45°, 90°, and 135° abduction and external rotation.
  - His or her other hand presses from dorsal against the humeral head, pushing it ventrally into a subluxation position in order to provoke symptoms.
  - At 45°, one may test the stability of the fibers sent from the subscapularis muscle into the ventral capsule as well as the middle glenohumeral ligament.
  - At 90° and 135° the stability of the inferior glenohumeral ligament and the ventral capsule may be tested.
  - A positive drawer test due to ventral translation of the humeral head and/or an avoidance response of the patient are considered signs of instability.

> Normally, in the abduction position of the shoulder joint with maximum external rotation, there is no ventral translation of the head because the ventral portion of the capsule is under maximum tension.

*Knee Joint*

Deviation of the axis of the standing leg (genu valgus) results from medial collapse of the ligament structure of the knee joint.

Testing the stability of the medial collateral ligament and the dorsomedial capsule by performing a *valgus stress* test to examine the ligament (**Fig. 2.43a, b**):

- Starting position of the patient: Supine.
- Starting position of the therapist: Lateral to the patient's leg.
- Performing the test:
  - The therapist holds the lower leg firmly between her arm and body.
  - The wrist of her proximal hand is placed on the lateral knee joint and pushes the knee medially as she turns her body.
  - Accompanying rotation of the hip joint may be prevented by pre-positioning the leg with internal rotation.
  - The valgus stress test is performed with the knee fully extended.
  - Given that the collateral ligament and capsule are under maximum tension, there should be no gapping.
  - For pain provocation of the medial collateral ligament, the valgus stress test is performed with

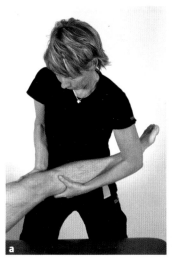
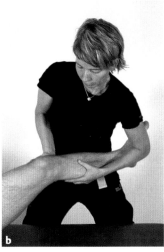

Fig. 2.43a, b Valgus stress test of the knee joint (fully extended and with 15° bending).

about 15° of knee bending. The dorsolateral portion of the capsule relaxes and thus mainly the lateral ligament comes under tension.
– The provocation position is held for about 30 seconds; the therapist should observe whether pain is reproduced.

## Examination of Periarticular Structures

The periarticular structures, also known as gliding structures, include the bursae and tendon sheaths. These may be damaged by the following:
- Rheumatic or metabolic disorders, for example, primary chronic polyarthritis (PCP) or gout
- Hormonal or vitamin imbalance, for example, during periods of extreme hormonal fluctuation (menopause or in patients with vitamin E deficiency)
- Single or repeated microtrauma

Typical signs include local tenderness and swelling over the bursae and around the tendon sheaths. Pain often occurs after excessive stress or repetitive strain or if there is compression of a bursa. A severe pulling, tearing pain with movement is typical.
   **Example:** If there is decentering of the humeral head, when the arm is passively abducted in the shoulder joint with fixation of the scapula, the bursa will be compressed cranially and respond with pain.

### Specific Examination for Dysfunctions of the Periarticular Structures

#### Examining Swelling
- Local swelling about the bursae.
- Due to swelling, the bursae are suddenly palpable during palpation.
- The pain worsens with pressure.
- There is crepitation around the tendon sheaths with movement.

#### Examining Pain
- Movement is painful and usually limited in certain directions (e.g., in subacromial bursitis, shoulder abduction would be most limited).
- Decompression reduces pain with movement (e.g., in subacromial bursitis, shoulder abduction is less painful if there is tension on the humerus, as this frees up the subacromial space).

**Pain Provocation**
- Pain affecting the bursa may be provoked by compression:

**Example:** Subacromial bursitis is provoked by movement of the humeral head cranially. Compression via the humerus toward the acromion triggers pain.

- The tendon sheaths respond with pain to local pressure (palpation) as well as to pressure produced by tension:

**Example:** The tendon sheaths of the finger flexors provoke pain with passive dorsal finger extension. This may be increased with elbow extension.

## Examining the Musculature

| Testing of muscle function was discussed in section
2.1.2 and will be described in more detail in Chapter 3.

### Muscle Elasticity

A muscle of normal length allows the joint to move to its end range without pain or an increase in tension. For multi-joint muscles, the position of the adjacent joint must be taken into account. End-range movements cannot be made simultaneously in both joints. This is prevented by the total length of the multi-joint muscle. This condition is referred to as a *physiological passive insufficiency*.

| In single-joint muscles, passive insufficiency is always
pathological.

Polyarticular movements always lead to loss of elasticity of the muscles involved. At the end of increased polyarticular tension, greater resistance due to increased muscle tension is normal. This is an expression of an end-range need for extension of the muscle. There should be no restriction on freely using the movement combination in everyday life, however.

### Increased Stretch Sensitivity of the Muscle—Muscle Shortening

Persistently elevated active muscle tonus (Laube 2004) and immobility may make the muscle more sensitive to being stretched. Due to its plasticity, the longer the condition persists, the greater are the changes within the muscle leading to reduced elasticity:

- *Reflexive shortening:* There is still no structural change in the muscle. It has an increased sensitivity to being stretched (neurophysiological process).
- *Reversible structural shortening:* Reversible transformation processes have begun. If the muscles are in a shorter position, for instance, due to long-term immobilization, although the number of muscle fibers remains constant, they lose motor units so that the fibers actually become shorter. If many lengthening stimuli act on the muscle, additional sarcomeres are added onto the fibers, causing them to lengthen. This is more of a lengthening of the muscle rather than stretching. Following immobilization, in the first 4 weeks of the healing process water-soluble *cross-links* form. With repeated movements in the pain-free range, these are easily influenced. If the collagen tissue is immobilized for more than 6 weeks in a short

position, water-insoluble pathological cross-links form.
- *Irreversible structural shortening:* This is when there is a contracture. Contractile units have been converted into noncontractile units.

### Alteration of the End-feel Due to Muscle Shortening

The end-feel occurs prematurely and tension in the muscle begins to increase before the end of the movement path. In reflexive shortening of the muscle, that is, before there are any structural changes to the muscle, the end-feel is *firm/springy*. Movement may be enhanced with relaxation techniques (e.g., postisometric relaxation).

A *firm* end-feel indicates structural shortening; relaxation techniques cannot lengthen the muscle. Possible articular causes of movement limitation must be ruled out using translational tests of the joint. Two different types of shortening may be distinguished:

- *Irreversible structural changes:* For example, myositis ossificans (muscular inflammation with calcium deposits in the muscle).
- *Reversible muscle shortening:* This is due to deposition of cross-links (hydrogen bonds or pathological water-insoluble cross-links).

### Muscular Causes of Pain

**Potential Causes of Painful Muscles**

- Reflexive changes to muscle tonus to protect a lesion (e.g., in joint degeneration or blockage)
- Overloading or straining the muscle, often due to deviations in terms of constitutional factors and static stability
- Following trauma (e.g., torn muscle)

**Pain Localization**

- Local pain affecting the muscle, which increases during contraction or stretching:
  - Contraction often causes an increased cramping tendency in the muscle.
  - The sensitivity of the muscle to stretching is significantly increased.
- Pain in the region of the entire muscle synergy, that is, in all muscles forming a functional unit. This leads to *chain reactions*.

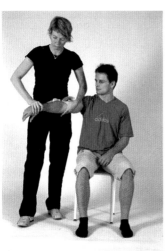 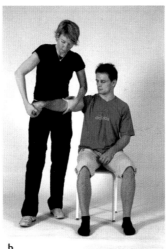

**Fig. 2.44a, b** Pain provocation of the hand extensors.

## Quality of Pain
- Pain coming from the muscles is felt as diffuse, dull, or piercing.
- A "bright," sharp pain occurs at trigger points (locally circumscribed muscle hardening):
  - Activated trigger points demonstrate radiating pain in their typical reference area.
  - Latent trigger points respond to pressure with local, dull pain.

## Onset of Pain
- Pain after inactivity such as long-term immobilization (e.g., morning pain) and staying in one position for a longer period of time.
- The pain worsens during contraction or stretching.
- Ischemic pain with static contraction.

## Specific Tests in Patients with Pain
- In longer-term pain, there is muscle atrophy or more pronounced muscle contours with extreme hardening.
- When testing movement, there is an altered quality of motion. There may be increased resistance, and often there is cogwheel rigidity. Movement may be limited.
- Active movement (especially with eccentric muscle activity) triggers pain.
- Passive movement is pain free. At the end of the movement, there is sensitivity to stretching.
- The affected muscles are tender. The tenderness may increase when the muscle contracts or stretches. Local areas of muscle hardening respond to pressure with referred pain with active trigger points.

## Pain Provocation
- Palpation of the muscle belly with pressure application, as well as of the musculotendinous junction, and the tenoperiosteal junction trigger pain. In the region of the belly of the muscle, there are often activated trigger points that respond to pressure with referred pain.
- Static contraction from the middle position and dynamic concentric and eccentric contraction cause pain. Strength is diminished.
- *Muscle selection test:* Several muscles in a muscle group often have the same function. By testing individual muscles, one can identify the affected muscle. The following questions must first be answered:
  - What are the individual muscles in the group?
  - How do they differ in terms of course and function? Are there additional functions of other muscles in the group?
  - Which antagonistic functions may be used for differentiation?

### *Example: Muscle selection of the hand extensors (Fig. 2.44a, b)*
Active wrist extension against resistance is painful throughout the entire course of the muscle group. Tender points may be found in the belly of the muscle and on its origin in the area of the lateral epicondyle. The extensor carpi radialis brevis and the extensor digitorum both originate on the lateral epicondyle. They are active during extension of the wrist. They may be differentiated from one another by the additional function of the extensor digitorum (finger extension).

When testing the extensor carpi radialis brevis, the extensor digitorum is inhibited by holding onto an object.

The extensor digitorum (finger extension) is tested against resistance while the patient presses the surface of his or her hand against a table. There is reciprocal inhibition of the activity of the antagonists of the extensor carpi radialis brevis.

- Static resistance from a "pre-stretched" position: If tension occurs from a middle position, in muscles with mild irritation, there will not be a response. The intensity of the provocation is significantly increased by using a pre-stretched position. First, static tension is produced. If the patient still fails to respond, the provocation may be increased to its maximum by using dynamic eccentric and concentric contraction against resistance from a pre-stretched position.

> *Muscle selection is used here the same as for testing from the middle position.*

**Examples:**
- *Test of the extensor carpi radialis brevis muscle:*
  – The starting position is palmar bending with elbow extension and forearm pronation, keeping the fingers relaxed.
  – From this position, the patient actively performs dorsal extension of his or her hand, keeping their fingers relaxed.
- *Test of the extensor digitorum muscle:*
  – The starting position is finger bending with palmar bending with simultaneous elbow extension and pronation.
  – From this position, the patient actively extends his or her fingers.

# References

Bialosky JE, Bishop MD, et al. The mechanisms of manual therapy in the treatment of musculoskeletal pain: a comprehensive model. Man Ther 2009;14(5):531–538

Bogduk N. Clinical Anatomy of the Lumbar Spine and Sacrum. 3rd ed. Melbourne: Churchill Livingstone; 1997

Hüter-Becker A, Dölken M. Physiotherapie in der Orthopädie. Stuttgart: Thieme; 2009

Kaltenborn F. Manuelle Therapie der Extremitätengelenke. 6th ed. Oslo: Norlis; 1982

Laube W. Leistungsphysiologie. In: Hüter-Becker A, Dölken M (Hrsg.). Biomechanik, Bewegungslehre, Leistungsphysiologie, Trainingslehre. Stuttgart: Thieme; 2004

Laube W. Sensomotorisches System; Physiologisches Detailwissen für Physiotherapeuten. Stuttgart: Thieme; 2009

Panjabi MM. The stabilizing system of the spine. Part II. Neutral zone and instability hypothesis. J Spinal Disord 1992;5(4):390–396

Rajadurai V. Wirksamkeitsvergleich einer kaudalen Gleitmobilisationstechnik in endgradiger und mittelgradiger Schulterabduktion bei Capsula adhaesiva. Physiosci 2011;7(3):121–125

Sahrmann SA. Diagnosis and Treatment of Movement Impairment Syndromes. St Louis: Mosby; 2002

Spirgi-Gantert I, Suppé B. FBL Klein-Vogelbach Functional Kinetics: Die Grundlagen. 6th ed. Berlin: Springer; 2007

Westerhuis P, Wiesner R. Klinische Muster in der Manuellen Therapie; Stuttgart: Thieme; 2011

## 2.1.6 Integration of Peripheral Nerves in the Examination of the Locomotor System
*Brigitte Tampin*

### Introduction

The clinical presentation of peripheral nerve lesions and their causes varies widely. Mechanical causes are common and include pressure, crush injuries or nerve strain. These may be acute one-off events, or they may occur as chronic or repeated events. Typical examples include compression syndromes such as carpal tunnel syndrome or supinator syndrome, spinal radiculopathy due to spinal foraminal stenosis, traumatic plexus lesions, scalenus syndrome, and space-occupying processes.

On the other hand, the influence of biochemical and inflammatory processes are increasingly important (Olmarker et al 1993; Yabuki et al 1998; Eliav et al 1999, 2001; Harrington et al 2000; Takahashi et al 2003). Metabolic diseases and toxic damage should also be taken into consideration (e.g., diabetic neuropathy).

Pain caused by a lesion or disease of the somatosensory nervous system is referred to as neuropathic pain (Jensen et al 2011; Treede et al 2008). It is generally characterized by pain and sensory abnormalities in the area corresponding to the innervation territory of the damaged nerve structure (Jensen and Baron 2003). In addition to pain, the core signs include sensory deficits, indicating a loss of function due to the reduction of afferent input caused by the nerve lesion. However, various other sensory symptoms, indicating a gain of function, can be present, including paresthesia or dysesthesia, spontaneous (not stimulus-induced) ongoing pain, spontaneous electric shock like sensations and evoked pain (hyperalgesia, allodynia). Pain associated with peripheral nerve lesions may be relatively easily diagnosed. More difficult are diffuse pain syndromes of unknown origin that may arise due to minimal nerve injury or nerve irritation with preserved nerve conduction (Greening and Lynn 1998). The cause of painful movement limitations may be sensitization of the nerves and associated heightened mechanosensitivity. Heightened nerve mechanosensitivity is a feature of nerve trunk pain which is regarded as a nociceptive pain (Bennett 2006; Marchettini et al, 2006). Nerve trunk pain typically occurs along the course of the corresponding nerve.

## Peripheral Nerve Innervation and Blood Circulation

The peripheral nervous system must adapt to all movements of the body. It is therefore constantly subject to mechanical forces. This task corresponds to its anatomical structure. The individual nerve fibers of a peripheral nerve are surrounded by layers of connective tissue (endoneurium, epineurium, perineurium). These allow gliding of the nerve fibers as well as the whole nerve and also act as a diffusion barrier. Normal nerve function (axonal transport, impulse conduction) is dependent on a continuous supply of energy/oxygen, which is ensured by an extensive system of blood vessels. An outer vessel system anastomoses with an inner system, which provides vessels to all connective tissue layers. The endoneurial blood vessels act as a "blood–nerve barrier" and protect the axon from being penetrated by chemical substances.

A certain pressure gradient in and around the nerve is necessary (Sunderland 1976) to maintain intrafascicular circulation. The pressure must be greatest in the epineurial arteriole and increasingly reduced in the capillary, fascicle, the epineurial vein, and in the surrounding tissue. Increased pressure in surrounding tissue can reduce venous backflow and thus influence metabolic activity.

> Nerve roots are much more vulnerable to injury than peripheral nerves, as, for example, they do not possess strong tissue layers such as an epineurium or perineurium (Sunderland 1991), nor do they have a lymphatic system.

The innervation of the peripheral nerves is supplied by the "nervi nervorum" (Hromada 1963), which are located in the connective tissue layers of the nerves. These may act as nociceptors, responding to mechanical, chemical, and thermal stimuli (Bove and Light 1997). The nervi nervorum contain neuropeptides such as substance P that play a role in neurogenic blood vessel dilation/inflammation (Sauer et al 1999). Presumably, disorders such as increased intraneural pressure, electrolyte imbalance, or altered nerve mechanics, may stimulate the nociceptors and thus cause pain (Murphy 1977; Bove and Light 1997).

## Causes of Neural Disorders

### Stretching

Lengthening and stretching of a nerve does effect its blood supply. With increasing stretch, the blood vessel diameter decreases and blood flow is obstructed. Microscopic studies demonstrated that stretching a healthy peripheral nerve 8% beyond its resting length led to slower venous flow in the epineurium and perineurium while a 15% stretch caused the blood flow in all intraneural vessels to come to a complete standstill (Lundborg and Rydevik 1973; Ogata and Naito 1986).

With release of the stretch, blood flow returned to normal after 30 minutes, but venous flow was only partially restored. Within 30 to 90 minutes after the onset of ischemia, nerve function began to decline (Lundborg 1975). One may assume that if a healthy nerve is strained to or beyond its elastic limit, the nerve conduction becomes compromised. The elastic limit of the peripheral nerves lies around a 20% stretch (Sunderland and Bradley 1961a), and that of the spinal nerves around 15% (Sunderland and Bradley 1961b). This limit is presumably much lower if nerves are inflamed (Murphy 1977).

### Friction

Constant friction on a nerve against a rough surface, or between two closely positioned surfaces, may lead to repetitive trauma (e.g., nerve entrapment syndrome, pronator syndrome, irritation of the ulnar nerve at the medial condyle). This may result in an inflammatory reaction (Triano and Luttges 1982) and the development of friction fibrosis. On one hand, this may cause the nerve to adhere to the site, while on the other it may compress the nerve fibers and impair the blood flow. As a response to the trauma, regenerating axons grow into the scar tissue, which are extremely mechanosensitive. Thus, movement of the nerve may cause increased impulse activity that is perceived as pain (S. Sunderland 1981; Asbury and Fields 1984; Woolf 1987; P. Sunderland 1991).

### Compression

The effect of compression on peripheral nerves depends on the amount of compression and the duration. Microscopic studies demonstrated that compression levels of 30 mmHg reduced intraneural blood flow and that compression levels of 50 to 80 mmHg caused a complete standstill of intraneural circulation (Rydevik et al 1981; Ogata and Naito 1986).

Lundborg (1970) showed that after 8 to 10 hours of ischemia, blood flow was restored within 5 to 20 minutes after the compression was removed. However, microvascular congestion developed so that 1 hour after removal of the compressive force only half of the arterioles and capillaries demonstrated good circulation. The restoration of venous flow was incomplete and microthrombuses and emboli were present.

Compression traumas can significantly change the vascular permeability of the endoneurium and thus impair nerve function (Lundborg 1970, 1975). Damage to the endoneurial blood vessels leads to collapse of the blood–nerve barrier, and as a consequence to the development of endoneurial edema (Rydevik et al 1984). This influences nerve function either directly as a result of altered ionic balance or indirectly through increased endoneurial fluid pressure. The increased pressure impairs microcirculation, resulting in post-traumatic ischemia. With long-term intraneural edema, fibroblast proliferation occurs, leading to the formation of fibrotic scar tissue.

Compression of a nerve may cause structural changes such as segmental demyelination (Fowler et al 1972) and thinning of the axon, leading to axonal degeneration (Sunderland 1981).

In healthy persons, compression pressure of 30 mmHg in the carpal tunnel decreased nerve conduction velocity and caused paresthesia of the hand (Lundborg et al 1982). At 50 to 60 mmHg, motor and sensory conduction were totally blocked and intraneural circulation stopped.

Gelberman et al (1981) measured tissue pressure of around 30 mmHg in the carpal tunnel in patients with signs of median nerve compression. In comparison, the pressure in the carpal tunnel in healthy persons was 2.5 mmHg. This suggests that compression may disrupt blood flow, vascular permeability, axonal transport, and impulse conduction.

The compression of a healthy peripheral nerve often causes a feeling of numbness, but normally does not cause any pain (Lindahl 1966; Sunderland 1981; Rydevik et al 1984). Pain may occur, however, if blood flow is significantly impaired (Hida et al 2003) or in the event of inflammation (Garfin et al 1991).

Experimental studies have shown that inflamed nerve fibers spontaneously discharged action potentials and were hypersensitive to mechanical stimuli or deformation. Any additional irritation of the nerve may cause ectopic discharge and thus pain (Porter and Wharton 1949; Parke 1991). This hyper-

sensitivity/sensibility of inflamed nerves to normal mechanical stimuli (increased mechanosensitivity) has also been found in patients with symptoms of nerve root irritation (Smyth and Wright 1958; Kuslich et al 1991; Owen et al 1994).

## Biochemical Processes/Inflammation

There is increasing evidence that pathological changes to nerves may be caused not only by mechanical forces, but also by purely biochemical processes in the absence of any mechanical impairment. The placement of autologous intervertebral disk material near the lumbar or sacral nerve roots led to signs of inflammation in the nerve root region as well as reduced blood flow (Olmarker et al 1993; Yabuki et al 1998).

In an experimental study by Eliav et al on rats (1999), treatment of the sciatic nerve with inflammatory mediators triggered local and distal pain and caused heat and mechanical hyperalgesia, mechanical allodynia (painful response to a normal mechanical stimulus), and cold hyperalgesia. No motor deficits were present. This suggests that the inflammation of the sciatic nerve without axonal damage can cause pain in distal regions.

In addition, an inflammatory stimulus around the saphenous nerve in rats caused spontaneous activity of action potentials and increased mechanosensitivity of the nerve without compromise of the nerve conduction (Eliav et al 2001).

The results of these studies have clinical implications. They support the notion that patients without signs of neurological deficits may have nerve pain and painfully limited movement due to heightened neural mechanosensitivity. In other words, findings in clinical neurological examinations and electrodiagnostic tests would be normal (Dyck 1990).

The principle of the examination of mechanosensitivity of the peripheral nerves is to deliver a mechanical stimulus (e.g., stretching or pressure) and to observe the response. In a healthy person, nerves can adapt to a range of body movements that in pathological conditions would elicit pain. Various anatomical positions of the peripheral joints can influence the peripheral nerve trunks in different ways. The clinician may use this knowledge to test individual nerve trunks.

*The following presentations of nerve-related pain disorders are possible:*
- *Disorders with primarily sensibility/sensitivity of the nerves and associated heightened nerve mechanosensitivity without nerve conduction impairment*

- Disorders with primarily nerve conduction
  impairment and no or only slightly increased
  mechanosensitivity
- Mixed types

## Examination of the Peripheral Nerves

One goal of a clinical examination is to determine the primary source of pain so that later targeted treatments may be performed. Thus, the physical examination must include provocation tests of the nerves (described on the following pages) as well as other tests of the neuromusculoskeletal system to rule out involvement of additional structures as pain triggers. (These tests are described in 2.1.5 Examining the Joint and the Surrounding Structures.)

### Subjective Assessment

The subjective assessment is an important part of the examination. A *body chart* is used to record the location and intensity of pain/symptoms as well as their quality and intensity. This information may sometimes provide useful clues.

The quality of neuropathic pain is often described as a shooting or burning quality, with tingling or electrical sensations and numbness (Bouhassira and Attal 2011) whereas nociceptive nerve trunk pain is often described as a deep, dull pain like a toothache, which increases with movement, stretching of the nerve, and pressure on the nerve. Nerve trunk pain occurs along the course of the corresponding nerve, and presumably arises due to increased activity of sensitized nervi nervorum (Asbury and Fields 1984). Both types of pain, neuropathic and nociceptive nerve trunk pain, may be present at the same time.

> Subjective reports of symptoms should not be over-estimated. Pain and paresthesia due to spinal radiculopathy are not always in the dermatome corresponding to the nerve root (Henderson et al 1983; Dalton and Jull 1989; Rankine et al 1998; Gifford 2001).

The patient's history provides information about potential mechanisms of injury or causes leading to pain and progression of the disorder. In addition, potential associations between prior injury/disease and the patient's current presentation may be revealed (e.g., double-crush phenomenon; Upton and McComas 1973). Information on the 24-hour symptom behavior is important for planning the structural examination. It provides information on the irritability (Maitland 2001) of the pain disorder

and also on painful and pain-relieving movement directions.

The subjective assessment concludes with further questions such as those related to overall health status, medication use, and the results of previous medical examinations (e.g., x-rays, computed tomography, magnetic resonance imaging [MRI] and nerve conduction studies; Maitland 2001).

> The information obtained during the subjective assessment should be interpreted in light of the findings of the structural examination and should correlate with them.

### Examination of the Peripheral Nerves

The structural examination of peripheral nerves is based on the same principles as the examination of other body structures. For instance, in a patient with a muscle tear, numerous tests are performed that must correlate/correspond with one another in order to arrive at the correct diagnosis. Testing includes tests of active movements, isometric muscle contraction, muscle stretching, and palpation of the muscle. These tests provoke the injured muscle mechanically, that is, these are provocation tests.

None of the tests alone are sufficient for arriving at a precise diagnosis. The physical findings must also be considered in relation to the subjective assessment. Do the subjective findings correspond with the objective findings? The final diagnosis is made on the basis of a thorough clinical reasoning process, taking into account all examination findings (subjective, objective, and the results of any available medical tests).

This procedure may be transferred to the examination of the peripheral nerves. For example, in order to diagnose a lumbar radiculopathy, it is not enough to say the straight leg raise test (SLR) is positive or negative. The result has to be seen in relation to numerous other tests, and these must correspond with each other before a diagnosis can be made.

In patients with nerve sensitization and signs of heightened mechanosensitivity, the physical examination should demonstrate the following findings (Hall and Elvey 1999):
- Antalgic posture
- Dysfunction of active movements
- Dysfunction of passive movements that, in terms of range of motion, corresponds with the active movement dysfunction
- Abnormal response to a neural provocation test
- Mechanical hyperalgesia in response to palpation of peripheral nerve trunks
- Detection of a local cause of the neural disorder

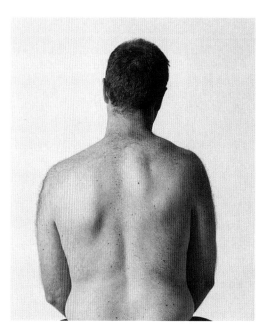

Fig. 2.45 Protective posture with severe symptoms on the right side affecting the cervical spine, shoulder, and arm.

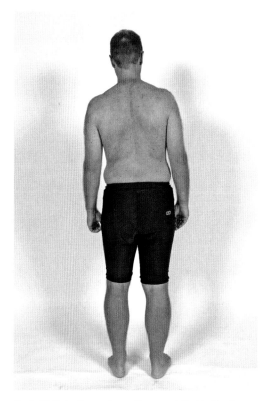

Fig. 2.46 Protective posture with severe left-sided lumbar spine symptoms, which are radiating into the left leg.

### Antalgic Posture

Depending on the severity of the pain disorder, an antalgic posture can be observed. The patient adapts a posture that reduces tension on the affected nerves.

### Examples:

- Right-sided cervical spine, shoulder, and arm symptoms. The corresponding protective posture involves elevation of the shoulder girdle, cervical ipsilateral sidebending, and possibly even elbow bending (**Fig. 2.45**).
- Left-sided pain in the lumbar spine, radiating to the posterior aspect of the left leg. Slight knee bending and lumbar sidebending lateral reduce mechanical provocation of the sensitive L5 nerve root (**Fig. 2.46**).

### Dysfunction Affecting Active Movements

Active movements requiring lengthening of the relevant nerves are limited by pain.

*During the examination, the therapist should observe the reproduction of symptoms as well as the quality and quantity of movement.*

In the case of heightened nerve mechanosensitivity in the upper limb, shoulder abduction is usually limited by pain, given that abduction leads to lengthening of the peripheral nerves (Kleinrensink et al 1995) as well as increased tension in the brachial plexus (Ginn 1988) and the C5–C7 nerve roots (Elvey 1988) (**Fig. 2.47**). Typical compensatory movements include cervical ipsilateral sidebending, shoulder girdle elevation, and elbow bending.

Cervical contralateral sidebending is also painfully limited, given that this movement causes increased tension in the C5–T1 nerve roots (Selvaratnam et al 1988, 1989) and further distally in the brachial plexus (Reid 1987; Wilson et al 1994) and the median nerve (McLellan and Swash 1976).

Of course, painful limitation of shoulder abduction may also be caused by a local shoulder pathology. In order to structurally differentiate between a local shoulder pathology and increased neural mechanosensitivity, *sensitizing movements* may be performed that produce increased tension on the nerves but do not have any influence on the local joint, such as cervical contralateral sidebending and/ or wrist extension. Wrist extension causes increased tension on the median nerve (Kleinrensink et al 1995; Wright et al 1996) and brachial plexus (Selvaratnam 1991; Wilson et al 1994). If shoulder abduction is further limited in range with addition

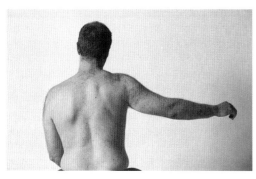

Fig. 2.47 Active shoulder abduction with compensatory movements.

of wrist extension (**Fig. 2.48**), this suggests that the cause is more likely to be neural rather than a shoulder pathology. The same applies to additional cervical contralateral sidebending (**Fig. 2.49**).

> *When performing any of these movements, the position of the shoulder girdle must remain constant. Elevation of the shoulder girdle would cause relaxation of the nerves. The therapist can control the elevation with gentle fixation of the shoulder girdle and at the same time sense any compensatory movements (**Fig. 2.48, Fig. 2.49**).*

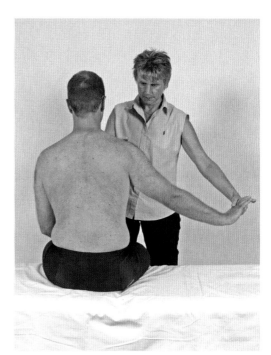

Fig. 2.48 Active shoulder abduction with wrist extension and shoulder girdle fixation.

### Example: Differentiation between neural and non-neural pathologies

Pain on the palmar aspect of the hand raises suspicion of carpal tunnel syndrome or a local non-neural pathology (e.g., ligament injury). In either case, wrist extension would provoke symptoms. Yet, if pain increases with additional shoulder abduction and cervical contralateral sidebending, a neural pathology is rather assumed.

> *The extent of movement limitation depends on the severity of heightened nerve mechanosensitivity. In some patients, only a slight movement restriction is present.*

Examinations of the lower quadrants use the same principles as already described. Lumbar bending, hip bending, knee and dorsal extension of the foot cause increased tension on the sciatic nerve, its distal branches, and the L4–S3 nerve roots. In painfully limited lumbar bending, additional dorsal extension of the foot may be used for differentiation (**Fig. 2.50**). If neural structures are affected, the movement (lumbar bending) is more painful, or pain occurs earlier in the range, and the range of motion reduces.

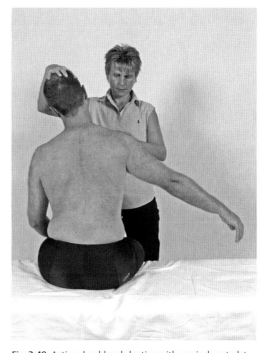

Fig. 2.49 Active shoulder abduction with cervical contralateral sidebending and shoulder girdle fixation.

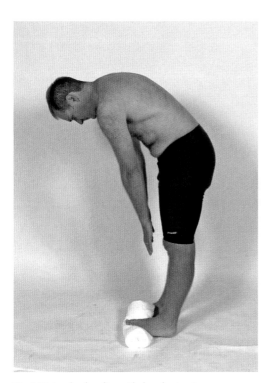

**Fig. 2.50** Lumbar bending with dorsal extension.

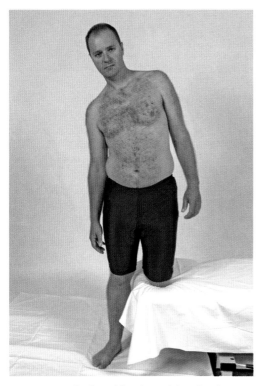

**Fig. 2.51** Active lumbar sidebending with knee bending.

Unlike the sciatic nerve, the femoral nerve runs along the anterior aspect of the hip joint. In patients with symptoms affecting the lumbar spine and the anterior thigh, the examination should be altered accordingly (contralateral lumbar sidebending, hip extension, knee bending; **Fig. 2.51**).

### Dysfunction Affecting Passive Movements

Active and passive movements have the same, or at least similar, effects on the nerves. Thus, in patients with heightened neural mechanosensitivity, the range of motion of passive movements should correspond to the range of motion of active movements. If there is any discrepancy (e.g., painfully limited active shoulder abduction, but no or only minimal symptoms with passive abduction), then the hypothesis of heightened mechanosensitivity as the cause of movement restriction is disproved.

### Abnormal Responses to Neural Provocation Tests

Neural provocation tests were first reported at the end of the 19th century. Lazarevic reported in 1880 on the Lasègue test (today: straight leg raise test, SLR) (Supik and Broom 1994) and Poore (1887) described examination methods for the median nerve, the radial nerve, and the ulnar nerve.

The importance of these tests has grown over the last 25 years. They are now part of the standard patient examination, although their interpretation has changed. The original terms, such as *brachial plexus tension test* (Elvey 1986), *upper limb tension test* and *adverse mechanical tension* (Butler 1989; Yaxley and Jull 1993), suggested that the underlying disorders were neural disorders due to a mechanical problem of abnormal tension. This view has changed over time (Butler 1998; Elvey 1998). The provocation tests are not tests of tension, but rather aim to examine the mechanosensitivity of the nerves. Thus, the nomenclature has also been adjusted, and these are now known as the *neural tissue provocation test* (NTPT; Hall et al 1998), *neurodynamic tests* (Shacklock 1995), the *upper limb neurodynamic test* (ULNT; Butler 2000), and the *brachial plexus provocation test* (BPPT; Sterling et al 2002).

> *For simplicity's sake, the term neural provocation test (NPT) is used in the following.*

**Neural Provocation Tests**
- NPT via median nerve (**Table 2.13, Table 2.14; Figs. 2.52–2.54**)
- NPT via radial nerve (**Table 2.15; Fig. 2.55, Fig. 2.56**)
- NPT via ulnar nerve (**Table 2.16; Fig. 2.57, Fig. 2.58**)
- Other NPTs of the upper extremity (**Table 2.17**):
  - Musculocutaneous nerve
  - Axillary nerve
  - Suprascapular nerve
- SLR test (**Table 2.18; Fig. 2.59**)
- NPT of the lower extremity (**Table 2.19**):
  - Femoral nerve (**Fig. 2.60, Fig. 2.61**)
  - Lateral cutaneous femoral nerve
  - Obturator nerve (**Fig. 2.62**)
  - Saphenous nerve
- Slump test (**Table 2.20; Fig. 2.63, Fig. 2.64**)

*Movement Patterns of Provocation Tests*
- The neural provocation tests use sequences of passive joint movements, which cause increased movement, elongation and tension, and finally stretching of a nerve.
- The individual movement directions vary, depending on which nerves are to be tested.
- The final position of a test is the position in which there is maximum tension on the nerve.

**Example:** Provocation test via median nerve (**Fig. 2.52**), which includes abduction, external rotation, fixation of the shoulder girdle, extension and supination of the elbow, and wrist extension and finger extension.

- The "final position" does not necessarily mean that full range of motion is obtained in all joints in the respective direction.

**Example:** Middle sequence of the NPT via median nerve (**Table 2.13, Table 2.14; Fig. 2.53**).

*Responses to Neural Provocation Tests*
Mechanical provocation of a nerve may provoke pain in a healthy person (**Tables 2.13–2.20**). Some people have a more sensitive nervous system than others, and hence the responses vary a lot. However, the provoked pain response is a normal physiological response (similar to a pain response upon stretching a muscle).

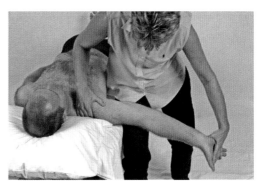
Fig. 2.52 Provocation test via median nerve (final position).

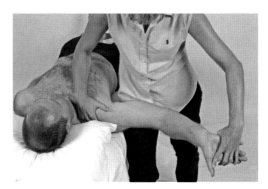
Fig. 2.53 Provocation test via median nerve (middle sequence).

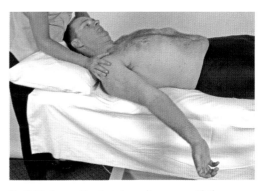
Fig. 2.54 Provocation test via median nerve, with the arm positioned and cervical contralateral sidebending.

**Table 2.13** Provocation test via median nerve (middle sequence)

| *(R) FROM, Norm* | *= (right), full range of motion, normal* |
|---|---|
| (L) Shoulder abduction √ | = left full range of motion, no pain |
| External rotation √ | = full range of motion, no pain |
| Extension of wrist/fingers √ | = full range of motion, no pain |
| Elbow: 60° extension deficit P1 pS, 50° P2 | = P1 pS onset shoulder pain<br>= P2 pain tolerance |
| Hand bending: ↓ pS | = Diminished shoulder pain |
| Shoulder girdle depression: ↑ pS | = Increased shoulder pain |
| Contralateral sidebending of cervical spine: ↑ pS | = Increased shoulder pain |
| Ipsilateral sidebending of cervical spine: ↓ pS | = Diminished shoulder pain |

> *In the case of nerve sensitization, the test movements will cause a pathological pain response as the nerves are hypersensitive to mechanical stimuli. The quality of the pain, and sometimes its localization, differ from a normal response; often the patient's exact symptoms are reproduced. It is therefore extremely important to compare responses between symptomatic and asymptomatic sides.*
> *It is best to thoroughly examine the healthy side first to see what a normal response entails in that particular patient.*

As already mentioned, it may not be possible to perform all test movements to their fullest range due to pain. Depending on the degree of pain irritability, one should determine prior to the examination how much pain should/can be provoked. Usually, individual movements are performed to the end of the movement, to the onset of pain (P1), or, if there is constant pain, to an increase in pain. Once a joint position is taken up, the movement is then taken back a little before the next movement component is added. The last movement is performed to P1, or to pain tolerance (P2), or to a pain-free end of movement, if possible. If there is pain during the test, the patient should report whether it corresponds to their specific pain complaint.

If pain is provoked, sensitizing or desensitizing maneuvers are performed to differentiate between neural or other structures.

**Example:** The provocation test via median nerve reproduces the patient's shoulder pain at the final test position. Depression of the shoulder girdle or cervical contralateral sidebending are sensitizing maneuvers. If the pain increases with sensitizing maneuvers, then the cause is presumably due to a neural disorder rather than to a shoulder joint disor-

der. Similarly, hand bending or ipsilateral sidebending of the cervical spine are desensitizing maneuvers and should reduce the pain. It is important to avoid altering the position of the shoulder joint.

> *Abnormal responses include pain that differs from the normal sensory responses on the healthy side or reproduction of the exact symptoms with greater movement limitation compared to the healthy side.*
> *When interpreting the results it is important to consider that a certain difference in range of motion between sides is normal (Table 2.14).*

Several authors have reported that the movement tests provoke muscular responses that may be seen as a type of protective mechanism or reflex movement (Bragard 1929; Elvey 1979; Quintner 1989; Hall et al 1998). Such responses occur in the antagonistic muscles of the respective movement direction (e.g., in the hamstring muscles during hip bending of SLR test). In patients with heightened mechanosensitivity the responses are stronger and occur earlier in range during the movement than in healthy people. This has been shown in the lower extremity in patients with lumbar radiculopathy (Hall 1996; Hall et al 1998) or lumbar back pain (Göeken and Hof 1993, 1994).

For the upper extremity, there is evidence that the trapezius muscle may play an important role (Balster and Jull 1997; van der Heide et al 2000, 2001a). In patients with cervical radiculopathy, muscle activity occurred earlier in range compared to healthy persons (van der Heide et al 2002).

Coppieters et al (1999, 2001b) demonstrated that in healthy persons during the NPT test via median nerve, the degree of shoulder girdle elevation increased with increased neural provocation. In

**Table 2.14** Provocation tests via median nerve (C[5], 6, 7, 8, T1; Figs. 2.52–2.54)

| | From proximal to distal | From distal to proximal | Middle sequence | Final position of the arm, cervical contralateral sidebending |
|---|---|---|---|---|
| Sequence of individual movements | • Shoulder abduction and external rotation<br>• Fixation of the shoulder girdle<br>• Supination<br>• Elbow extension<br>• Extension of wrist and fingers (emphasizing the extension of thumb and index finger) | • Fixation of the shoulder girdle<br>• Extension of fingers and wrist<br>• Supination<br>• Elbow extension<br>• Shoulder external rotation<br>• Shoulder abduction with fixation of the shoulder girdle | • Shoulder abduction and external rotation<br>• Fixation of the shoulder girdle<br>• Supination<br>• Extension of fingers and wrist<br>• Elbow extension | • Shoulder abduction and external rotation<br>• Elbow extension, supination, extension of wrist and fingers, fixation of the shoulder girdle, cervical contralateral sidebending |
| Sensitizing maneuvers | • Depression of shoulder girdle<br>• Cervical contralateral sidebending | • Depression of shoulder girdle<br>• Cervical contralateral sidebending | • Depression of shoulder girdle<br>• Cervical contralateral sidebending | |
| Examination | • Pain reproduction<br>• Muscle activity (elevation of shoulder girdle, elbow bending) | • Pain reproduction<br>• Muscle activity (elevation of shoulder girdle, elbow bending) | • Pain reproduction<br>• Muscle activity (elevation of shoulder girdle, elbow bending)<br>• Onset of pain (P1)<br>• Pain tolerance (P2; van der Heide et al 2000; Coppieters et al 2002) | • Pain reproduction<br>• Muscle activity (shoulder girdle elevation, cervical ipsilateral sidebending) |
| Normal responses | • Painful stretch in anterior shoulder<br>• Painful stretch in volar elbow region, radiating to forearm<br>• Tingling sensation in hand and forearm (Kenneally 1985; Rubenach 1985; Bell 1987)<br>• Sensory responses increase with cervical contralateral sidebending and decrease with cervical ipsilateral sidebending<br>• No difference between arms in regard to sensory responses<br>• Full range of motion with extensor of elbow and wrist<br>• Responses independent of age and sex | • Average 72° ± 21° abduction (Lohkamp and Small 2011) or 36.7° ± 8.5° (Reisch et al 2005) | • Sensory responses similar to proximal–distal (van der Heide et al 2000)<br>• Elbow extension deficit of 16.5–53.2° and a difference between sides of up to 8° is normal (Pullos 1986)<br>• No significant difference between both arms<br>• In combination of hand extension and cervical contralateral sidebending; average deficit of 40° for elbow extension (standard deviation 16.1°; Coppieters et al 2001a)<br>• The stronger the provocation the stronger the elevation of the shoulder girdle (Coppieters et al 2001b) | |
| Reliability | | • Good inter-therapist and intra-therapist reliability for range of movement of shoulder abduction (Kelley and Jull 1998; Lohkamp and Small 2011), moderate inter-therapist reliability (Schmid et al 2009) | • Good to excellent inter-therapist and intra-therapist reliability for onset of pain (P1) and pain tolerance (P2; van der Heide et al 2000; Coppieters et al 2002; Vanti et al 2010; Lohkamp and Small 2011), moderate inter-therapist reliability (Schmid et al 2009)<br>• Increased range of motion of 7.5° is significant after treatment | |

**Table 2.15**  Provocation tests via radial nerve (C5, 6, 7, 8 [T1]; **Fig. 2.55, Fig. 2.56**)

| | *From proximal to distal* | *From distal to proximal* | *Middle sequence (ULNT 2; Butler 2000)* | *Final position of the arm, cervical contralateral sidebending* |
|---|---|---|---|---|
| Sequence of individual movements | • Depression and fixation of shoulder girdle (Elvey and Hall 1997)<br>• Shoulder abduction<br>• Internal rotation<br>• Elbow extension<br>• Pronation<br>• Bending of wrist and fingers | • Finger and wrist bending<br>• Pronation<br>• Elbow extension<br>• Shoulder internal rotation<br>• Depression and fixation of the shoulder girdle<br>• Shoulder abduction | • Depression and fixation of shoulder girdle<br>• Elbow extension<br>• Shoulder internal rotation<br>• Wrist and finger bending<br>• Shoulder abduction | • Arm in shoulder abduction, internal rotation, pronation, elbow extension, pronation, wrist bending<br>• Movement in cervical contralateral sidebending |
| Sensitizing maneuvers | • Cervical contralateral sidebending<br>• Depression of shoulder girdle | • Cervical contralateral sidebending<br>• Depression of shoulder girdle | • Cervical contralateral sidebending<br>• Depression of shoulder girdle | • Depression of shoulder girdle |
| Examination | • Pain reproduction<br>• Muscle activity (shoulder elevation, elbow bending) | • Pain reproduction<br>• Muscle activity (shoulder elevation, elbow bending) | • Pain reproduction<br>• Muscle activity (shoulder elevation, elbow bending) | • Pain reproduction<br>• Muscle activity (shoulder elevation, cervical ipsilateral sidebending) |
| Normal responses | No publication | No publication | • Painful stretch on radial aspect of proximal forearm, often with painful stretch on lateral aspect of upper arm<br>• Strong stretch over biceps brachii muscle and occasionally in dorsal aspect of hand<br>• Other areas of symptoms: finger, thumb, back of hand, elbow, olecranon, neck (Petersen et al 2009)<br>• No difference between sides<br>• Symptoms worsen with cervical contralateral sidebending<br>• Abduction: 41.45° ± 4.06° (Yaxley and Jull 1991) | No publication |
| Reliability | Good intra-therapist reliability for measuring resistance (Petersen et al 2010) | No publication | • Good inter-therapist and intra-therapist reliability for measuring shoulder abduction with the help of a fixation device (Yaxley and Jull 1991)<br>• Moderate inter-therapist reliability without fixation device (Schmid et al 2009) | No publication |

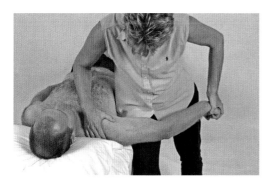

Fig. 2.55 Provocation test via radial nerve (middle sequence).

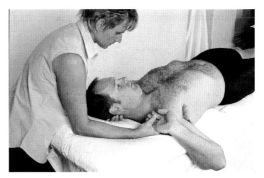

Fig. 2.58 Provocation test via ulnar nerve, arm positioned, cervical contralateral sidebending.

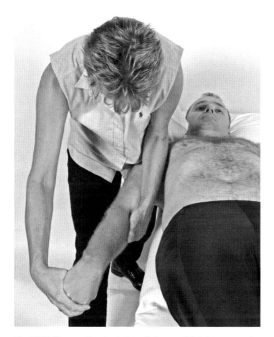

Fig. 2.56 Provocation test via radial nerve (distal sequence).

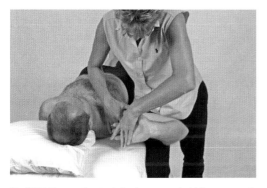

Fig. 2.57 Provocation test via ulnar nerve (middle sequence).

patients with cervicobrachial pain, the degree of elevation increased even further and it diminished after specific treatment (Coppieters et al 2003a). It is possible that the elevation was due to the activation of trapezius muscle and other shoulder girdle elevators (levator scapulae muscle).

Although scientific evidence is lacking for most NPTs that muscle reactions occur to protect the nerves, many clinicians report sensing a certain resistance while the movement is being performed (Bragard 1929; Kenneally et al 1988; Butler 1989; Butler and Gifford 1989; Quintner 1990; Yaxley and Jull 1993; Selvaratnam et al 1994; Vanti et al 2010). The resistance usually occurs during the movement at onset of pain (or when pain worsens in patients with constant pain). This has been confirmed by the author's own experience (**Tables 2.14–2.20**).

The therapist is free to choose the order of the individual joint movements in a given test: from distal to proximal, from proximal to distal, middle sequence, or positioning the arm in a symptom-provoking position and then performing cervical contralateral sidebending (**Figs. 2.52–2.58**). In certain situations the sequence may be determined by the localization and irritability of the pain.

The distal–proximal sequence of the NPT via radial nerve (**Fig. 2.56**) is suitable, for instance, for differentiating between De Quervain syndrome and a neural pathology. The hand is held in bending with ulnar abduction. In proximal symptoms the therapist begins with proximal movements followed by distal movements to aid differentiation.

If heightened neural mechanosensitivity is present, this should be evident in all tests irrespective of the order in which the movements are performed. The author often prefers the middle sequence, because it is the easiest to perform and to document.

**Table 2.16**   Provocation tests via ulnar nerve (C7, 8, T1; ULNT 3; Butler 2000; **Fig. 2.57, Fig. 2.58**)

| | From proximal to distal | From distal to proximal | Middle sequence | Final position of the arm, cervical contralateral sidebending |
|---|---|---|---|---|
| Sequence of individual movements | • Abduction of shoulder, depression and fixation of the shoulder girdle, external rotation<br>• Elbow bending<br>• Pronation<br>• Hand and finger extension (emphasizing extension of the little finger) | • Wrist and finger extension<br>• Pronation<br>• Elbow bending<br>• External rotation<br>• Depression and fixation of the shoulder girdle<br>• Shoulder abduction | • Abduction and external rotation of shoulder<br>• Depression and fixation of the shoulder girdle<br>• Pronation<br>• Wrist and finger extension<br>• Elbow bending | • Abduction and external rotation of shoulder<br>• Depression of the shoulder girdle<br>• Elbow bending<br>• Pronation<br>• Wrist and finger extension, fixation of shoulder girdle<br>• Test movement: contralateral sidebending of cervical spine |
| Sensitizing maneuvers | • Depression of the shoulder girdle<br>• Contralateral sidebending of cervical spine | • Depression of the shoulder girdle<br>• Contralateral sidebending of cervical spine | • Depression of the shoulder girdle<br>• Contralateral sidebending of cervical spine | |
| Examination | • Pain reproduction<br>• Muscle activity (elevation, elbow extension) | • Pain reproduction<br>• Muscle activity (elevation, elbow extension) | • Pain reproduction<br>• Muscle activity (elevation, elbow extension) | • Pain reproduction<br>• Muscle activity (elevation, ipsilateral sidebending of cervical spine) |
| Normal responses | No publication | • Sensory response and tingling in hypothenar and both medial fingers (Flanagan 1993) | No publication | No publication |
| Reliability | Moderate intra-therapist reliability for measuring resistance (Petersen et al 2009) | Moderate inter-therapist reliability (Schmid et al 2009) | No publication | No publication |

An example of documenting responses to the NPT via median nerve (middle sequence) in a patient with shoulder pain (pS) on the left side is provided above in **Table 2.13**.

The principles of examination apply to all NPTs. Thus, only selected tests are discussed in the following. (The movement components of the tests, sensitizing maneuvers, normal responses, and information on reliability are documented in **Tables 2.14–2.20**).

Except for the SLR test, the validity of most provocation tests has not yet been documented (Xin et al 1987; Thelander et al 1992; Vucetic and Svensson 1996). The use of the slump test for diagnosing a herniated disk was not convincing compared to other physical tests (Stankovic et al 1999).

Kleinrensink et al (2000) demonstrated that the NPT via median nerve is specific for the median nerve. The movement components of the test cause most tension in the median nerve and not in other peripheral nerves. The NPTs via radial nerve and ulnar nerve have not been shown to be specific for those nerves.

However, in one case study, findings of the NPT via ulnar nerve suggested a pathology affecting the nerve that indeed was later confirmed during surgery (Shacklock 1996).

Coveney (1997) reported a sensitivity of 82% and a specificity of 75% for the NPT via median nerve for diagnosing carpal tunnel syndrome. However, only the reproduction of symptoms was used as a positive test response. Wainner et al (2003) reported a sensitivity of 97% and a specificity of 22% for diagnosing cervical radiculopathies and carpal tunnel syndrome, however their criteria for a "positive" test are debatable. Only one of the following three criteria was required for a positive test response: (1) reproduction of the patient's symptoms, (2) a difference between arms in elbow range of motion, or (3) contralateral neck sidebending increased symptoms

**Table 2.17** Additional neural provocation tests for the upper extremity (Butler 2000)

| | Musculocutaneous nerve (C5–C7) | Axillary nerve (C5, C6) | Suprascapular nerve (C5, C6) |
|---|---|---|---|
| Sequence of individual movements | • Depression and fixation of shoulder girdle<br>• Elbow extension<br>• Extension of shoulder<br>• Ulnar deviation of the hand | • Shoulder internal rotation<br>• Depression of shoulder girdle<br>• Elbow extension<br>• Extension of shoulder<br>• Ulnar deviation of the hand | • Therapist on opposite side<br>• Horizontal adduction<br>• Cervical contralateral sidebending<br>• Depression of shoulder girdle<br>• Rotation of scapula |
| Sensitizing maneuvers | • Cervical contralateral side-bending<br>• Shoulder abduction<br>• Shoulder external rotation | • Cervical contralateral side-bending | |
| Examination | Pain reproduction | Pain reproduction | Pain reproduction |
| Normal responses | No publication | No publication | No publication |
| Reliability | No publication | No publication | No publication |

Source: Butler (2000).

**Table 2.18** SLR (L4–S2; **Fig. 2.59**)

| | | Differentiation | Differentiation | Differentiation |
|---|---|---|---|---|
| Movement components | • Knee extension<br>• Hip bending | | | |
| Sensitizing maneuvers | • Dorsal extension (Boland and Adams 2000)<br>• Hip internal rotation<br>• Hip adduction (Breig and Troup 1979)<br>• Clinical significance of cervical spine bending is questionable (Hall et al 1998) | • Sural nerve: dorsal extension of foot with inversion | • Tibial nerve: dorsal extension of foot with eversion | • Peroneal nerve (superficial cutaneous branches): plantar bending of foot with inversion |
| Examination | • Pain reproduction<br>• Onset of muscle activity in hamstrings (Hall et al 1998) | • Pain reproduction | • Pain reproduction | • Pain reproduction |
| Normal responses | • Range of motion with hip bending of 50–120°<br>• Pain or discomfort in posterior leg<br>• No difference between sides (Slater et al 1994; Herrington et al 2008) | • Symptoms in calf muscle and postero-lateral malleolus, lateral aspect of foot, radiating to back of knee and posterior thigh (Molesworth 1992) | | • Stretching pain in antero-lateral lower leg and foot with plantar bending and inversion of foot (Shacklock 1989; Molesworth 1992)<br>• Increased pain with hip bending<br>• Referred to posterior thigh and back of knee<br>• Possible pain in calf muscles |
| Reliability | • Very good inter-therapist reliability (Boland and Adams 2000)<br>• Very good intra-therapist reliability (Herrington et al 2008)<br>• Improved range of motion on SLR of more than 13° after treatment may be considered a treatment effect | | | |

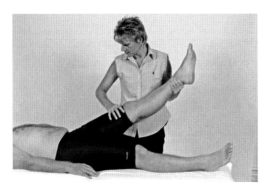

Fig. 2.59 Straight leg raise test.

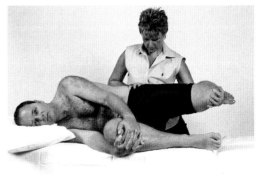

Fig. 2.61 Provocation test via femoral nerve with an extended cervical spine and hip joint.

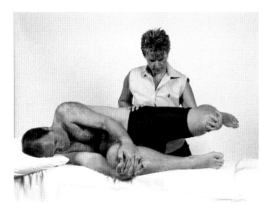

Fig. 2.60 Provocation test via femoral nerve, cervical spine bending, hip extension.

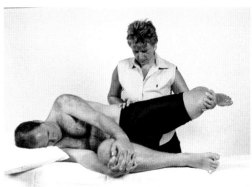

Fig. 2.62 Provocation test via obturator nerve.

Table 2.19 Additional neural provocation tests for the lower extremity (Figs. 2.60–2.62)

|  | Femoral nerve (L2–L4) | Lateral cutaneous femoral nerve (L2, L3) | Obturator nerve (L2, L3) | Saphenous nerve |
|---|---|---|---|---|
| Movement components | • Side-lying position<br>• Spinal bending<br>• Hip bending of bottom leg, hip extension top leg | • Side-lying position<br>• Spinal bending<br>• Hip bending of bottom leg, hip extension top leg<br>• Test movement: abduction of hip (Butler 2000) | • Side-lying position<br>• Spinal bending,<br>• Hip bending of bottom leg, hip extension top leg<br>• Test movement: abduction of hip (Butler 2000) | • Prone<br>• Knee extension<br>• Dorsal extension and inversion of foot<br>• Hip external rotation (Butler 2000) |
| Sensitizing maneuvers | • Bending of cervical spine<br>• Contralateral bending of lumbar spine | • Bending of cervical spine | • Bending of cervical spine<br>• Contralateral bending of lumbar spine | • Bending of cervical spine |
| Examination | • Pain reproduction<br>• Movement limitation with hip extension | • Pain reproduction<br>• Movement limitation with hip adduction | • Pain reproduction<br>• Movement limitation with hip abduction | • Pain reproduction |
| Normal responses | • Pulling sensation in anterior thigh<br>• Cervical extension reduces symptoms, bending worsens symptoms (Davidson 1987) |  | No publication |  |
| Reliability | No publication | No publication | No publication | No publication |

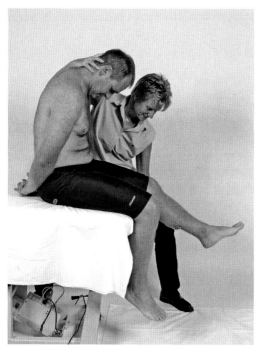

Fig. 2.63 Slump test with cervical spine bending.

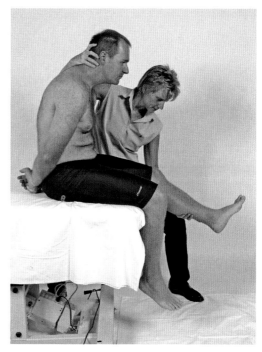

Fig. 2.64 Slump test with cervical spine extension.

**Table 2.20** Slump test (**Fig. 2.63, Fig. 2.64**)

| Movement components | • Sitting, arms behind back<br>• Bending of lumbar spine<br>• Bending of cervical spine<br>• Knee extension<br>• Finally, eliminate cervical spine bending |
|---|---|
| Sensitizing maneuvers | • Dorsal extension of the foot<br>• Bilateral extension of the knees<br>• Plantar bending of the foot with inversion |
| Examination | • Pain reproduction<br>• Muscle activity (extension of cervical spine, knee bending) |
| Normal responses | • Pain in middle thoracic spine region and back of knee (Maitland 1986)<br>• Increased leg pain with bending of the cervical spine<br>• Increased range of motion of dorsal extension of the foot and extension of the knee with cervical extension (Maitland 1986; Fidel et al 1996) |
| Reliability | • Good reliability for knee extension and pain changes when altering cervical spine position (Lew and Briggs 1997)<br>• Good inter-therapist and intra-therapist reliability (Yeung et al 1997)<br>• Very good intra-therapist reliability (Herrington et al 2008) |

or ipsilateral neck sidebending decreased symptoms.

The diagnostic accuracy of NTP via median nerve for detecting carpal tunnel syndrome was also assessed by Vanti et al (2010), using only one of the three criteria used by Wainner and colleagues (2003). Sensitivity was estimated as 92% and speci-ficity as 15%. The sensitivity and clinical validity of the test are supported by two additional case studies (van der Heide et al 2002). In patients with a C6 or C7 radiculopathy, the test reproduced the patients' exact symptoms. This suggests that the test does cause mechanical irritation of these nerve roots.

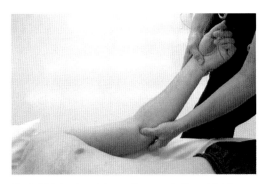

Fig. 2.65 Palpation of the median nerve in the cubital fossa.

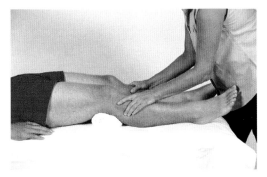

Fig. 2.66 Palpation of the peroneal nerve.

### Mechanical Hyperalgesia as a Response to Palpation of Peripheral Nerve Trunks

Specific nerve palpations are (similar to other soft-tissue palpations) part of the routine examination (**Fig. 2.65, Fig. 2.66**) and may aid further in the assessment of mechanical nerve sensitivity. The first reports on palpation of nerve trunks were published in 1887 (Poore 1887). As previously explained, healthy nerves are not sensitive to harmless mechanical stimuli (Kuslich et al 1991; Hall and Quintner 1996). Yet inflamed nerve roots are extremely mechanosensitive and the entire length of the nerve may be sensitive (Hall and Quintner 1996). Spreading of the sensitivity along the nerve is presumably due to axonal regeneration (Devor and Rappaport 1990) or possibly sensitization of the nervi nervorum due to neurogenic inflammation (Quintner 1998).

> The nerves on the healthy side should always be examined first.

Normally, there is no difference between sides in terms of the responses to palpation (Sterling et al 2000) nor do the responses depend on the age of the patient. The inter-therapist reliability for the palpation of peripheral nerve trunks in the upper extremity (Schmid et al 2009) and the lower extremity (Walsh and Hall 2009) is well established.

Palpation of mechanosensitive nerves provokes either a pain response, if palpation on the symptom-free side fails to produce pain, or it causes a hyperalgesic response if palpation on the healthy side elicits a normal pain response.

Sometimes a nerve may be palpated as a distinct string (e.g., the ulnar nerve at the elbow). At other times, it must be palpated through the overlying muscles and soft tissues. In the latter case it is not felt as a distinct structure.

### Palpation of Peripheral Nerves

Palpation examination methods are listed in **Table 2.21** and **Table 2.22**.

### Identifying a Local Cause of a Neural Disorder

The findings described above may be associated with various causes of neural pain. This does not necessarily mean that the pain is treatable with manual techniques. Certain diseases, such as diabetic neuropathy or painful neuropathy due to a space-occupying mass, may as well exhibit the characteristics of increased neural mechanosensitivity and related movement restrictions.

> Before a decision about the choice of treatment or the indications and contraindications can be made, the cause and localization of the pain must be identified.

### Example: Radicular pain due to a spinal pathology

The examination of the spinal column includes the palpation of individual segments and passive segmental movement tests (**Fig. 2.67, Fig. 2.68**). Abnormal mobility and pain reproduction are considered pathological.

In the case of a C6 radiculopathy, one would expect to find a dysfunction affecting the motion segments C5–C6 or C6–C7. In this case, this would likely be the source/location of the radicular pain.

For diagnosing patients with cervicobrachial pain syndrome, the examination methods described by Hall and Elvey (1999) have been proven to be of value (Hall et al 1997; van der Heide et al 2001b; Allison et al 2002; Cowell and Phillips 2002; Coppieters et al 2003a, b).

> Another important aspect related to neural pain is the examination of nerve function. The neurological examination is the only clinical tool for determining whether there are signs of impaired nerve conduction and clinical signs suggestive of peripheral nerve damage.

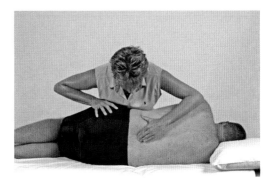

**Fig. 2.67** Segmental motion test of the cervical spine.

**Fig. 2.68** Segmental motion test of the lumbar spine.

**Table 2.21** Nerve palpation in the upper extremity

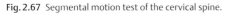

| Trunks of the brachial plexus | Neurovascular bundle | Median nerve | Radial nerve | Ulnar nerve | Axillary nerve | Suprascapular nerve | Dorsal scapular nerve |
|---|---|---|---|---|---|---|---|
| Posterior triangle between the anterior and middle scalene muscles | • Below the coracoid process<br>• In the axilla | In axilla superior to the brachial artery | In the intermuscular septum (radial sulcus) | In axilla inferior to the brachial artery | Through posterior part of deltoid muscle | • Scapular notch<br>• Infraspinatus fossa | Between thoracic spine and medial border of the shoulder blade |
| • Upper trunk C5 and C6<br>• Middle trunk C7 | | In the elbow, medial to the tendon of the biceps brachii muscle and the brachial artery | In forearm, between the extensor carpi radialis longus and brevis muscles | At the olecranon | Lateral border of shoulder blade | | |
| • Lower trunk C8 and T1 | | In the carpal tunnel | In the anatomic "snuff box" | Between the pisiform and hamulus of hamate | | | |

**Table 2.22** Nerve palpation in the lower extremity

| Sciatic nerve | Common peroneal nerve | Posterior tibial nerve | Peroneal nerve (deep) | Tibial nerve | Sural nerve (continuation of tibial nerve) | Femoral nerve | Lateral femoral cutaneous nerve |
|---|---|---|---|---|---|---|---|
| P: Between trochanter major and ischial tuberosity | S: Fibular neck just below the head of the fibula | S: Posterior to the medial malleolus and arterial pulse | S: Between the first and second metatarsals | • Lateral to the popliteal artery<br>• 3 cm proximal to the knee fold | S:<br>• Posterior to the lateral malleolus<br>• Lateral side of the dorsum of the foot | S: Lateral to the femoral artery | S: Somewhat medial and 2 cm inferior to the anterior superior iliac spine |
| Just before it branches into the tibial nerve and peroneal nerve | | | | | | | |

Note: P = Prone, S = Supine.

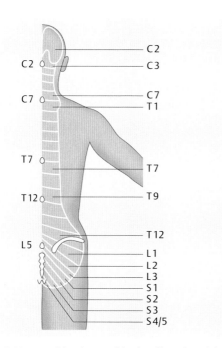

**Fig. 2.69** Areas of distribution of the dorsal branches of the spinal nerves.

## Peripheral Neurological Examination

The clinical examination includes an analysis of nerve conduction of afferent and efferent nerve trunks and sensory and motor nerve roots. For routine screening, the examination covers the following aspects:

- Sensation testing:
  - Tactile sensitivity (sensitivity to touch, sharp/blunt)
- Myotatic (stretch) reflexes
- Muscular strength

Detailed examinations also include tests of temperature (test tube) and vibration (tuning fork) sense, two-point discrimination tests, and proprioceptive testing. These are, however, not further discussed in this chapter.

Sensory and motor deficits may occur due to disorders of the sensory/motor nerve root in the region of the spinal nerve roots, or they may be due to distal disorders. Hence thorough knowledge of the dermatomes/myotomes innervated by the nerve roots and the peripheral nerves is vital for differentiating between deficits due to nerve root pathologies and those caused by distal peripheral nerve lesions (see **Fig. 2.70** and **Fig. 4.8**).

> The healthy side should always be examined first to allow an immediate comparison of whether the results on the symptomatic side are normal or not.

### Sensation Testing
**Sensitivity to Touch and Pinprick**
A cotton swab or cotton wool can be used to examine the function of the A-beta fibers. The patient should not be allowed to see the areas being touched. For the examination of dermatomes of the limbs the assessment begins proximally with two circles each around the upper arm or thigh, and then the forearm or lower leg, and one circle around the hand or foot. The fingers and dermatomes in the foot should be assessed individually on their dorsal and ventral aspects. The patient should indicate whether he or she feels the touch and whether the sensation is equally strong for every area. The same procedure is performed using a pointy object (e.g., toothpick, end of a paperclip) to examine the A-delta fibers.

> Changes in tactile sensation include increased or diminished sensation or total loss of sensation.

The area of abnormal sensation should be precisely identified and recorded on a body chart. The borders of altered sensation may be assessed from either perspective—that is, from the abnormal or healthy region:

- For reduced sensation: The test instrument is moved from the region of diminished sensation toward that of normal sensation.
- For increased sensation: Testing is performed from the region of normal sensation toward that of increased sensation.

*Abnormal Perceptions*
- Analgesia: Numbness or reduced sensation
- Hypoalgesia/hypoesthesia: Reduced sensation
- Hyperalgesia: Increased sensation
- Dysesthesia: Discomfort
- Allodynia: Painful perception

Injury/disease affecting the sensory fibers of the dorsal branch of the spinal nerve (ramus dorsalis) may cause sensory disturbances affecting the corresponding area on the back (**Fig. 2.69**).

The ventral branch of the spinal nerve (ramus ventralis) provides sensory, motor, and autonomic innervation to the anterior region of the body and the extremities. Compression of the nerve roots (e.g., due to a herniated disk) may cause classic radicular symptoms with radiating pain and sensory loss affecting the dermatomes. During the neurological examination of patients with suspected nerve root

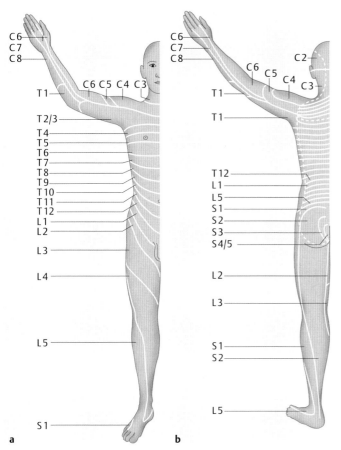

**Fig. 2.70a, b** Dermatomes.
**a** From ventral.
**b** From dorsal.

a

b

compression, sensation in the areas of the dermatomes is evaluated (sensitivity to touch, pinprick, and perception of temperature) (**Fig. 2.70a, b**).

To assess neuropathic pain, sensory testing has to be performed in the patient's main area of pain and findings compared to the contralateral mirror side (unilateral pain) or to a proximal or distal pain-free site (bilateral pain) (Treede et al 2008). Sensory testing should include mechanical (touch, pinprick, vibration) as well as thermal (warm/cold) stimulation.

### Reflexes

Percussion with a reflex hammer causes a quick stretch of the relevant muscles or tendons. The muscle being examined should be in a lengthened position and the point of contact of the hammer should be at a right angle to the tendon or muscle fibers.

In the upper extremity reflexes of the deltoid muscle (C5), biceps brachii muscle (C5, C6), brachioradialis muscle (C6), triceps brachii muscle (C7,

C8), and the pronator reflex (C6, C7) are tested; in the lower extremity reflexes of the adductor brevis, longus, and magnus muscles are tested (L2, L3) as well as the rectus femoris muscle (L3, L4), semimembranosus and semitendinosus muscle (L5), biceps femoris muscle (L5, S1), and the Achilles tendons reflex (S1).

*Classification of Reflex Responses (Petty and Moore 2001)*

- 0 = absent
- 1 = diminished
- 2 = normal
- 3 = increased
- 4 = clonus

*A side comparison should always be performed. Absent or weakened reflexes are not necessarily pathological. If the muscle reflex is always absent or weakened while all other muscles exhibit normal reflexes, this may be considered an abnormality.*

**Table 2.23** Assessment of key muscles (myotomes) of the upper quadrant

| Muscle | Nerve root | Method |
|---|---|---|
| | | *Sitting or standing* |
| Rectus capitis anterior muscle | C1 | Bending of the head |
| Rectus capitis posterior major and minor with obliquus capitis superior muscle | C2 | Extension of the head |
| Scalene muscles | C3 | Sidebending of the cervical spine |
| ▪ Trapezius muscle<br>▪ Levator scapulae muscle | C4 | Elevation of the shoulder girdle |
| | | *Supine* |
| Deltoid muscle | C5 | ▪ Arm in approximately 45° abduction<br>▪ Resistance against abduction at the elbow |
| Biceps brachii muscle | C6 | ▪ Elbow flexed to 90° and supinated<br>▪ Resistance against bending at the forearm |
| Triceps muscle | C7 | ▪ Elbow flexed to 90°<br>▪ Resistance against extension at the forearm |
| Extensor pollicis longus muscle | C8 | ▪ Elbow flexed to 90°<br>▪ Thumb extended<br>▪ Resistance against extension at the thumbnail |
| Flexor digitorum profundus muscle | C8 | ▪ Elbow flexed to 90°<br>▪ Therapist places fingers on the volar aspect of the patient's fingers<br>▪ Patient closes fist<br>▪ Resistance against finger bending |
| Lumbrical muscle | T1 | ▪ Lumbrical grip<br>▪ Therapist tries to spread the patient's fingers apart |

Source: Maitland (2001).

### Muscle Strength

For isometric muscle strength testing of relevant key muscles (myotomes) (**Table 2.23, Table 2.24**), the muscle being examined should be tested in its mid-position. The resistance should increase gradually; the amount of resistance should be applied according to the specific muscle group and the individual patient.

> With suspicion of a peripheral nerve lesion, the strength of all individual muscles supplied by the affected nerve has to be assessed.

Examples of peripheral nerve examinations are found in various publications (Shacklock 1995, 1996; Elvey 1997; Elvey and Hall 1997; Hall and Elvey 1999).

Nerve-related pain disorders are heterogeneous with clinical signs and symptoms; patterns of pain and sensory and motor abnormalites vary widely between individuals. Even though patients can present with very similar pain characteristics and sensory symptoms, the pathophysiology, the pain type (nociceptive/neuropathic) and the underlying pain mechanism do likely differ (Tampin et al 2012). A thorough clinical examination, including the examination of the peripheral nervous system (as outlined previously) and sound clinical reasoning are crucial for diagnosing the underlying cause of the pain disorder and targeted treatment. The following two brief case studies outline some of the clinical reasoning processes in patient examination.

**Table 2.24** Assessment of key muscles (myotomes) of the lower quadrant

| Muscle | Nerve root | Method |
|---|---|---|
| | | *Standing* |
| Gastrocnemius muscle | S1 | Patient stands on one leg and rises onto toes |
| | | *Supine* |
| Iliopsoas muscle | L2 | ▪ 90° bending of knee and hip<br>▪ Resistance against hip bending above the knee |
| Quadriceps muscle | L3 | ▪ Therapist passes his or her arm under the thigh and places her hand on the opposite thigh<br>▪ Patient extends the knee<br>▪ Resistance against extension |
| Tibialis anterior muscle | L4 | ▪ Foot in dorsal extension and inversion<br>▪ Resistance at medial margin of foot against extension |
| Extensor hallucis longus muscle | L5 | ▪ Foot and first toe in extension<br>▪ Resistance against extension |
| Extensor digitorum longus muscle | ▪ L5<br>▪ (S1) | ▪ Foot and toes in extension<br>▪ Resistance against extension |
| Peroneus longus and brevis muscles | S1 | ▪ Foot in extension and eversion<br>▪ Resistance at lateral margin of foot |
| Toe bending | | ▪ Patient flexes toes<br>▪ Resistance against bending |
| | | *Prone* |
| ▪ Biceps femoris muscle<br>▪ Semitendinosus muscle<br>▪ Semimembranosus muscle | ▪ L5<br>▪ S1 | ▪ Knee flexed around 90°<br>▪ Resistance against bending |
| Gluteus maximus muscle | ▪ L4<br>▪ L5<br>▪ (S1)<br>▪ (S2) | ▪ Hip extended and knee flexed<br>▪ Resistance against hip extension |

Source: Maitland (2001).

**Case Study 2: Subjective Assessment**

A 16-year-old girl attended the clinic with a constant deep, dull pain in the region of the right supraspinatus muscle that she referred to as shoulder pain. The intensity of the pain was high (8/10). She did not report any symptoms of numbness or paresthesia.

The pain started about a month ago. The patient was unaware of any specific incident, although she said the pain may have started during a tennis match. Since then it had increasingly worsened, and for the past two days she had kept her arm in a sling.

Two weeks prior a computed tomography (CT) scan of the shoulder had been performed; the results were normal. Since pain onset, treatment consisted of taking anti-inflammatory medication. This relieved the pain somewhat, but the patient's overall condition did not improve.

The pain was movement and position dependent. Activities such as lifting an object, extending the arm, or letting it hang down aggravated the pain immediately, and it remained aggravated for some time. Immobilization was the only effective pain reduction.

Further reports with regard to the patient's overall health were normal.

The information from the subjective assessment was suggestive of a muscular injury (supraspinatus muscle). Yet, the continually worsening pain seemed to contradict this. A healing process should be expected within 4 weeks. Certain findings pointed towards a neural disorder. The pain was localized in the region of the subscapular nerve, and the quality of the pain appeared to correspond to nerve trunk pain. Pain-provoking movements or positions would all produce a mechanical stimulus on neural structures.

*Physical Examination*

1. **Antalgic posture:** The patient sat on the treatment bench supporting the right arm, with bending of the elbow.

2. **Dysfunction with active movements:**
   a) Active movements of the cervical spine appeared normal at first, but on closer examination (with fixation of the shoulder girdle) cervical contralateral sidebending was painfully restricted.
   b) Active shoulder bending was painfully limited at about 120°, and an increase in shoulder pain occurred. The patient performed shoulder bending with simultaneous elbow bending. When asked to leave the elbow extended, shoulder bending was already restricted at 90°.
   c) Active shoulder abduction was also painfully limited; compensatory movements such as elevation of the shoulder girdle occurred quite early during the movement, and the range of motion was significantly reduced with shoulder girdle fixation. Even elbow extension alone (with neutral positioning of the shoulder) increased shoulder pain.
   d) Active movements on the asymptomatic side were normal.

3. **Dysfunction with passive movements:** Similar to the examination of active movement dysfunction, passive shoulder bending and abduction on the symptomatic side were painfully limited (abduction already at 60–70°). The movement was normal on the healthy side.

4. **Abnormal respones to an NPT:**
   a) As already mentioned, abduction of 60 to 70° exacerbated the shoulder pain. While maintaining exactly this shoulder position, the elbow was extended, which led to further pain exacerbation. A similar response occurred with wrist extension.
   b) Such a response would not be expected in a purely muscular injury as movements of the hand and elbow have no direct influence on the supraspinatus muscle. The pain increase with cervical contralateral sidebending further confirmed the findings.
   c) This patient illustrates that NPTs cannot always be performed to their full extent due to painful movement restrictions and irritability of the pain disorder.

5. **Mechanical hyperalgesia as a response to peripheral nerve trunk palpation:** Palpation of the subscapular nerve, the dorsal scapular nerve, and the neurovascular bundle were painful on the symptomatic side.

6. **Detection of a local cause of the neural disorder:** The examination of the cervical spine revealed movement dysfunctions affecting the segments C4–C5 and C5–C6 with localized pain provocation.

Continued ▷

## Case Study 2: Subjective Assessment (Continued)

*Neurological Examination*
Findings of the neurological examination were normal.

*Clinical Reasoning*
The pain localization, pain quality, pain behavior, the patient's antalgic posture, and the correspondence between passive and active movement limitations relating to movements that cause a mechanical stimulus on the nerves, as well as abnormal responses to the NPT and nerve palpation, led to a hypothesis of the presence of a neural disorder associated with heightened nerve mechanosensitivity. Sensitized neural structures would thus be the cause of pain. However, this patient did not present with neuropathic pain as no sensory alterations were found in the main pain area.

Various factors may explain the pathogenesis. It could be speculated that a specific movement that occurred while playing tennis caused a muscular injury. The related inflammatory process could have led to an irritation of the subscapular nerve. Yet, the problem could also have been due to a direct local irritation of the subscapular nerve, as demonstrated in conjunction with shoulder abduction and external rotation in baseball pitchers (Ringel et al 1990) and volleyball players (Witvrouw et al 2000). Finally, an irritation of the spinal nerves C5 or C6 could have occurred.

**Case Study 3: Subjective Assessment**

A 69-year-old woman reported intermittent, sometimes severe pain in the right buttock, which radiated into the posterior aspect of the right thigh and calf. She often experienced a simultaneous tingling sensation in that area.

The pain had started 1 month ago for no apparent reason. The symptoms had gradually worsened (presumably related to travel: a flight from Europe to Asia as well as travelling around). At times the pain was so intense that the patient could hardly walk. The pain was provoked immediately when standing up or when walking. Sitting (shifting the weight onto the left side) and lying down (on her back with support under her knee) quickly relieved the pain.

The patient reported that she often had back pain in the past, although she had never needed treatment. The patient was otherwise in good health.

*Physical Examination Results*

1. **Antalgic posture:**
   a) The patient stood with a slightly tilted pelvis and a relatively straight lumbar spine. Slight atrophy of the calf muscles and hamstrings was evident on the right side. The patient's weight was primarily on her left leg.
   b) Shifting the weight over the right leg provoked immediately the pain in her leg, while posterior pelvic tilt slightly relieved it.
2. **Dysfunction with active movements:**
   a) Extension of the lumbar spine and sidebending to the right worsened the symptoms immediately and thus movements were severely limited by pain.
   b) Bending of the lumbar spine and sidebending to the left were asymptomatic.
3. **Dysfunction with passive movements:**
   a) Passive extension of the lumbar spine and sidebending to the right provoked the same pain as active movements.
   b) Passive bending of the lumbar spine and sidebending to the left reduced the pain.
4. **Abnormal responses to an NPT:**
   a) The findings of the slump and SLR test were normal.
   b) Range of motion was normal on both sides, and the sensitizing maneuvers did not provoke any pathological pain.
5. **Mechanical hyperalgesia as a response to palpation of the peripheral nerve trunks:** Palpation of the peripheral nerve trunks did not reveal any abnormalities.
6. **Detection of a local cause of the neural disorder:**
   a) Intervertebral movements of the lumbar spine were extremely limited in all directions and in all segments.
   b) Palpation over the right facet joint L5–S1 immediately provoked the leg pain.

*Neurological Examination*

The neurological examination revealed myotomal weakness of the key muscle for S1 (gastrocnemius muscle). The Achilles tendon reflex could not be elicited on the right side. Light touch and pinprick sensation was reduced on the lateral border of the foot (S1 dermatome) and in the area of the leg pain.

*Clinical Reasoning*

The hypothesis was the presence of a neural disorder, that is, S1 compression radiculopathy on the right side with loss of sensory and motor nerve function and presence of neuropathic pain, but normal neural mechanosensitivity. This was supported by the following: pain localization (dermatome S1), pain behavior (triggered by compression, improvement in nonweight-bearing position), antalgic posture, a corresponding dysfunction of passive and active movements, as well as concurrence between the subjective symptoms and objective findings, the absence of abnormal responses to neural provocation tests (palpation and movement), the localization of a local movement disorder (with reproduction of the exact symptoms during palpation of L5–S1), and neurological deficits related to the S1 nerve root. The provisional diagnosis was later confirmed by CT studies. The CT scan demonstrated an asymmetrical disk protrusion at L5–S1 that was more pronounced on the right side. Overlying this was a focal posterolateral disk herniation on the right, which extended up to 7 mm behind the posterior contour of the intervertebral disk and was displacing the right S1 nerve root.

# References

Allison GT, Nagy BM, et al. A randomized clinical trial of manual therapy for cervico-brachial pain syndrome—a pilot study. Man Ther 2002;7(2):95–102

Asbury AK, Fields HL. Pain due to peripheral nerve damage: an hypothesis. Neurology 1984;34(12):1587–1590

Balster SM, Jull GA. Upper trapezius muscle activity during the brachial plexus tension test in asymptomatic subjects. Man Ther 1997;2(3):144–149

Bell A. The upper limb tension test—bilateral straight leg raising—a validating manoeuvre for the upper limb tension test. In: Dalziel BA, Snowsill JC, eds. Proceedings of the Fifth Biennial Conference of the Manipulative Therapists Association of Australia. Melbourne: Manipulative Therapists Association of Australia; 1987

Bennett GJ. Can we distinguish between inflammatory and neuropathic pain? Pain Res Manag 2006;11: 11–15

Boland RA, Adams RD. Effects of ankle dorsiflexion on range and reliability of straight leg raising. Aust J Physiother 2000;46(3):191–200

Bouhassira D and Attal N. Diagnosis and assessment of neuropathic pain: The saga of clinical tools. Pain 2011;152: S74–S83.

Bove GM, Light AR. The nervi nervorum—missing link for neuropathic pain? Pain Forum 1997;6:181–190

Bragard K. Die Nervendehnung als diagnostisches Prinzip ergibt eine Reihe neuer Nervenphänomene. Munch Med Wochenschr 1929;76:1999–2003

Breig A, Troup JD. Biomechanical considerations in the straight-leg-raising test. Cadaveric and clinical studies of the effects of medial hip rotation. Spine 1979;4(3):242–250

Butler DS. Adverse mechanical tension in the nervous system: a model for assessment and treatment. Aust J Physiother 1989;35:227–238

Butler DS. "Adverse neural tension" reconsidered. Aust J Physiother 1998;3:33–36

Butler DS. The Sensitive Nervous System. Melbourne: Noigroup Publications; 2000

Butler DS, Gifford L. The concept of adverse mechanical tension in the nervous system. Physiotherapy 1989;75: 622–636

Coppieters MW, Stappaerts KH, et al. A qualitative assessment of shoulder girdle elevation during the upper limb tension test 1. Man Ther 1999;4(1):33–38

Coppieters MW, Stappaerts KH, et al. Addition of test components during neurodynamic testing: effect on range of motion and sensory responses. J Orthop Sports Phys Ther 2001a;31(5):226–235, discussion 236–237

Coppieters MW, Stappaerts KH, et al. Shoulder girdle elevation during neurodynamic testing: an assessable sign? Man Ther 2001b;6(2):88–96

Coppieters MW, Stappaerts KH, et al. Reliability of detecting "onset of pain" and "submaximal pain" during neural provocation testing of the upper quadrant. Physiother Res Int 2002;7(3):146–156

Coppieters MW, Stappaerts KH, et al. Aberrant protective force generation during neural provocation testing and the effect of treatment in patients with neurogenic cervicobrachial pain. J Manipulative Physiol Ther 2003a;26(2): 99–106

Coppieters MW, Stappaerts KH, et al. The immediate effects of a cervical lateral glide treatment technique in patients with neurogenic cervicobrachial pain. J Orthop Sports Phys Ther 2003b;33(7):369–378

Coveney B. The upper limb tension test response in subjects with a clinical presentation of carpal tunnel syndrome. Proceedings of the 10th Biennial Conference of the Manipulative Physiotherapists Association of Australia. Melbourne: Manipulative Physiotherapists Association of Australia; 1997

Cowell IM, Phillips DR. Effectiveness of manipulative physiotherapy for the treatment of a neurogenic cervicobrachial pain syndrome: a single case study—experimental design. Man Ther 2002;7(1):31–38

Dalton PA, Jull GA. The distribution and characteristics of neck-arm pain in patients with and without a neurological deficit. Aust J Physiother 1989;35(1):3–8

Davidson P. Prone knee bend: an investigation into the effect of cervical flexion and extension. 5th Biennial Conference. Melbourne: Manipulative Therapists Association of Australia; 1987

Devor M, Rappaport HZ. Pain and pathophysiology of damaged nerve. In: Fields HL, ed. Pain Syndromes in Neurology. Oxford: Butterworth-Heinemann; 1990

Dyck PJ. Invited review: limitations in predicting pathologic abnormality of nerves from the EMG examination. Muscle Nerve 1990;13(5):371–375

Eliav E, Benoliel R, et al. Inflammation with no axonal damage of the rat saphenous nerve trunk induces ectopic discharge and mechanosensitivity in myelinated axons. Neurosci Lett 2001;311(1):49–52

Eliav E, Herzberg U, et al. Neuropathic pain from an experimental neuritis of the rat sciatic nerve. Pain 1999;83(2): 169–182

Elvey RL. Painful restriction of shoulder movement—a clinical observation study. Proceedings of a Conference on Disorders of the Knee, Ankle and Shoulder. Brisbane: Manipulative Therapists Association of Australia; 1979

Elvey RL. Treatment of arm pain associated with abnormal brachial plexus tension. Aust J Physiother 1986;32(4): 225–230

Elvey RL. The clinical relevance of signs of adverse brachial plexus tension. Proceedings of the International Federation of Orthopaedic Manipulative Therapists. Cambridge: International Federation of Orthopaedic Manipulative Therapists; 1988

Elvey RL. Physical evaluation of the peripheral nervous system in disorders of pain and dysfunction. J Hand Ther 1997;10(2):122–129

Elvey RL. "Adverse neural tension" reconsidered. Aust J Physiother 1998;3:13–18

Elvey RL, Hall T. Neural tissue evaluation and treatment. In: Donatelli RA, ed. Physical Therapy of the Shoulder. New York: Churchill Livingstone; 1997

Fidel C, Martin E, et al. Cervical spine sensitizing maneuvers during the slump test. J Manual Manip Ther 1996;4:16–21

Flanagan M. Normative responses to the ulnar nerve bias tension test [unpublished thesis]. Adelaide: University of South Australia; 1993

Fowler TJ, Danta G, et al. Recovery of nerve conduction after a pneumatic tourniquet: observations on the hind-limb of the baboon. J Neurol Neurosurg Psychiatry 1972;35(5): 638–647

Garfin SR, Rydevik BL, et al. Compressive neuropathy of spinal nerve roots. A mechanical or biological problem? Spine 1991;16(2):162–166

Gelberman RH, Hergenroeder PT, et al. The carpal tunnel syndrome. A study of carpal canal pressures. J Bone Joint Surg Am 1981;63(3):380–383

Gifford L. Acute low cervical nerve root conditions: symptom presentations and pathobiological reasoning. Man Ther 2001;6(2):106–115

Ginn K. An investigation of tension development in upper limb soft tissues during the upper limb tension test. Proceedings of the International Federation of Orthopaedic Manipulative Therapists. Cambridge: International Federation of Orthopaedic Manipulative Therapists; 1988

Göeken LN, Hof AL. Instrumental straight-leg raising: results in healthy subjects. Arch Phys Med Rehabil 1993;74(2): 194–203

Göeken LN, Hof AL. Instrumental straight-leg raising: results in patients. Arch Phys Med Rehabil 1994;75(4):470–477

Greening J, Lynn B. Minor peripheral nerve injuries: an underestimated source of pain. Man Ther 1998;3(4): 187–194

Hall T. Neuromeningeal involvement in the straight leg raise test identified by electromyography [unpublished thesis]. Perth: Curtin University of Technology; 1996

Hall T, Elvey RL. Nerve trunk pain: physical diagnosis and treatment. Man Ther 1999;4(2):63–73

Hall T, Quintner J. Responses to mechanical stimulation of the upper limb in painful cervical radiculopathy. Aust J Physiother 1996;42(4):277–285

Hall T, Elvey RL, et al. Efficacy of manipulative physiotherapy for the treatment of cervicobrachial pain. Proceedings of the 10th Biennial Conference of the Manipulative Physiotherapists Association of Australia. Melbourne: Manipulative Physiotherapists Association of Australia; 1997

Hall T, Zusman M, et al. Adverse mechanical tension in the nervous system? Analysis of straight leg raise. Man Ther 1998;3(3):140–146

Harrington JF, Messier AA, et al. Herniated lumbar disc material as a source of free glutamate available to affect pain signals through the dorsal root ganglion. Spine 2000;25(8):929–936

Henderson CM, Hennessy RG, et al. Posterior-lateral foraminotomy as an exclusive operative technique for cervical radiculopathy: a review of 846 consecutively operated cases. Neurosurgery 1983;13(5):504–512

Herrington L, Bendix K, et al. What is the normal response to structural differentiation within the slump and straight leg raise tests? Man Ther 2008;13(4):289–294

Hida S, Naito M, et al. Intraoperative measurements of nerve root blood flow during discectomy for lumbar disc herniation. Spine 2003;28(1):85–90

Hromada J. On the nerve supply of the connective tissue of some peripheral nervous system components. Acta Anat (Basel) 1963;55:343–351

Jensen TS, Baron R. Translation of symptoms and signs into mechanisms in neuropathic pain. Pain 2003;102: 1–8

Jensen TS, Baron R, et al. A new definition of neuropathic pain. Pain 2011;152: 2204–2205

Kelley S, Jull GG. Breast surgery and neural tissue mechanosensitivity.The Australian Journal of Physiotherapy. 1998; 44:31–37

Kenneally M. The upper limb tension test. Proceedings of the 4th Biennial Conference of the Manipulative Therapists Association of Australia. Brisbane: Manipulative Therapists Association of Australia; 1985

Kenneally M, Rubenach H, et al. The upper limb tension test: the straight leg raise test of the arm. In: Grant R, ed. Physical Therapy of the Cervical and Thoracic Spine. New York: Churchill Livingstone; 1988

Kleinrensink GJ, Stoeckart R, et al. Mechanical tension in the median nerve. The effects of joint positions. Clin Biomech (Bristol, Avon) 1995;10(5):240–244

Kleinrensink GJ, Stoeckart R, et al. Upper limb tension tests as tools in the diagnosis of nerve and plexus lesions. Anatomical and biomechanical aspects. Clin Biomech (Bristol, Avon) 2000;15(1):9–14

Kuslich SD, Ulstrom CL, et al. The tissue origin of low back pain and sciatica: a report of pain response to tissue stimulation during operations on the lumbar spine using local anesthesia. Orthop Clin North Am 1991;22(2):181–187

Lew PC, Briggs CA. Relationship between the cervical component of the slump test and change in hamstring muscle tension. Man Ther 1997;2(2):98–105

Lindahl O. Hyperalgesia of the lumbar nerve roots in sciatica. Acta Orthop Scand 1966;37(4):367–374

Lohkamp M, Small K. Normal response to upper limb neurodynamic test 1 and 2A. Man Ther 2011;16(2):125–130

Lundborg G. Ischemic nerve injury. Experimental studies on intraneural microvascular pathophysiology and nerve function in a limb subjected to temporary circulatory arrest. Scand J Plast Reconstr Surg Suppl 1970;6:3–113

Lundborg G. Structure and function of the intraneural microvessels as related to trauma, edema formation, and nerve function. J Bone Joint Surg Am 1975;57(7):938–948

Lundborg G, Rydevik B. Effects of stretching the tibial nerve of the rabbit. A preliminary study of the intraneural circulation and the barrier function of the perineurium. J Bone Joint Surg Br 1973;55(2):390–401

Lundborg G, Gelberman RH, et al. Median nerve compression in the carpal tunnel—functional response to experimentally induced controlled pressure. J Hand Surg Am 1982;7(3):252–259

Maitland GD. Vertebral Manipulation. 5th ed. London: Butterworth-Heinemann; 1986

Maitland GD. Vertebral Manipulation. 6th ed. London: Butterworth-Heinemann; 2001

Marchettini P, Lacerenza M, et al. Painful peripheral neuropathies. Curr Neuropharmacol 2006;4: 175–181

McLellan DL, Swash M. Longitudinal sliding of the median nerve during movements of the upper limb. J Neurol Neurosurg Psychiatry 1976;39(6):566–570

Molesworth J. The effect of chronic inversion ankle sprains on the dorsiflexion-inversion straight leg raise test and the plantarflexion-inversion straight leg raise test [unpublished thesis]. Adelaide: University of South Australia; 1992

Murphy RW. Nerve roots and spinal nerves in degenerative disk disease. Clin Orthop Relat Res 1977; Nov–Dec(129): 46–60

Ogata K, Naito M. Blood flow of peripheral nerve effects of dissection, stretching and compression. J Hand Surg Br 1986;11(1):10–14

Olmarker K, Rydevik B, et al. Autologous nucleus pulposus induces neurophysiologic and histologic changes in porcine cauda equina nerve roots. Spine 1993;18(11):1425–1432

Owen JH, Kostuik JP, et al. The use of mechanically elicited electromyograms to protect nerve roots during surgery for spinal degeneration. Spine 1994;19(15):1704–1710

Parke WW. The significance of venous return impairment in ischemic radiculopathy and myelopathy. Orthop Clin North Am 1991;22(2):213–221

Petersen, CM, Zimmermann CL, et al. Upper limb neurodynamic test of the radial nerve: a study of responses in symptomatic and asymptomatic subjects. J Hand Ther 2009; 22(4):344–353

Petty NJ, Moore A. Neuromusculoskeletal Examination and Assessment. 2nd ed. London: Churchill Livingstone; 2001

Poore GV. Clinical lecture on certain conditions of the hand and arm which interfere with the performance of professional acts, especially piano-playing. BMJ 1887;1(1365):441–444

Porter EL, Wharton PS. Irritability of mammalian nerve following ischemia. J Neurophysiol 1949;12(2):109–116

Pullos J. The upper limb tension test. Aust J Physiother 1986;32:258–259

Quintner JL. A study of upper limb pain and paresthesiae following neck injury in motor vehicle accidents: assessment of the brachial plexus tension test of Elvey. Br J Rheumatol 1989;28(6): 528–533

Quintner JL. Stretch-induced cervicobrachial pain syndrome. Aust J Physiother 1990;36:99–103

Quintner JL. Peripheral neuropathic pain: a rediscovered clinical entity. Annual General Meeting of the Australian Pain Society. Hobart: Australian Pain Society; 1998

Rankine JJ, Fortune DG, et al. Pain drawings in the assessment of nerve root compression: a comparative study with lumbar spine magnetic resonance imaging. Spine 1998;23(15):1668–1676

Reid SA. The measurement of tension changes in the brachial plexus. In: Dalziel BA, Snowsill JC, eds. Proceedings of the 5th Biennial Conference of the Manipulative Therapists Association of Australia. Melbourne: Manipulative Therapists Association of Australia; 1987

Reisch R, Williams K, et al. ULNT2—median nerve bias: examiner reliability and sensory responses in asymptomatic subjects. J Manual Manip Ther 2005;13:44–55

Ringel SP, Treihaft M, et al. Suprascapular neuropathy in pitchers. Am J Sports Med 1990;18(1):80–86

Rubenach H. The upper limb tension test—the effect of the position and movement of the contralateral arm. Proceedings of the 4th Biennial Conference of the Manipulative Therapists Association of Australia. Brisbane: Manipulative Therapists Association of Australia; 1985

Rydevik B, Brown MD, et al. Pathoanatomy and pathophysiology of nerve root compression. Spine 1984;9(1):7–15

Rydevik B, Lundborg G, et al. Effects of graded compression on intraneural blood blow. An in vivo study on rabbit tibial nerve. J Hand Surg Am 1981;6(1):3–12

Sauer SK, Bove GM, et al. Rat peripheral nerve components release calcitonin gene-related peptide and prostaglandin E2 in response to noxious stimuli: evidence that nervi nervorum are nociceptors. Neuroscience 1999;92(1):319–325

Schmid AB, Brunner F, et al. Reliability of clinical tests to evaluate nerve function and mechanosensitivity of the upper limb peripheral nervous system. BMC Musculoskelet Disord 2009;10:11

Selvaratnam PJ. The brachial plexus tension test in patients and cadavers [unpublished doctoral dissertation]. Melbourne: Monash University; 1991

Selvaratnam PJ, Glasgow EF, et al. The strain at the nerve roots of the brachial plexus (abstr.). J Anat 1988;161:260

Selvaratnam PJ, Glasgow EF, et al. Differential strain produced by the brachial plexus tension test on C5 to T1 nerve roots. In: Jones HM, Jones MA, Milde M, eds. Proceedings of the 6th Biennial Conference of the Manipulative Therapists Association of Australia. Adelaide: Manipulative Therapists Association of Australia; 1989

Selvaratnam PJ, Matyas TA, et al. Noninvasive discrimination of brachial plexus involvement in upper limb pain. Spine 1994;19(1):26–33

Shacklock M. The plantarflexion/inversion straight leg raise test. An investigation into the effect of cervical flexion and order of component movements on the symptom response [unpublished thesis]. Adelaide: University of South Australia; 1989

Shacklock, M. Neurodynamics. Physiotherapy 1995;81:9–16

Shacklock M. Positive upper limb tension test in a case of surgically proven neuropathy: analysis and validity. Man Ther 1996;1(3):154–161

Slater H, Butler DS, et al. The dynamic nervous system: examination and assessment using tension tests. In: Boyling JD, Palastanga N, eds. Grieve's Modern Manual Therapy. 2nd ed. Edinburgh: Churchill Livingstone; 1994

Smyth MJ, Wright V. Sciatica and the intervertebral disc; an experimental study. J Bone Joint Surg Am 1958;40-A(6):1401–1418

Stankovic R, Johnell O, et al. Use of lumbar extension, slump test, physical and neurological examination in the evaluation of patients with suspected herniated nucleus pulposus. A prospective clinical study. Man Ther 1999;4(1):25–32

Sterling M, Treleaven J, et al. Pressure pain thresholds of upper limb peripheral nerve trunks in asymptomatic subjects. Physiother Res Int 2000;5(4):220–229

Sterling M, Treleaven J, et al. Responses to a clinical test of mechanical provocation of nerve tissue in whiplash associated disorder. Man Ther 2002;7(2):89–94

Sunderland P. Nerve Injuries and Their Repair. London: Churchill Livingstone; 1991

Sunderland S. The nerve lesion in the carpal tunnel syndrome. J Neurol Neurosurg Psychiatry 1976;39(7):615–626

Sunderland S. Stretch-compression neuropathy. Clin Exp Neurol 1981;18:1–13

Sunderland S, Bradley KC. Stress-strain phenomena in human peripheral nerve trunks. Brain 1961a;84(1):102–119

Sunderland S, Bradley KE. Stress-strain phenomena in human spinal nerve roots. Brain 1961b;84(1):120–124

Supik LF, Broom MJ. Sciatic tension signs and lumbar disc herniation. Spine 1994;19(9):1066–1069

Takahashi N, Yabuki S, et al. Pathomechanisms of nerve root injury caused by disc herniation: an experimental study of mechanical compression and chemical irritation. Spine 2003;28(5):435–441

Tampin B, Slater H, et al. Quantitative sensory testing somatosensory profiles in patients with cervical radiculopathy are distinct from those in patients with nonspecific neck–arm pain. Pain 2012; 153: 2403–2414

Thelander U, Fagerlund M, et al. Straight leg raising test versus radiologic size, shape, and position of lumbar disc hernias. Spine 1992;17(4):395–399

Triano JJ, Luttges MW. Nerve irritation: a possible model of sciatic neuritis. Spine 1982;7(2):129–136

Treede R-D, Jensen TS, et al. Neuropathic pain. Redefinition and a grading system for clinical and research purposes. Neurology 2008;70: 1630–1635

Upton AR, McComas AJ. The double crush in nerve entrapment syndromes. Lancet 1973;2(7825):359–362

van der Heide B, Allison GT, et al. Physiologische Reaktionen auf einen Provokationstest der Neuralstrukturen in der oberen Extremität. Krankengymnastik 2000;52:816–828

van der Heide B, Allison GT, et al. Pain and muscular responses to a neural tissue provocation test in the upper limb. Man Ther 2001a;6(3):154–162

van der Heide B, Allison GT, et al. Physiologische Reaktionen auf einen Provokationstest der Neuralstrukturen bei Patienten mit klinischer Diagnose einer zervikalen Radikulopathie–3 Fallstudien. Manuelle Therapie 2002;6: 131–138

van der Heide B, Elvey R. et al. Pain and muscular responses to a neural tissue provocation test in patients with cervicobrachial pain. Inaugural International Physiotherapy Congress of the World Confederation for Physical Therapy, Asia Pacific Region, Singapore; 2001b

Vanti C, Conteddu L, et al. The upper limb neurodynamic test 1: intra- and intertester reliability and the effect of several repetitions on pain and resistance. J Manipulative Physiol Ther 2010;33(4):292–299

Vucetic N, Svensson O. Physical signs in lumbar disc hernia. Clin Orthop Relat Res 1996; (333):192–201

Wainner RS, Fritz JM, et al. Reliability and diagnostic accuracy of the clinical examination and patient self-report measures for cervical radiculopathy. Spine 2003;28(1): 52–62

Walsh J, Hall T. Reliability, validity and diagnostic accuracy of palpation of the sciatic, tibial and common peroneal nerves in the examination of low back related leg pain. Man Ther 2009;14(6):623–629

Wilson S, Selvaratnam P, et al. Strain at the subclavian artery during the upper limb tension test. Aust J Physiother 1994;40(4):243–248

Witvrouw E, Cools A, et al. Suprascapular neuropathy in volleyball players. Br J Sports Med 2000;34(3):174–180

Woolf CJ. Physiological, inflammatory and neuropathic pain. Adv Tech Stand Neurosurg 1987;15:39–62

Wright TW, Glowczewskie F, et al. Excursion and strain of the median nerve. J Bone Joint Surg Am 1996;78(12): 1897–1903

Xin SQ, Zhang QZ, et al. Significance of the straight-leg-raising test in the diagnosis and clinical evaluation of lower lumbar intervertebral-disc protrusion. J Bone Joint Surg Am 1987;69(4):517–522

Yabuki S, Kikuchi S, et al. Acute effects of nucleus pulposus on blood flow and endoneurial fluid pressure in rat dorsal root ganglia. Spine 1998;23(23):2517–2523

Yaxley GA, Jull GA. A modified upper limb tension test: an investigation of responses in normal subjects. Aust J Physiother 1991;37(3):143–152

Yaxley GA, Jull GA. Adverse tension in the neural system. A preliminary study of tennis elbow. Aust J Physiother 1993;39(1):15–22

Yeung E, Jones M, et al. The response to the slump test in a group of female whiplash patients. Aust J Physiother 1997;43(1):245–252

## 2.2   Testing of General Functions

*Jan Cabri*

### 2.2.1   Amundsen's Ordinal Scale for Activities of Daily Living (ADL)

*The ordinal scale developed by Amundsen (1990) allows the therapist to assess the abilities of the patient in terms of his or her ability to perform everyday activities.*

Various activities, such as transferring from lying on the back to sitting up, from sitting to standing, and going up or down stairs, are rated on a scale of 1 to 4 (**Table 2.25**).

**Table 2.25** Amundsen's ordinal scale for activities of daily living (ADL)

| Points | Tasks |
|---|---|
| 1 | Patient can accomplish the function with maximum assistance |
| 2 | Patient can accomplish the function with moderate assistance |
| 3 | Patient can accomplish the function with minimal assistance |
| 4 | Patient can accomplish the function without any assistance |

### The Roland–Morris Questionnaire (Roland and Morris, 1983)

When your back hurts, you may find it difficult to do some of the things you normally do.

The following list contains statements that people have used to describe their back pain. As you read these sentences, you may find that some of them describe exactly how you feel **today**. While you read the list, think of how you feel **today**. If a sentence applies to you today, place an "x" in the box to the left of it. If a statement does not apply, do not mark the box. Skip it and continue to the next one. Please note that you should only mark those statements that you are certain apply to you **today**.

☐ I stay at home most of the time because of my back.
☐ I change position frequently to try to get my back more comfortable.
☐ I walk more slowly than usual because of my back.
☐ Because of my back, I am not doing any jobs that I usually do around the house or yard.
☐ Because of my back, I use a handrail to get upstairs.
☐ Because of my back, I lie down to rest more often.
☐ Because of my back, I have to hold onto something to get out of an easy chair.
☐ Because of my back, I try to get other people to do things for me.
☐ I get dressed more slowly than usual because of my back.
☐ I only stand up for short periods of time because of my back.
☐ Because of my back, I try not to bend or kneel down.
☐ I find it difficult to get out of a chair because of my back.
☐ My back is painful almost all of the time.
☐ I find it difficult to turn over in bed because of my back.
☐ My appetite is not very good because of my back.
☐ I have trouble putting on my socks (or stockings) because of my back.
☐ I can only walk short distances because of my back pain.
☐ I sleep less well because of my back.
☐ Because of my back pain, I get dressed with the help of someone else.
☐ I sit down for most of the day because of my back.
☐ I avoid heavy jobs around the house or in the yard because of my back.
☐ Because of my back pain, I am more irritable and bad-tempered with people than usual.
☐ Because of my back, I go upstairs more slowly than usual.
☐ I stay in bed most of the time because of my back.

**Fig. 2.71** The Roland Morris questionnaire. (From: Beyerlein 2002.)

## 2.2.2 The Functional Status Index (FSI)

The FSI is an ordinal survey that was developed by Alan Jette (1987). The survey is completed independently by the patient. It covers 18 aspects from the following areas: mobility, manual tasks, self-care, household, and social activities. The patient has about 30 minutes to complete the survey.

Using the FSI, patients may grade their ability as well as the severity of their pain and the degree of difficulty in accomplishing various tasks.

## 2.2.3 The Roland-Morris Questionnaire

The Roland-Morris questionnaire (**Fig. 2.71**) is primarily used by patients with low back pain (Roland and Morris 1983; Waddell 1998). It mainly covers current impairments, with 24 statements on activities that can no longer be performed due to low back pain. The patient should mark those statements that apply to his or her current situation.

The Roland-Morris questionnaire is considered one of the best surveys for clinical research on patients with low back pain.

### 2.2.4  The Barthel Index (Mahoney 1965)

> *The Barthel Index evaluates the patient's ability to take care of him or herself.*

The index (**Fig. 2.72**) is based on an operational definition of impairment. The Barthel Index is not a diagnostic instrument.

A professional examiner should perform the test, which consists of 10 activities graded on a two-point or three-point ordinal scale. The point scores are weighted so that the total index is between 0 (dependent activity) and 15 (independent activity). It takes about 1 hour to complete the test.

### 2.2.5  Functional Performance Evaluation (FPE)

> *The FPE measures the patient's general abilities and limitations.*

Using a standardized procedure, a trained examiner observes specific physical activities as they are performed by the patient. The FPE is easy to use, requires little technical effort, and yields reliable results:

**Example: Patient with chronic back pain**
- Five minutes walking:
  - Distance covered by the patient in 5 minutes of walking back and forth between two markings 20 m apart, without any assistance.
  - The walls may be used for support, but no handrails may be used.
  - The floor should not be slippery.
  - A chair should be available in case the patient would like to rest.
  - At the end of each lap, or every minute, the patient is told whether he or she is getting slower.
  - Average: 185 m.
- One minute stair climbing:
  - Number of stairs the patient can go up and down in 1 minute.
  - The stairs should be normal and straight (no curves), with the handrail on one side and the wall within reach on the other.
  - A chair should be available in case the patient would like to rest.
  - Average: 48 steps.

- One minute standing up from sitting:
  - How many times can the patient get up from a chair in 1 minute?
  - The chair should be straight, with a cushioned seat, but no armrests, and 45 cm high.
  - The patient may not use his or her arms for support.
  - Average: Standing up 11 times.

### 2.2.6  Hand-held Devices (HHD)

The patient's strength may be determined with hand-held measurement instruments. The HHD tests appear suitable for large and strong muscle groups, but are less so for dynamic testing. The grip strength dynamometer is an example of an HHD, which measures grip strength (kg) using a voltage meter (**Fig. 2.73**).

### 2.2.7  Isokinetic Dynamometry

The isokinetic dynamometer uses electronic data processing to display dynamic muscle contractions as data/numbers (**Fig. 2.74**). This instrument allows one to measure muscle strength as a value. This enables a comparison with the contralateral side or an assessment of training/therapy improvements. The device controls the angular velocity using reaction force over the full range of joint movement.

One advantage is that it can measure maximum (deliberate) rotational movements of one lever arm with (relatively) constant angular velocities, given that it matches the resistance it provides to the movement to the momentary and specific muscular ability of the individual person.

## The Barthel Index

Date    ...........................................................................................................................

Patient    .......................................................................................................................

Examiner ........................................................................................................................

| | Points |
|---|---|
| **Eating** | |
| • Independently, eats on his own, uses dishes and tableware | 10 |
| • Needs some assistance, e.g., cutting bread or meat | 5 |
| • Not independent, even with assistance (see above) | 0 |
| **Bed/wheelchair or chair transfer** | |
| • Independent in all phases of action | 15 |
| • Minimal assistance or surveillance needed | 10 |
| • Significant assistance needed for transfer, changing position, lying/sitting alone | 5 |
| • Not independent, even with assistance (see above) | 0 |
| **Washing** | |
| • Independently washes face, hands; combs hair, brushes teeth | 5 |
| • Cannot do the above independently | 0 |
| **Use of toilet** | |
| • Independent in all phases of action (including cleansing) | 10 |
| • Needs assistance, e.g., due to inadequate stability or with dressing or undressing/cleansing | 5 |
| • Not independent, even with assistance (see above) | 0 |
| **Bathing** | |
| • Independent in all phases of action in shower or bath | 5 |
| • Cannot bathe or shower independently | 0 |
| **Walking on same floor or using a wheelchair** | |
| • Walks independently over 50 m, possibly with assistance, but not walker | 15 |
| • Minimal assistance or surveillance needed, can walk 50 m with assistance | 10 |
| • Cannot walk independently, but can use wheelchair independently, also around corners and pulling up to a table; distance of at least 50 m | 5 |
| • Cannot walk or use a wheelchair independently | 0 |
| **Stair climbing** | |
| • Can independently climb (several) stairs | 10 |
| • Needs assistance or should be watched when climbing stairs | 5 |
| • Cannot independently climb stairs, even with assistance (see above) | 0 |
| **Dressing/Undressing** | |
| • Independently gets dressed/undressed (also with corset or hernia support) | 10 |
| • Needs assistance, but can perform 50% of the activity independently | 5 |
| • Not independent, even with assistance (see above) | 0 |
| **Bowel control** | |
| • Always continent | 10 |
| • Occasionally incontinent, maximum 1×/week | 5 |
| • Often/always incontinent | 0 |
| **Bladder control** | |
| • Always continent, possibly independent with long-term care catheter/Cystofix | 10 |
| • Occasionally incontinent, maximum 1×/day, assistance with external urinary catheter | 5 |
| • Often/always incontinent | 0 |

**Sum:**

Fig. 2.72 The Barthel Index. (From: Wulf 2004.)

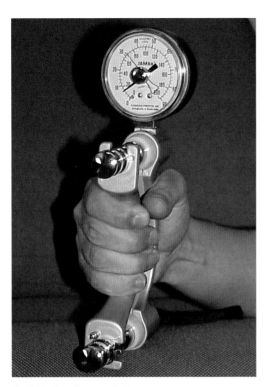

**Fig. 2.73** The grip strength dynamometer.

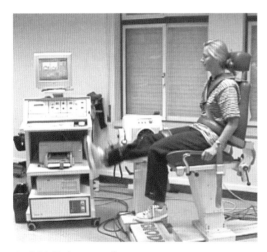

**Fig. 2.74** Biodex system 3.

## References

Amundsen L. Muscle Strength Testing—Instrumented and Non-instrumented Systems. New York: Churchill Livingstone; 1990

Beyerlein C. Klinische Behandlung nicht-spezifischer chronischer Kreuzschmerzen: ein strukturierter Ansatz zur Einschätzung psychosozialer Risikofaktoren. Manuelle Therapie 2002;6:151–163

Jette AM. The functional status index: reliability and validity of a self-report functional disability measure. J Rheumatol Suppl 1987;14(Suppl 15):15–21

Katz P. Measures of adult general functional status. Arthritis and Rheumatism 2003;49(S5):S15–S27

Mahoney FI, Barthel DW. Functional evaluation: the Barthel index. Md State Med J 1965;14:61–65

Roland M, Morris R. A study of the natural history of back pain. Part I: development of a reliable and sensitive measure of disability in low-back pain. Spine 1983;8(2):141–144

Waddell G. The Back Pain Revolution. Edinburgh: Churchill Livingstone; 1998

Wulf D. Physiotherapeutische Untersuchung, Behandlungsprinzipien und Planung. In: Hüter-Becker A, Dölken M (Hrsg.). Physiotherapie in der Neurologie. Stuttgart: Thieme; 2004

# 3 Examining Posture and Muscle Balance

# 3 Examining Posture and Muscle Balance

*Salah Bacha*

Musculoskeletal problems are usually complex in nature. Clinically active physical therapists need a range of skills that will allow them to examine and treat patients with problems resulting from dysfunctions of various tissues.

This chapter focuses on the musculoskeletal system, and in particular, an analysis of posture and muscles, as well as their contribution to the development and persistence of dysfunctions affecting the locomotor system. Using a system that was developed for examination, one can identify any deviations from the "norm" in terms of posture and muscle function. The results obtained on this basis can thus be clinically interpreted for treatment planning and implementation.

## 3.1 Posture

Posture is often viewed as a static position. Yet experience shows that it may be static or dynamic in nature. In static posture, the body's segments are lined up over each other or in relation to each other; they are held in this position and stabilized (e.g., upright standing, sitting, and lying down). A dynamic posture contains positions in which the body's segments move and change their relationship to one another in space (e.g., walking).

Upright standing is usually considered to be the classic posture and is thus most often analyzed. In the context of dynamics, however, posture is also a preparatory position for the next movement (dynamic posture). A typical example would be standing on one leg.

### 3.1.1 Static Posture

A comprehensive definition of posture has been established by the Posture Committee of the American Academy of the Orthopaedic Surgeons (1947). The idealized posture is described as a condition of skeletal and muscular balance (at rest or during movement) that protects the body's load-bearing structures against injury or excessive loading, irrespective of a person's position (standing, sitting, lying down). Thus, it allows for the best possible muscular efficiency and offers optimal space for the thoracic and abdominal organs.

*This definition is important for two reasons: on the one hand, it points to the relevance of the interaction between posture and neuromusculoskeletal dysfunction, and on the other it includes the relationship to the functioning of the internal organs. It is clear that optimal posture, as a structural support, is essential for proper breathing function.*

*An example of dysfunction is diminished respiratory volume in patients with thoracic kyphosis.*

### 3.1.2 Posture and Gravity

Posture, in relation to gravity, is the organization of the body's segments over the supporting surface. This includes all supporting surfaces, and thus the body's structures as well as the environment, from the feet to the skull base. Each segment is balanced on the part of the body (or the environmental surface) below it. When standing, the feet balance on the floor; finally, the cranium balances on the atlas.

When standing upright, there is a small surface forming the body's base of support. Klein-Vogelbach et al (1990) defined this as "the smallest surface that frames the contact points between the body's segments with the supporting surface." The contact between the feet and the floor forms the supporting surface. When the body is in a neutral position, the center of gravity is approximately at the level of the second sacral vertebra, and it is relatively far away from the supporting surface. The body is thus in a position of unstable balance. This has the advantage of high mobility, but the disadvantage of a constant risk to stability. On all fours, the center of gravity is lower and there is a larger supporting surface and hence greater stability.

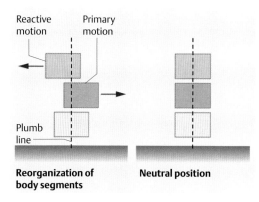

**Reorganization of body segments**        **Neutral position**

**Fig. 3.1** Balance response.

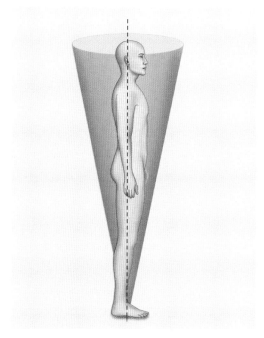

**Fig. 3.2** Oscillations represented by a funnel, with the body swaying inside of it.

> *Parameters for postural efficiency in relation to gravity are a low center of gravity, a wide supporting surface, and the vertical line of gravity (plumb line) passing through the center of the supporting surface.*

Every movement reorganizes the body's segments in relation to one another and in space. It thus changes the distribution of weight within the body and over the supporting surface. In an effort to maintain balance, the muscles are proactively and reactively activated; this is to reorganize the body's segments and at the same time to stabilize it against gravity, preventing a fall (Klein-Vogelbach 2000) (**Fig. 3.1**).

**Practical Relevance**

In terms of movement behavior, the supporting surface should always be enlarged in the direction of movement. The necessary readjustment of body segments is smaller, and thus there is greater postural stability.

### 3.1.3  Posture and the Sensory System

Balance may be threatened either by intrinsic impulses (coordinated movements resulting from muscle force and respiration) or extrinsic impulses (external parameters, e.g., unstable supporting surface, gravity). In a person standing still and on a firm surface, the breathing and continuous gravitational pull force the body to continually organize its segments using alternating oscillations. These subtle movements are invisible to the naked eye and do not require voluntary active control. The amount of sway is about 12° posteriorly and anteriorly, and about 16° laterally and medially (Nashner 1989). Afferents from the receptors in the inner ear, the eyes, and the various somatosensory structures (skin, muscle, joint capsule) regulate these movements.

These oscillations are proactively and reactively regulated by alternating muscular activity to prevent a fall. In addition to postural control, the reactively alternating tension appears mainly to prevent fatigue of the leg muscles and to promote blood circulation. The geometric depiction of the movements, using a linear projection from down to up, produces a funnel shape that is known as the *sway envelope* (**Fig. 3.2**).

Visible oscillations are a sign of inadequate balance or stability. They are often seen in older people or after an injury of a weight-bearing joint (e.g., upper ankle joint).

▮ *Posture is minimized movement.*

### 3.1.4  Posture and Bone Loading

Forces arising from static conditions and the musculature may change the shape of the bone and its articular surfaces. The forces arising from the changed spinal curve (scoliosis) mold the shape of the joint surfaces. These changes may occur in the form of erosion or exostosis. An example of such deformities is genu recurvatum.

A comparison of radiographs of the normal knee joint (**Fig. 3.3a**) and genu recurvatum shows the following changes associated with the deformity:
- Curvature of the tibia in the sagittal plane dorsally (recurvatum deformity of the leg; **Fig. 3.3b**).
- Instead of the normal horizontal position of the tibial plateau, there is a visible ventral and caudal tilt of the joint surface.

This structural change points to a likely long-term varus deformity. Based on the *law of transformation of the bones* (Wolff [1892] 1991), the shape and the consistency of a bone reflect the quality and quantity of the forces shaping it.

### 3.1.5    Posture and the Rotary Moment of the Joints

The interaction between the body's segments and gravity (shown through a vertical line of gravity) is essential to kinematics (the description of movement) and kinetics (the description of the forces that cause a movement; **Fig. 3.4a, b**). Whether or not a movement occurs in a joint depends, for instance, on the distance between the center of the joint (rotational center) and the vertical line of gravity. If the line of gravity passes through the rotational center, the joint partners are in balance (rotary moment = 0). In this centered position, intra-articular pressure is evenly distributed over the joint surface, and the muscle activity is at a minimum since there is no tendency to fall. Thus, less muscle activity is needed to stabilize the lever against gravity.

If the vertical line of gravity is some distance from the rotational center, there is a rotary moment in the joint. The cranial lever has a tendency to fall in the direction of the vertical line of gravity. This results in an uneven distribution of intra-articular weight.

*The position of a vertical line of gravity in relation to the joint is clinically relevant for postural analysis. The closer the joint center is to the vertical line of gravity, the smaller is the rotary moment in the joint.*

**Clinical Relevance**

The interpretation of posture in relation to the rotary moment (falling tendency) shows which muscles are constantly active against gravity. These in turn may correlate with symptom localization in the standing patient.

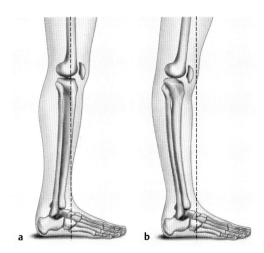

**Fig. 3.3a, b**
**a** Normal knee joint.
**b** Genu recurvatum: dorsal curvature of the tibia in the sagittal plane and tilting of the tibial joint surface ventrally and caudally.

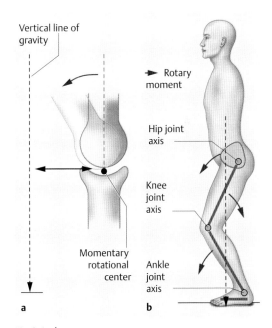

**Fig. 3.4a, b**
**a** Interaction between a vertical line of gravity and rotary moment. Normal position without a rotary moment.
**b** Tilting of the lever with rotary moment.

### 3.1.6   Posture and Muscle Adaptation

Postural deviations lead to muscular imbalance (**Fig. 3.5a, b**). If a muscle shortens, its antagonist lengthens. In accordance with the principle of functionality, the contractile (muscle fibers) and noncontractile elements of the muscles adjust to the changed posture. The contractile elements adapt the length of their sarcomeres to produce maximum strength in a given position. The ratio of connective tissue to muscle fibers in shortened muscles increases in favor of the noncontractile portion. The muscle becomes firmer; in terms of movement behavior, the adaption is evidenced by increased resistance of the muscle to lengthening.

**Clinical Relevance**
Within a kinematic chain, movement impulses follow a path of least resistance. Changes in muscle stiffness mean that some joints move less and others move more.

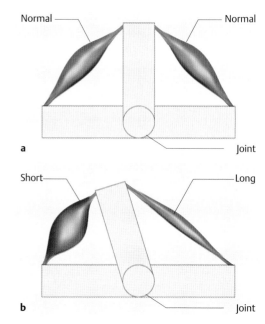

**Fig. 3.5a, b** Muscle adaptation.
**a** Muscle balance.
**b** Muscle imbalance.

## 3.2   Diagnosis

To better understand human movement, one must begin with an analysis of posture. This is a basic tool for prevention and also for identifying the cause of dysfunction and treatment planning.

Impairments of posture are often at the root of neuromusculoskeletal syndromes. These may be myofascial, periarticular, and/or neural. Dysfunctions due to trauma and/or systemic disease are not included in this category. Yet, postural deficits may exacerbate or promote related symptoms.

Neuromusculoskeletal syndromes often result from consecutive microtraumas. The stress theory defines microtrauma as *repetitive submaximal stress*, which exceeds the adaptation and regeneration ability of the tissue. A requirement for properly functioning elements of the locomotor system, such as biomechanics, the function of the internal organs, and respiration, is idealized posture and muscle balance.

With regard to the relationship between pain and posture, one may wonder why, on the one hand, "poor" posture does not always lead to pain, while on the other hand people with "good" posture sometimes have problems. One possible explanation is the lack of movement variation, in other words, maintaining a fixed posture. This can result in strain. Another possibility might be the above-mentioned stress theory as it relates to the tissues.

**Example:** A competitive athlete, with "poor" posture (when standing upright) compared to the "norm" nevertheless has no pain. Due to his athletic activity, his movement repertoire varies, while the ability to withstand strain increases the adaptation of the tissue. Nevertheless, he may have a dysfunction given the one-sidedness of his athletic activity.

### 3.2.1   Idealized Posture as a Reference

A postural evaluation is based on the hypothesis that for every posture there is an "idealized variant." Its principles are characterized by the parameters: economy (efficiency), balance control (stabilization within the field of gravity), and lack of pain (**Fig. 3.6**). Understanding its interaction means recognizing the foundation for understanding locomotor system function and thus for increasing objectivity in the evaluation of posture and muscle function.

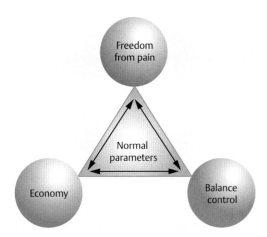

**Fig. 3.6** The triad of movement control: regulating, interactive parameters of idealized variants between posture and movement.

Idealized posture is not the norm. Rather, it is a reference that renders comparable evaluations possible. There is thus no such thing as abnormal posture, but rather there are deviations from set parameters that characterize an "idealized posture."

> *There is no norm, but rather only an idealized variant of posture.*

## Postural Reference or Idealized Variant

The idealized upright posture is defined as how the body deals with gravity to assume a position in which the body's segments are optimally aligned on top of one another. It is characterized by economy, minimal use of energy, and maximum efficiency. If these parameters are met, the idealized variant requires little energy, is pain-free, and nonfatiguing (**Fig. 3.7a, b; Table 3.1**).

## Observational Parameters for Evaluating Posture

Visual examination and palpation require a great deal of clinical experience. It is therefore all the more important to use observational parameters. These enhance the objectification of the observation and inter-therapist reliability (agreement between different therapists on the results of observation). In addition, using a type of system allows for comparable results in the various stages of the examination.

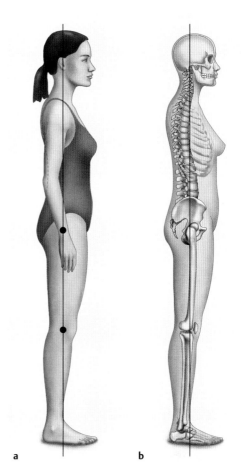

a                              b

**Fig. 3.7a, b** Idealized postural variant.

*Example: Observational parameters*
- Arbitrarily selected body points and lines, which serve as visual guide for the therapist (**Fig. 3.8a, b**)
- Flexible ruler to evaluate spinal statics (**Fig. 3.9**)
- Inclinometer or plurimeter, which show relatively precise movement amplitudes and torsion (**Fig. 3.10**)

## 3.2.2   Examination of Posture

The following factors are evaluated:
- Position of the *joints* and structural deviations of the *bones.*
- *Muscle activity:* In potential rotary moments ask the question "who is holding what?" (Klein-Vogelbach et al 1990). To determine the rotary moments in the joints, the evaluation parameters relate to the position of a vertical line of gravity in relation to the load-bearing joints.

**Table 3.1**  The interaction between a vertical line of gravity and the rotary moment along with their effect on passive structures

| Vertical line of gravity through joint | Rotary moment | Active FV[a] | Passive FV |
|---|---|---|---|
| C0–C1 | Ventral—bending | Extensors | Nuchal ligament |
| Cervical spine | Dorsal—extension | – | Anterior longitudinal ligament |
| Thoracic spine | Ventral—bending | Extensors | • Posterior longitudinal ligament<br>• Ligamentum flavum<br>• Supraspinal ligament |
| Lumbar spine | Dorsal—extension | – | Anterior longitudinal ligament |
| Sacroiliac joint | Ventral—bending | – | • Sacrotuberous ligament<br>• Sacrospinal ligament<br>• Iliosacral ligament |
| Hip joint | Dorsal—extension | Iliopsoas muscle | Iliofemoral ligament |
| Knee joint | Ventral—extension | – | Dorsal capsule |
| Upper ankle joint | Ventral-dorsal—extension | Soleus muscle | – |

Source: Levangie and Norkin (1992).
Note: [a] FV = force vectors.

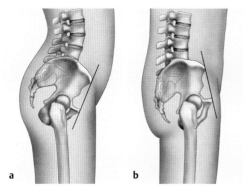

**Fig. 3.8a, b**  Parameters for observing posture. In this instance, a connecting line between the anterior superior iliac spine (ASIS) and the symphysis.

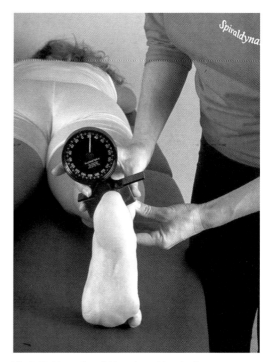

**Fig. 3.10**  Measuring tibial torsion with an inclinometer. (From: Larsen C. Füße in guten Händen. Stuttgart: Thieme; 2003.)

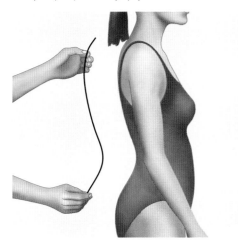

**Fig. 3.9**  Evaluation of the spinal column with a flexible ruler.

- *Muscle length:* "Is the muscle in an elongated or shortened position?" (Kendall et al 1993).
- *Muscle architecture:* "How does the muscle act on the joint in question?"

This is followed by the clinical interpretation, which is based on the following criteria:

### Kinematics

Kinematics describes additional movements in the kinetic chain. Any deviation in static conditions from the idealized variant changes the position of the axes of movement in space. Thus, the joint movements change within the kinematic chain (**Fig. 3.11a, b**).

**Example:** Genu varum due to medial rotation of the femur in the hip joint and eversion of the lower ankle joint
The movement axis for knee bending/extension is diagonal to the frontal plane. Extension must therefore occur in a posterolateral direction, leading to genu varum.

### Kinetics

Kinetics describes the forces involved in initiation and transmission of movement. Deviations from the idealized variants change the relationship of the position of the muscle fibers relative to the joint and thus the effect of the resulting force vector on the joint (**Fig. 3.12a, b**).

**Example:** Muscle fibers lateral to the rotational center of the hip joint cause a rotary moment in the direction of abduction. Pelvic anteversion displaces some of the abductor muscle fibers ventral to the hip joint, and it reduces the number of fibers involved in abduction. The abductors increase their bending activity.

## Standard Deviations

The following four figures with their accompanying checklists describe typical deviations seen in the musculoskeletal system:

- Swayback (**Fig. 3.13a, b**)
- Flat back (**Fig. 3.14a, b**)
- Swayback with kyphosis (**Fig. 3.15a, b**)
- Pelvic obliquity (**Fig. 3.16a, b**)

*Clinical Interpretation*
- The primary deviation is in the pelvis.
- Further along the kinetic chain, retroversion causes bending of the lower lumbar spine (increased dorsal strain on the intervertebral disks).

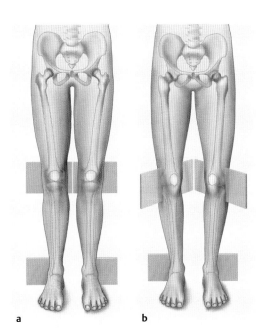

a                              b

Fig. 3.11a, b  Interaction between malposition of the joints and its effect on movement.
a  Neutral position of the axes of movement.
b  The movement axes are diagonal to the frontal plane and cause genu recurvatum (Kendall et al 1993).

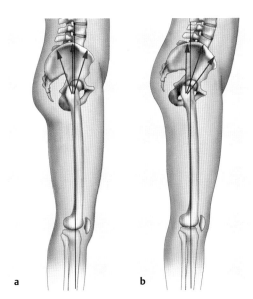

a                              b

Fig. 3.12a, b  The interaction between changed posture and the direction of force of a muscle. Here, the example of the gluteus medius muscle is shown with pelvic bending at the hip joint.

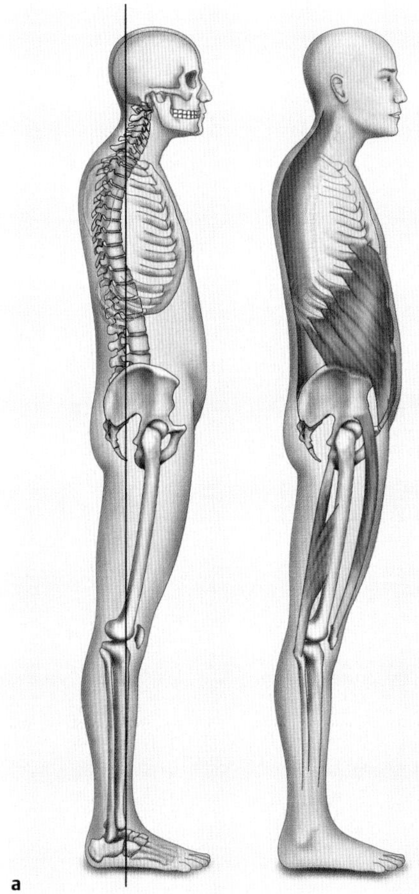

| Upper ankle joints | Usually in an ideal position |
|---|---|
| Knee joints | Extension from the thigh |
| Hip joints | Extension from both levers (the thigh is tilted forward and the pelvis backward) |
| Pelvis | Ventral translation (causes increased extension of the hip joint) |
| Lumbar spine | Flattened (– lower lumbar spine) In the kinetic chain, pelvic retroversion leads to increased lumbar bending |
| Thoracic spine | Increased kyphosis (+ thoracic spine) Dorsal translation of the rib cage in response to ventral translation of the pelvis |
| Cervical spine | Usually there is extension of the middle/upper cervical spine or lordosis (+ middle, upper cervical spine) |
| Head | In response to the rib cage, usually there is ventral translation |
| Relevant rotary moments | Hip extension Thoracic spine bending Cervical spine extension |
| Elongated muscles | Hip joint flexors (monoarticular) External abdominal oblique muscle Upper extensors of the thoracic spine Cervical spine flexors |
| Shortened muscles | Hamstring muscles Gluteus maximus muscle Upper fibers of the internal abdominal oblique muscle Suboccipital |

**Fig. 3.13a, b**
**a** Swayback (comfortable posture) with changed muscle lengths. **b** Checklist.

- Retroversion and ventral translation of the pelvis potentiate the decentering of the head of the hip ventrally. As a result, the load-bearing surface of the femoral head is smaller.
- To maintain its balance, the body responds by moving the thorax backward and the head forward.
- In the long term, the inactive gluteal musculature leads to atrophy and reduced stiffness (visible as flattening of the buttock contours; on palpation, the gluteal muscles feel soft).
- In the long term, the shortened position of the hamstring muscles leads to their adaptive shortening, which has consequences for movement behavior. This is relevant, for example, for forward bending. The activity of the hamstrings in an eccentric mode is needed to hold the spinal column in a neutral position.

*Considerations for Further Examination*
The gluteal muscles should be tested for selective tension and the hamstrings for their ability to shorten. Given that both muscles act to extend the hip, it is especially important to examine their synergistic coordination. Due to their superficial position, the hamstring muscles cause a higher rotary moment than the gluteal muscles. Classified as *global* (as opposed to the deeper-lying local) mobilizers, they tend toward shortening and hyperactivity. If they are dominant, every time they are activated, there is ventral translation of the head of the hip.

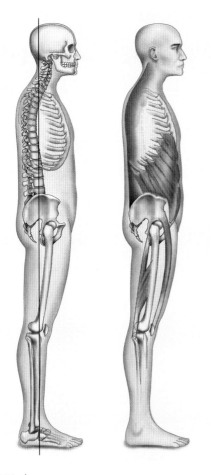

| Upper ankle joints | + Plantar bending or neutral position |
|---|---|
| Knee joints | + Extension or neutral position |
| Hip joints | + Extension (from the pelvis) |
| Pelvis | Retroversion (extension position in the hip joint) |
| Lumbar spine | Flattened (– lumbar spine) |
| Thoracic spine | Lower: flat (– lower) Upper: kyphotic (+ upper) |
| Cervical spine | + Extension |
| Head | Mild translation |
| Relevant rotary moments | Upper ankle joint plantar bending Knee joint bending Hip joint extension Cervical spine extension |
| Lengthened muscles | Psoas major muscle |
| Shortened muscles | Hamstring muscles Rectus abdominis muscle |

**a**

**b**

**Fig. 3.14a, b**
**a** Flat back and altered muscle length. **b** Checklist.

### Clinical Interpretation
- The dominant deviation is pelvic malalignment.
- In terms of the kinetic chain, retroversion causes bending of the lower lumbar spine (dorsal distraction of the intervertebral disks).
- There is potentiation of the force of the hamstring muscles and the rectus abdominis muscle. This increases the pelvic deviation with the same consequences as in patients with a *swayback*. The difference is in the smaller degree of hip joint extension.
- The elongated position of the psoas muscle leads to a "positional weakness" of the muscle (specific insufficiency in shortening).
- *Kinematics:* In terms of the kinetic chain, distally initiated hip joint bending causes lumbar bending.

- *Kinetics:* The positional weakness of the psoas muscle and the dominance of the rectus abdominis muscle lead to a loss of selective bending in the hip joint and premature lumbar spine motion. This movement may cause hypermobility of the lumbar spine (bending).

### Considerations for Further Examination
For active intervention, it is important to know about the positional weakness of the elongated muscles. To confirm possible adaptation, the affected muscles are tested with maximum shortening (e.g., examination of the psoas muscle and the serratus muscle, p. 138).

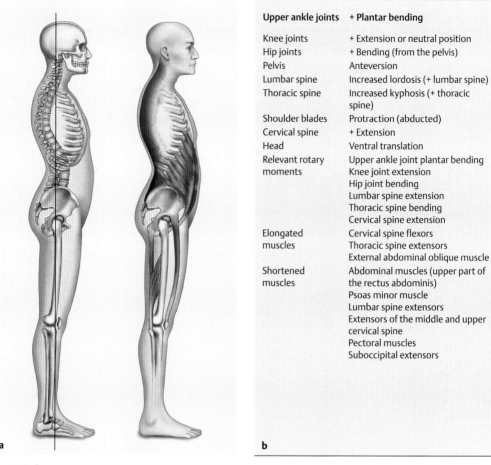

| Upper ankle joints | + Plantar bending |
| --- | --- |
| Knee joints | + Extension or neutral position |
| Hip joints | + Bending (from the pelvis) |
| Pelvis | Anteversion |
| Lumbar spine | Increased lordosis (+ lumbar spine) |
| Thoracic spine | Increased kyphosis (+ thoracic spine) |
| Shoulder blades | Protraction (abducted) |
| Cervical spine | + Extension |
| Head | Ventral translation |
| Relevant rotary moments | Upper ankle joint plantar bending<br>Knee joint extension<br>Hip joint bending<br>Lumbar spine extension<br>Thoracic spine bending<br>Cervical spine extension |
| Elongated muscles | Cervical spine flexors<br>Thoracic spine extensors<br>External abdominal oblique muscle |
| Shortened muscles | Abdominal muscles (upper part of the rectus abdominis)<br>Psoas minor muscle<br>Lumbar spine extensors<br>Extensors of the middle and upper cervical spine<br>Pectoral muscles<br>Suboccipital extensors |

a                                                                    b

**Fig. 3.15a, b**
**a** Swayback with kyphosis and altered muscle length. **b** Checklist.

### Clinical Interpretation

- The relevant deviations are pelvic anteversion and kyphosis of the thoracic spine.
- The elongated thoracic spine extensors and the bending position of the vertebral joints have a negative impact on the inspiratory mechanics of the ribs and may lead to respiratory dysfunction.
- *Kinematics:* The changed position of the vertebral joints prevents optimal rib excursion.
- *Kinetics:* Respiratory dysfunction is caused by active insufficiency of the elongated muscles (thoracic spine extensors) on the dorsal aspect of the body and the dominance of the shortened pectoral muscle and rectus abdominis muscle on its ventral aspect.

### Considerations for Further Examination

Basically, it is important to know whether—and to what extent—the deviation is permanent. It is useful to compare it to the posture in the supine patient. If deviations are still evident in this position, this is suggestive of fixation of the posture or adaption of structures.

With regard to a possible respiratory dysfunction, along with an examination of the joints, one should also test muscle function in order to identify the role of the muscles. Shortening of the rectus abdominis muscle, for instance, may not only hold the rib cage in a lower position, but may also inhibit the diaphragm.

> *In elevated shoulder, there is shortening of the musculature on the side that is raised.*

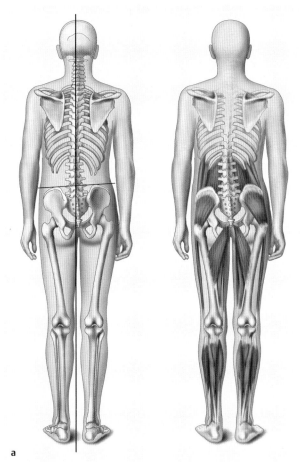

| Feet | Asymmetry of the longitudinal arch and/or upper ankle joint is commonly seen. In this example the longitudinal arch is flattened and/or the left foot is everted (– longitudinal arch and + eversion left side) |
|---|---|
| Knee joint | Unilateral valgus shortens the leg (on the left in this example) |
| Hips | Adduction on right Abduction on left |
| Pelvis | Pelvis is tilted laterally upward on right (may be associated with translation of the pelvis to the right) |
| Lumbar/thoracic spine | Compensatory scoliosis, usually concave to the right in the lumbar region |
| Shoulder girdle | Usually compensation with higher left side |
| Cervical spine/head | Various forms of compensation |
| Relevant rotational moments | Possible left sidebending in the lumbar spine with rotation |
| Elongated muscles | Posterior tibialis (with eversion) Tensor fascia latae (right) Adductors (left) Gluteus medius (right) Quadratus lumborum (left) |
| Shortened muscles | Tensor fascia latae (left) Abductors (left) Adductors (right) Quadratus lumborum (right) |

**a** **b**

**Fig. 3.16a, b**
**a** Pelvic obliquity and altered muscle length. **b** Checklist.

### Clinical Interpretation
- The asymmetry is an important factor in sustaining the pelvic obliquity.
- *Kinematics:* Asymmetry of the feet translates to other body segments.
- *Kinetics:* Asymmetrical muscle strength has a potentiating effect on the malalignment.
- The shortening of the adductors and the lengthening of the abductors on the right side exacerbates the lateral pelvic tilt.

### Considerations for Further Examination
Precise testing of muscle functioning is essential to objectify the asymmetry. Hypothetically elongated muscles, in particular, should be tested at the shortest range (abductors on right side and quadratus lumborum on left side).

### Summary
At present there are no direct studies proving the correlation between musculoskeletal symptoms and malalignment. Clinical experience shows, however, that malalignment due to deviations can exacerbate or prolong the pathological condition. The largely subjective nature of the examination procedures is problematic. Their value depends on the clinical experience of the therapist. It is all the more important to systematically use the few available parameters that can help make the results objectifiable.

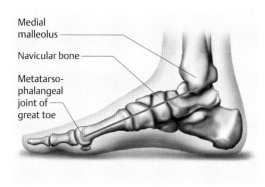

Medial
malleolus

Navicular bone

Metatarso-
phalangeal
joint of
great toe

**Fig. 3.17** Assessment of the longitudinal arch of the foot with the Feiss line.

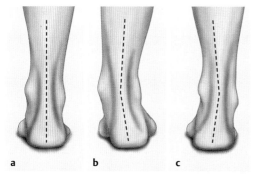

a        b        c

**Fig. 3.18a–c** Assessment of the back of the foot.
**a** Normal.
**b** Calcaneus valgus. **c** Calcaneus varus.

### 3.2.3   Observational Parameters for Assessing Joint Position

**Examination of the Foot**

*Longitudinal Arch*

- Observational parameter: The Feiss line that connects the medial malleolus, navicular bone, and the first metatarsophalangeal joint (**Fig. 3.17**).
- Pes planus: Flattening of the longitudinal arch (flat foot):
  - Characteristic: The navicular bone is located below the Feiss line.
  - Weight-bearing produces a valgus deformity at the knee, internal rotation, and/or adduction of the hip joint.
  - Deficient shock absorption in the stance phase places excessive stress on the weight-bearing joints. In the kinetic chain, the adductors are often insufficient.

- Pes cavus: Higher longitudinal arch of the foot (high arch):
  - Characteristic: The navicular bone is above the Feiss line.
  - *Kinematics:* Pes cavus is often found coupled with reduced dorsal extension in the upper ankle joints. During the stance phase, there may be compensatory hyperextension of the knee joint.
  - *Kinetics:* Plantar bending of the upper ankle joint when standing upright causes hyperactivity and thus places excess stress of the tibialis anterior muscle:
  - There is usually tightening of the plantar flexors due to the reduced range of motion.
  - Walking on a soft, uneven surface elicits pain.

*Back of Foot*

- Observational parameters: Visible longitudinal axes of the heel and distal lower leg (**Fig. 3.18a–c**).
- Idealized position:
  - Longitudinal axis of the lower leg and heel are in a vertical line.
  - Angle tolerance: 0 to 10°.
- Deviations:
  - Valgus position of the calcaneus.
  - Line of the heel deviates laterally.
- *Kinetics:*
  - Increased medial stress at the heel may ascend up the kinetic chain and affect the knee joint with increased intra-articular stress on the lateral aspect of the knee joint and periarticular stress medially.
  - Asymmetrical deviation usually causes a functional leg-length discrepancy.
- *Kinematics:* **Table 3.2**.

**Table 3.2** Calcaneus valgus

| *In weight-bearing positions, the effects of calcaneus valgus continue up the kinematic chain of the leg:* | |
| --- | --- |
| Hip | - Internal rotation<br>- Bending<br>- Adduction |
| Knee | Valgus (external rotation) |
| Foot | Pes planus (flattening of the longitudinal arch) |
| Forefoot | Pressure against the floor causes supination of the forefoot |

## Examination of the Knee Joint

- Observational parameters: Functional longitudinal axis of the leg, or mechanical axis, which creates a connecting line between the center of the hip joint, knee joint, and upper ankle joint.
- Idealized position: Plumb line through the center between the malleoli.
- Aids: String or yardstick to help visualize the line.
- Deviations:
  - Genu varum (bowlegs): Plumb line is lateral to the malleoli.
  - Genu valgum (knock knees): Plumb line is medial to the malleoli.

### Clinical Relevance

The line represents a plumb line in a weight-bearing situation and provides important information on the distribution of forces and stability. A comparison of the result when the patient is standing upright with the result when the patient is prone is highly clinically relevant. If the plumb line lies outside of the malleoli only when the patient is standing, this indicates instability in weight-bearing positions.

- Kinematics:
  - Deviations in static posture change the position of the axes of motion. In patients with genu valgum and varum, the bending-extension axis of the knee joint is at an angle to the fontal plane. This changes the plane of movement in the legs (**Fig. 3.19a, b**).
  - Prolonged pes planus may produce or exacerbate genu valgum.
  - At more cranial sites in the body, pes planus may produce internal rotation/adduction of the hip joint.
  - Asymmetrical deviation causes a leg-length discrepancy with pelvic obliquity.
- Kinetics:
  - The abductors and outward rotators of the hip joint are usually insufficient.
  - Prior to possible intervention, one must determine whether there is adaptive lengthening of the abductors or asymmetrical shortening of the hamstrings (p. 137).

## Examination of the Hip Joint

- Observational parameters (**Fig. 3.20a–c**):
  - Connecting lines of the right and left anterior superior iliac spines.
  - Connecting lines of the right and left posterior superior iliac spines.

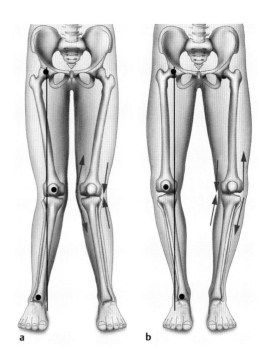

a          b

Fig. 3.19a, b  Valgus deviations.
**a** Lateral compression and medial stress.
**b** Medial compression and lateral stress.

- Tangential plane in which anterior superior iliac spine and symphysis lie.
- Deviations:
  - Anterior tilt of the pelvis: Anterior superior iliac spine is clearly caudal to the posterior superior iliac spine or ventral to the symphysis.
  - Posterior tilt of the pelvis: Anterior superior iliac spine is clearly cranial to the posterior superior iliac spine or dorsal to the symphysis.
- Kinematics:
  - Anterior tilting of the pelvis causes hip joint bending.
  - Above the level of the pelvis it leads to increased lumbar lordosis (especially in the lower segments).
- Kinetics:
  - Forward tilting of the pelvis leads to more muscle fibers of the abductors ventral to the bending-extension axis of the hip joint, which means the flexors predominate over the abductors.
  - There is insufficient stabilization of the pelvis when weight is placed on the leg. This is clearly demonstrated by, for example, a positive Trendelenburg sign and/or medial rotation of the thigh when walking.

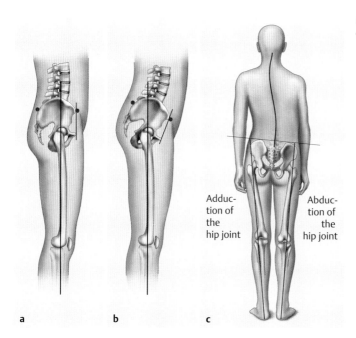

Fig. 3.20a–c Parameters for assessment of pelvic positions.

Adduc-
tion of
the
hip joint

Abduc-
tion of
the
hip joint

a                    b                    c

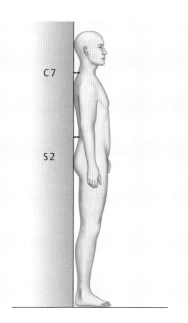

C7

S2

Fig. 3.21 Lateral view of the spine. The wall serves as a reference for assessing static spinal posture.

## Examination of the Spine

> *Without a radiograph it is difficult to objectify the ideal S-curve of the spine.*

Observation requires a great deal of experience. The therapist should have already examined as many patients as possible in order to have stored the maximum number of comparable images in his or her head.

- Idealized position: Most therapists develop a sense of this over time.
- Aids:
  - A flexible ruler is a useful means of assessing the curvature of the spinal column (**Fig. 3.9**). Clinical experience has shown relatively high concurrence with radiographs.
  - Radiographs are very important for the evaluation of static posture, but they are not always available.
  - A wall can be a useful visual aid as it provides an optical contrast. The patient should stand with his or her back to the wall while the therapist evaluates the points of contact and the distance between the back and the wall (**Fig. 3.21**).
- Typical deviations:
  - Swayback with kyphosis: The physiological curvature of the spinal column is increased in all three segments (hyperlordosis of the lumbar

spine, increased kyphosis of the thoracic spine, and hyperlordosis of the cervical spine).
- Flat back: The physiological curvatures of the spinal column are flattened in all three segments (flattened lumbar spine, thoracic spine, and cervical spine).
- Individual segments of the spine also may be affected in isolation and/or to various degrees. Example: Hyperlordosis of the lower lumbar spine.

- *Kinematics:*
  - The position of the pelvis directly influences the shape of the spine; in the same way, the individual spinal segments also influence one another.
  - The quality of motion in the chain depends on the mobility of the segments.
- *Kinetics:*
  - The muscular attachments of the extremities to the trunk strongly influence spinal stability.
  - The trunk muscles have a direct effect on the shape of the spine as well as its stability under stress (see 3.3.6 Interpretation of Posture).

## Examination of the Scapulae

- Observational parameters (see **Fig. 3.25**):
  - Reference line: Medial border of scapula, dorsal surface.
  - Body points: Inferior and superior angles, scapular surface, spinal processes of thoracic vertebrae.
- Aids:
  - Ruler.
  - Skin marker.
- Idealized position in the dorsal view: The medial border should be nearly vertical (the inferior angle may deviate by about 7° laterally):
  - The superior angle should be at the level of the second thoracic spinal process.
  - The scapular surface forms an angle of about 30° with a lateral plumb line.
- Deviations:
  - Caudal rotation of the scapula: The inferior angle is located cranio-medially to the superior angle. This malposition is characterized by the more caudal position of the glenoid cavity.
  - Ventral rotation of the scapula: Increased ventral and caudal tilt. The angle between the longitudinal axis of the scapula and a lateral plumb line of the body exceeds 30°.
  - Both deviations narrow the subacromial space (predisposition for irritation of the rotator cuff, especially of the supraspinatus muscle).

- *Kinematics:*
  - End-range movement amplitude of the shoulder joint includes mobility of the thoracic spine.
  - The position of the scapula depends directly on the shape of the rib cage (ventral rotation of the scapula with kyphosis of the thoracic spine).
- *Kinetics:*
  - A special feature is the presence of multiple attachments of the scapular muscles (cervical spine, thoracic spine, ribs, humerus, and pelvis). This constellation leads to direct interaction between body segments. Hence, arm strength depends on the stability of the thoracic spine and the quality of the muscular guiding of the scapula.
  - The timing of the muscle forces acting on the scapula ensures efficient movement.

## Examination of the Upper Arm

- Observational parameters:
  - Reference line: Longitudinal axis of the upper arm, lateral border of the acromion.
  - Body points: Olecranon, lateral contours of the head of the humerus, subacromial surface.
- Idealized position:
  - Vertical position of the longitudinal axis of the upper arm.
  - Olecranon points dorsally and somewhat laterally.
  - The head of the humerus is located, at most, one-third of its width ventral to the acromion.
- Deviations:
  - Olecranon clearly points dorsally and laterally, which is an indication of internal rotation of the arm at the shoulder joint (contributing factor in impingement syndrome).
  - Head of humerus is located more than one-third its width ventral to the acromion. This indicates ventral decentering of the head of the humerus (contributing factor in impingement syndrome).
- *Kinematics:*
  - The position of the humerus determines the quality of the movement of the scapula in the kinematic chain.
  - Active abduction is always coupled with external rotation.
  - The tuberculum majus glides behind the acromion and thus prevents impingement of the subacromial structures.
- *Kinetics:*
  - The ideal position of the humerus relative to the joint surface requires the coordinated use of

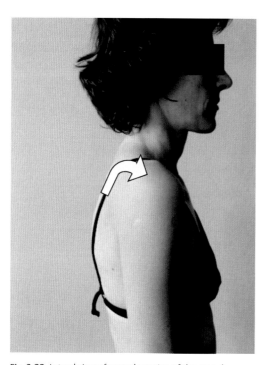

**Fig. 3.22** Lateral view of ventral rotation of the scapula.

several muscles. Dominance of internal rotators can prevent the necessary external rotation.

- The centering of the humeral head in the glenoid cavity during dynamic movement largely depends on the coordinated use of the scapular muscles. Relevant muscles include the anterior serratus (caudal portion) and the ascending part of the trapezius, which act synergistically, producing lateral rotation of the scapula with the glenoid cavity pointing cranially and laterally.
- Another function is lifting the weight of the arm against gravity: the weight of the arm when flexed causes ventral rotation of the scapula (forward and downward; **Fig. 3.22**).
- The descending part of the trapezius muscle and the anterior serratus muscle have a stabilizing effect in lifting the scapula against gravity.

### 3.2.4    Dynamic Posture

### Single-leg Stance

> *The most common dynamic posture occurring spontaneously during movement is the single-leg stance (**Fig. 3.23a–c**).*

Not just walking, but most athletic as well as everyday activities require asymmetric leg loading. To understand various musculoskeletal problems—especially those involving the lower back and the lower extremity—it is important to know the parameters of the idealized variant:

- Observational parameters:
  - The neutral posture of the back may be visualized using the following points on the body: the symphysis, navel, sternum, and chin. An imaginary connecting line between these points corresponds to the longitudinal axis. Ideally, it should remain vertical.
  - The neutral position of the pelvis is visualized by the right and left anterior superior iliac spines (ASIS). An imaginary line connecting these two should remain horizontal.
  - The evaluation of ideal leg loading is based on the following body points: the trochanter major, femoral condyle, and navicular bone. Ideally, the trochanter is a fixed point in space, the condyles remain in the same frontal plane, and the navicular maintains the same distance to the floor.
  - A central parameter is insufficiency of the standing leg abductors. This influences the position of the back as well as the leg.
  - Standing on one leg with the eyes closed can help evaluate the proprioceptive quality of the standing leg. The result is an approximate value.

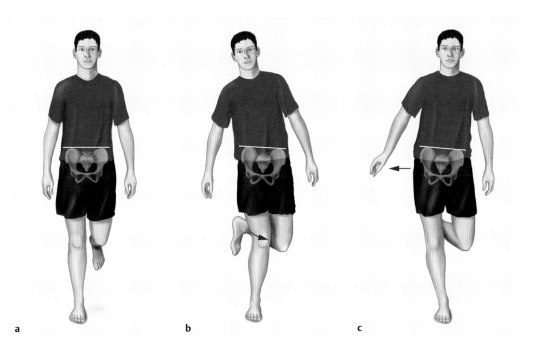

**Fig. 3.23a–c** Single-leg stance. **a** Normal. **b** Medial collapse. **c** With hip joint adduction.

## 3.3   Musculature

### 3.3.1   Basic Principles

The structural architecture of the musculature consists of tightly woven contractile (proteins) and non-contractile (connective tissue) elements. The muscle—including the fascicles and muscle fibers—is enclosed in the connective tissue. The connective tissue has different names, depending on where it is located:

- Endomysium: The connective tissue around the muscle fibers.
- Perimysium: The connective tissue around each fascicle.
- Epimysium: Connective tissue around the muscle.
- Between the muscles, there is a layer of fascia, a superficial connective tissue network that envelops the muscle.
- The muscle tissue and the connective tissue network (fascia) form the structural and functional unit called the *myofascial system.*

### 3.3.2   The Tasks of the Myofascial System

The myofascial system has various tasks related to movement behavior:

- Acting organ: It can initiate and limit (or control) movement. Movement control occurs on local and global levels. Global movement control consists of balance responses as the body deals with gravity. The body's segments are stabilized in relation to one another and/or their position in space (fall prevention).
- Protective organ: On a local level, movement control consists of intersegmental stabilization in order to protect the joint partner and the immediately surrounding pain-sensitive structures.
- Sensory organs: With their muscle spindles and mechanoreceptors, the muscle and the fascia possess an afferent feedback system that informs the central nervous system (CNS) about the length of the muscle fibers and the fascia as well as the tension on them.

*Note: The myofascial system fulfills the following different functions in terms of movement behavior*
- *Postural control: To maintain equilibrium and keep the center of gravity inside the supporting base*
- *To initiate and produce target-oriented movement through joint motion.*
- *To provide segmental stabilization by reactively recruiting the local muscles.*
- *To control the movement of the body segments (accelerate and decelerate body parts to interact with gravity)*
- *Sensomotor function in terms of biofeedback from the muscles (muscle spindles, Golgi receptors) and from the fascia layers (especially the fascia superficialis) to regulate muscle tonus and provide movement coordination.*

### 3.3.3   Functional Classification of the Musculature in the Myofascial System

The current basis for diagnosis and treatment intervention is founded on a classification of the musculature in the myofascial system, based on its function in movement behavior. This supplants the previous, customary classification of phasic and tonic musculature based on Janda (1979). It is still uncertain which muscles belong to which system, given that many variables (e.g., genes and individual functional status) play a role.

### Local or Primary Stabilizers

*Sources in the literature refer to the terms local and primary stabilizers. The following uses the term "local stabilizers."*

This refers to the deep muscles that are located near the joint. These are primarily (but not entirely) made up of slow-twitch (type I) fibers (slowly contracting motor units). They are characterized by continual low-intensity contraction (25% of active maximum force).

#### Examples:
- Multifidus muscle, medial part, on the spine
- Vastus medialis obliquus muscle in the lower extremity
- Rotator cuff in the upper extremity

The term *primary stabilizers* refers to the fact that, in terms of movement behavior, the muscles exhibit

pre-programmed, minimal contraction. This anticipatory activity protects the spinal joints from any movement of the extremities. Their activation is independent of the direction of movement (Hodges and Richardson 1997).

An important insight in terms of clinical practice is the close relationship between the type I fibers and the muscle spindles. In patients with back problems, along with dysfunction of the local stabilizers, there is a proprioception deficit. In addition to the symptoms, clinical signs include the inability to reproduce a neutral position of the spine, to maintain the position during dynamic movement, and the inability to select appropriate muscle tonus. They have a tendency toward global recruitment of mass co-contractions. This is seen as stiff, uncoordinated movement. Increased proprioceptive afference has a facilitating effect on the local system.

*The activation of the local stabilizers is part of the early phase of rehabilitation.*
*The activation of the proprioceptors has a facilitating effect on the local stabilizers.*

### Global or Secondary Stabilizers

*In the literature, the terms "global" and "secondary" stabilizers" are used. The following uses the term "global stabilizers."*

These are mainly monoarticular, more superficial muscles. The percentage of muscle fiber types, in terms of their composition, has not yet been clearly established, yet type I fibers appear to tend to dominate.

#### Examples:
- Vastus lateralis and intermedius muscles of the quadriceps muscle
- Internal and external abdominal oblique muscles
- Gluteus maximus and medius muscles (ventral fibers)

The muscles are pennate (feathered), with a wide anchor of fascia. Due to their architecture, they are made to produce strength. Given their anatomical position, they act selectively on the joint that they span. Their stabilizing function is specific. They respond to gravity to prevent falling. They are primarily recruited in a closed system and in an eccentric mode.

*Example: Descending stairs*

The gluteus medius muscle stabilizes the pelvis and controls its motion downward. The vastii muscles of the quadriceps control the bending of the knee joint during the eccentric phase. In terms of gravity, they act as a control to prevent the body segments that are located above the knee joint from falling. They also stabilize the spinal column during movements of the extremities. And, as the trunk changes position, they control the torso's body segments to prevent a fall due to gravity.

> *Corresponding to their function, the global stabilizers should preferably be selectively activated in a closed system.*

## Global Mobilizers

The global mobilizers are superficial multi-joint muscles. Their position (further away from the rotational center) and architecture (fusiform) predestines them to produce movement. Contraction of these muscles causes movement in various extremity joints and between the body segments in relation to the spinal column.

*Examples:*

- Rectus femoris muscle and tensor fasciae latae muscle, which simultaneously move the hip and knee
- Latissimus dorsi muscle, which acts on the shoulder blade and the humerus
- Rectus abdominis muscle, which can simultaneously move the thoracic and lumbar spines

The muscles primarily consist of (type II) fast-twitch fibers (rapidly contracting motor units), which are generally recruited concentrically in an open system with high-stress or rapid (ballistic) movements. Their activation depends on the direction of movement. Movement of the arm posteriorly and superiorly, with shoulder joint bending, is activated by the rectus abdominis muscle. If the arm extends anteriorly and inferiorly, it is mainly the erector spinae muscle group that tenses (Hodges and Richardson 1997). Movements performed in the sagittal plane primarily recruit the global system.

> *The following parameters facilitate the recruitment of the global stabilizers:*
> - *Rapid movements requiring a great deal of force*
> - *Movements in an open system and in the sagittal plane*
> - *Movements in the concentric phase*

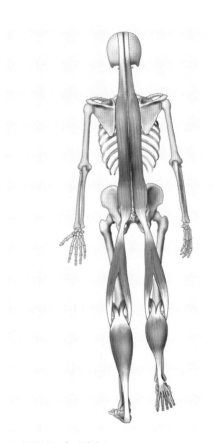

**Fig. 3.24** Myofascial chains.

**Clinical Relevance**

Initial rehabilitation exercises should be performed slowly; they should require little strength, and they should address perception.

## Global Structural Continuity of Myofascial Chains

On local and global levels, the musculature and the connective tissue form a structural and functional unit. A look at the anatomy reveals that the individual muscles are also continuous globally with the connective tissue that extends vertically and horizontally.

> *In the literature, this structural continuity is referred to by various terms. In the following, the term "myofascial chains" is used (**Fig. 3.24**).*

The creation of myofascial chains is based on the adaptive response of the musculature and the connective tissue to the specific requirements in the field of gravity in the development of locomotion. Gravity exerts constant pressure and tension on the body. The various structures respond by thickening, which is clearly seen on the surface anatomy (e.g., the thoracolumbar fascia with lumbosacral thickening).

This anatomical specificity is an economic response of the body to the interaction between gravity and body mass. In terms of movement behavior, the myofascial chains fulfill sensory, coordinative, and postural functions. They bring about a three-dimensional transmission of force between the head, the trunk, and the extremities, and they connect all body parts functionally and structurally with one another.

**Clinical Relevance**

Given its relationship to the fascia, every time local tension acts on a muscle, there is transmission of the impulse in the corresponding chain. In actual practice, this means that each local muscle shortening leads to compensation within the myofascial chain. Thus, when stretching an individual muscle, one should consider the entire chain.

### 3.3.4    Response to Dysfunction

**Local Stabilizers**

Musculoskeletal symptoms are closely associated with inhibition of the local stabilizers. There is biological adaptation with decreased circumference, mainly of type I fibers, as well as an increased ratio of fat and connective tissue. Insufficient segmental stabilization combined with the proprioception deficit, and thus inadequate myofascial anticipatory tension, increases the risk of injury of the surrounding structures during movement.

> The primary task in patient management is to diagnose the dysfunction of the local myofascial system.

**Global Stabilizers**

If there is a dysfunction, their response—albeit to a lesser extent—is similar to the local stabilizers, that is, with diminished strength and stamina. Because this system is highly involved in the body's response to gravity, weakness of the global stabilizers is evident as postural deviation and/or lacking control over the load-bearing joints (e.g., when walking).

> A characteristic feature of dysfunction of the global stabilizers is positional weakness in the inner core due to adaptive muscle elongation.

**Global Mobilizers**

When dysfunction occurs, there is a tendency toward hyperactivity and muscle shortening. In conjunction with irritation of the neural structures, there is hypersensitivity to stretching (e.g., shortening of the biceps femoris muscle related to irritation of the sciatic nerve).

> As a consequence, the global mobilizers should primarily be examined for shortening and sensitivity.

**Myofascial Chains**

Under extreme stress, the myofascial chains respond by thickening. Immobilization leads to water loss within the ground substance and thus to formation of cross-links between the collagen fibers.

### 3.3.5    Sources of Dysfunction

The causes of myofascial dysfunction vary. The biopsychosocial model of disease provides a useful foundation:

- Affective components (e.g., psychological stress) in an individual's social surroundings influence muscle tension.

**Example:** A classic clinical presentation is a raised shoulder with hyperactivity of the shoulder blade elevators. This is related to dysfunction of the complex consisting of the head, cervical spine, and shoulder girdle.

- Activity-specific stress resulting from work, sports, or leisure activities may exceed the biological adaptation ability of the musculature and fascia.
- Repetitive movements at work and/or during sports may lead to dominance of a myofascial system and thus to altered intramuscular and intermuscular coordination.
- Immobilization following trauma and illness can lead to an adaptive change in the biological and physiological properties of the myofascial structures. The duration of immobilization is the deciding factor: the longer it is, the more likely is a decrease in type I fibers.
- Diseases such as diabetes or unregulated hyperthyroidism promote a similar transformation.
- Along with naturally occurring atrophy, with increasing age the ratio of connective tissue to muscle tissue and type I to type II fibers changes (fewer type II muscle fibers).

**Clinical Relevance**

Prolonged illness and related bed rest may lead to the above-named changes. Prompt, adequate mobilization can minimize adaptation.

> Intramuscular coordination is related to the regulation of descending impulse frequency at the spinal cord level and the number or recruited motor units in the muscle.
> Intermuscular coordination relates to the synergistic cooperation of the agonists and antagonists. It is regulated by central and reflexive mechanisms.

### 3.3.6    Interpretation of Posture

The myofascial balance is the ability of the CNS to selectively activate the muscles in the right order and "dosage" in an efficient and action-oriented manner. Muscular control of joint mobility in its entire amplitude is a feature of normal contraction ability in both shortened and elongated muscle positions. For example, the strength of a muscle during an isometric contraction depends on its position or length. The position of maximum strength is the middle position. This is where there is the most optimal cross-bridging between the actin and myosin filaments.

Although there is virtually no overlap in a position of maximum elongation, the muscle tissue can still produce energy, albeit less than in the middle position. This also applies to maximum shortening in which the overlap is the greatest.

A deviation from the idealized posture necessarily alters the length of the muscle. Prolonged poor posture can lead to structural adaptation. This in turn alters the optimal tension/length relationship and results in a loss of control in a certain zone or diminished movement amplitude.

Performing an analysis of posture to determine which muscles are shortened and which are in an elongated position can provide a possible explanation about positional weaknesses of the affected muscles and/or their inability to shorten. An evaluation of posture in relation to the musculature may also help determine which muscles should be examined and how (e.g., testing contraction quality of a certain muscle in the neutral zero position, in a shortened position, or in an elongated position, or a test of stretching ability).

A given muscle may have normal ability in a neutral position, but may be weak in a shortened position. A *positional weakness* is present if biological adaptation (elongation of the muscle fibers in a series) occurred due to a fixed posture. The biologi-

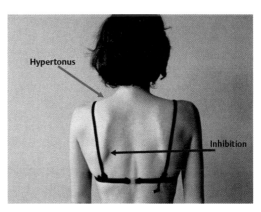

**Fig. 3.25** Hyperactivity of the musculus trapezius pars descendens.

cal stimulus to reverse the adaptation toward the norm would only be possible with activation of the affected muscle in the shortened position.

## Clinical Interpretation of Topography/Palpation

Diagnosis begins with the inspection. According to Janda (1979), inspection of the superficial anatomy of the body can provide helpful clues for the further examination. Hyperactive/hypertrophic muscles are recognizable due to elevation; inhibited/atrophied muscles may be seen as flattened. To test the hypothesis, and confirm or discard it, the therapist should palpate the relevant sites. When the myofascial structures are relaxed, passive tension is due to various connective tissue components, and active tension is due to the contractile elements.

*Examples:*

- *Hyperactivity of the descending part of the trapezius muscle* (**Fig. 3.25**):
  - Seen as elevation
  - Below the inferior angle, there is a visible indentation that suggests inhibition of the ascending part of the trapezius muscle.
  - Inspection is followed by palpation.
- *Inhibition and/or weakness of the transversus abdominis muscle* (**Fig. 3.26**):
  - Protruding lower abdomen as well as a transverse line at the level of the navel area suggestive of the hypothesis.
  - A vertical indentation is a clue to the dominance of the external abdominal oblique muscle.

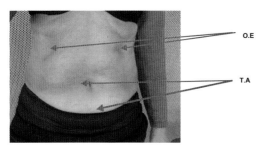

**Fig. 3.26** Inhibition and/or weakness of the transversus abdominis muscle.

### Clinical Relevance

The clinical interpretation of the topography may be based on the theory of the classification of the myofascial system. The musculus trapezius pars descendens, which is classified as a mobilizer, has a tendency toward hyperactivity and shortening. The ascending part of the trapezius muscle and the transversus abdominis muscle are stabilizers that have a tendency toward inhibition and/or weakness. This hypothesis requires a test of muscle functioning of the relevant muscle components.

> *A temporary or prolonged myofascial imbalance is an expression of a CNS disorder.*

### Diagnosis-based Classification

Based on current knowledge, there is a logical priority in terms of diagnosis, that is, priority is placed on diagnosing the primary stabilizers. Randomized clinical studies show a close correlation between their dysfunction and musculoskeletal lumbar spine symptoms. Their function actively ensures the neutral position (*neutral zone*) of the spinal segments. In this region, the passive structures are relaxed and there is the least resistance to intersegmental movements. The effectiveness of the stabilizers depends less on strength (25% of the maximum is sufficient) than on endurance and timely recruitment.

### Examples:

- Transversus abdominis muscle
- Multifidus muscle (medial portion)
- Diaphragm
- Pelvic floor musculature

> *In normal movement behavior, there is anticipatory activation of the muscles as a synergistic local unit.*

## Test of the Local Stabilizers

### *Transversus Abdominis Muscle*

- *Action:* Isolated activation of the transversus abdominis muscle without substitution of the global muscles.
- *Starting position:*
  - Supine or prone.
  - The legs are positioned in such a manner that they allow the spine to be in a neutral position.
- *Learning process:* Before the test, the patient should understand that he or she must locate the ASIS points using palpation. Visualization of the muscle position, for instance with pictures, may be helpful.
- *Patient instructions:*
  - Supine: "Draw your navel in toward your spine," or "Imagine bringing the two points of your pelvis (ASIS) closer together."
  - Prone: "Lift your belly off an imaginary air cushion."
  - "The pressure of the back against the underlying surface should remain the same; continue breathing."
  - To avoid substitution due to inhalation, the patient should hold their breath briefly after exhaling; then they should perform the movement and then immediately continue to breathe normally while holding the contraction for 10 seconds.
- *Control parameters:*
  - Palpation site: Roughly 2 cm medially and caudally to the ASIS; there should be no protrusion, but only an increase in tension.
  - Visual control in the supine patient: The epigastric angle remains about the same; normal breathing; the spine stays in the neutral position (visible at the body points: navel, tip of the sternum, and the symphysis).
  - Visual control in the prone patient: tapered, triangular-shape of the waist; the pelvis and spine remain constant; objective controls for the patient and the therapist are *pressure biofeedback* (air-filled pressure chamber connected to a pressure gauge, similar to a blood pressure unit) and *electromyograph (EMG) biofeedback.*
- *Norm:* The patient meets the above-named parameters and can hold the tension for 10 to 15 seconds and perform 10 repetitions.

The patient should understand that the test measures precision and stamina rather than strength. Minimal contraction is required. The prone position is a suitable starting position for the measurement of pressure biofeedback.

## Test of the Global Stabilizers

Corresponding to their classification, these muscles are tested in relation to their relevant functions:
- Ability to move the spine to a neutral position
- Fall-preventing stabilization of the neutral position in dynamic movement
- Fall-preventing control in the eccentric phase and isometric stabilization of the anchoring of the extremities to the trunk in a closed system
- Controlled isolated selective movement of the extremities with a stabilized trunk in an open system

### Placing the Trunk in the Neutral Posture (Fig. 3.27)
In the neutral posture, the passive structures contribute the least to stabilization of the spinal column segments. The local musculature ensures intersegmental stability by virtue of minimal tension and high responsiveness. Assuming a neutral position of the spine when sitting activates the trunk extensors.

Given their medial position on the spine, the multifidi muscles are suited for allowing lumbar lordosis from caudal. On the other hand, the superficial erector muscle produces extension primarily in the thoracolumbar region. Lacking extension of the lumbosacral junction may be a sign of dysfunction of the multifidi muscles and dominance of the erector muscle.

The test described in the following is based on models by Klein-Vogelbach (2000) and Hamilton and Richardson (1996). It examines the selective ability of the global stabilizers to maintain the neutral position of the spinal column and the vertical position:
- **Action:** Activation of the neutral position of the spinal column without substitution of the global mobilizers.
- **Starting position:**
  – Comfortably seated.
  – The leg position should allow the pelvis to move (ca. 90° bending in the hip joint), that is, the legs are hip-width apart with the feet under the knee joints.
- **Learning process:**
  – The patient should understand before the test that they should straighten their trunk and "grow" upward.

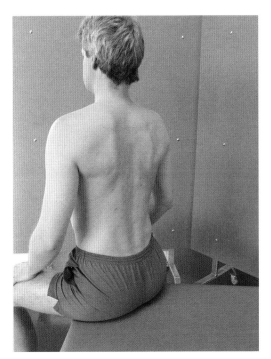

Fig. 3.27 Establishing the neutral posture of the spinal column: the synergistic activity in the shoulder girdle musculature can be seen. This supports the hypothesis of a dysfunction affecting the spinal column stabilizers.

  – The therapist should explain that the neutral position of the spinal column creates the optimal length of the trunk; exaggerated extension or bending shortens it. The therapist can also help the patient visualize and understand this by demonstrating on a model of the spine.
  – When performing the trunk movement, the patient should touch the crown of their head and their coccyx.
- **Patient instructions:**
  – "Think of growing by moving your coccyx and the crown of your head upward."
  – "Keep the pressure of the feet against the floor the same to avoid any tension in the legs."
- **Control parameters:** Ideally, the extension should begin in the lumbosacral region and move continually upward toward the head.

Beginning thoracolumbar lordosis is suggestive of dominant global mobilizers.

### The Building Block Game (Dynamic Stabilization; Fig. 3.28)
This test is progressively more difficult than the preceding one. It is based on the clinical observations by Klein-Vogelbach (2000) concerning the movement

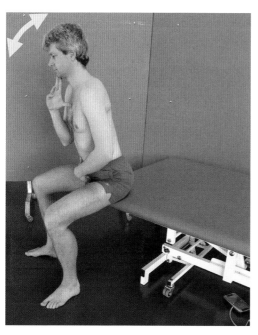

**Fig. 3.28** The Building Blocks (based on Klein-Vogelbach).

behavior that occurs with bending of the trunk. The author has found that, in patients with back dysfunction, when they bend their back forward there is often excessive extension of the thoracic spine to compensate for lacking lumbosacral extension.

> This is also suggestive of dominance of the dorsal global mobilizers.

- *Action:* Selective fall-preventing activation of the global stabilizers without substitution by the mobilizers.
- *Starting position:*
  - Comfortably seated.
  - The position of the legs should allow for movement of the pelvis (ca. 90° bending in the hip joint), that is, the legs should be placed hip-width apart with the feet underneath the knee joints.
- *Learning process:*
  - The patient should understand before the test that they should bend the trunk slightly forward while maintaining the neutral position of the spine. Here, too, visualization using a model of the spinal column may be helpful.
  - Only after the patient has bent their trunk a few times should the actual test begin.
  - The patient should move his or her pelvis without resistance.

- *Patient instructions:*
  - "Bend your trunk slightly forward and then back again to the starting position."
  - "Take care to keep your spine straight while you bend."
- *Control parameters:*
  - Ideally, the pelvis and the chest should move together as one unit.
  - The movement should take place in the hip joints only.
  - The therapist stands at the patient's side to observe the bending action.

> Placing sticky notes on the middle of the frontal plane of the pelvis and the chest can facilitate the evaluation.

### Test of the Global Stabilizers in a Closed System

The most important thing with regard to the various movements (e.g., bending down, going downstairs, or lifting an object) is the eccentric stabilization of the extremity segments in relation to each other and the trunk. This primarily involves selective use of the global stabilizers. This function may be assessed using the *single-leg squat test* (with one or two legs).

Another common movement variant in the interaction of the body with the environment leads to formation of a closed system (bridging), for example, when bracing oneself. In such events, the body's segments are specifically stabilized by fall-prevention activity. The ventral bridge test selectively tests this function of the global stabilizers.

### Single-leg Squat (Fig. 3.29a–c)

- *Action:* Selective activation of the global stabilizers of the leg, especially the gluteus medius muscle and the quadriceps vasti muscle.
- *Starting position:*
  - Standing on one leg.
  - The trunk is held vertically.
  - The arms are crossed over the sternum.
  - One leg is hanging with pelvic bending.
- *Learning process:*
  - Before the test, the patient should understand that this test evaluates the strength and endurance of the leg and pelvis muscles.
  - He should perform a squat.
- *Patient instructions:*
  - "Squat down a little and stay there for 10 seconds, and then come up again."
  - "Try to move your trunk as little as possible."

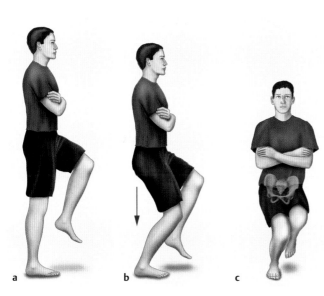

Fig. 3.29a–c Single-leg squat.
**a** Starting position.
**b** Beginning to squat.
**c** View from anterior.

- *Control parameters:*
  - The therapist evaluates the standing leg side.
  - Ideally, a connecting line between the spines should remain horizontal.
  - If the joints are centered, the *functional longitudinal leg axis* (axis of leg loading) should stay in the sagittal plane of the hip joint. The following points on the body are helpful landmarks: center of the hip joint, knee, and upper ankle joint.
  - Additional points on the body to observe: trochanter major, femoral condyles, patella, and navicular bone.

  *Signs of dysfunction:*
  - *Displacement of the trochanter posteriorly and/ or laterally.*
  - *The femoral condyles turn medially.*
  - *The navicular bone moves closer to the floor.*

- *Notes:*
  - Always compare sides.
  - Begin with the unaffected or better side.
  - If the patient wears inlays or inserts, perform the test with and without them.
  - Take the movement of the trunk into account as well, given that large swaying movements may signal inadequate proprioception and stabilization between the leg and trunk and/or within the trunk.
  - If endurance is being tested, the movement should be repeated 10–15 times.

### Ventral Bridge (Fig. 3.30)

The main feature of this test is that the entire body is involved in stabilization. This test is often used in everyday clinical practice:

- *Action:* Selective fall-prevention activation of the ventral global stabilizers without substitution by the mobilizers.
- *Starting position:*
  - Prone.
  - Support on forearms at chest level.
  - The tips of the feet are in contact with the floor.
- *Learning process:*
  - Before performing the test, the patient should understand that they should lift their entire body off the floor.
  - It is best if they attempt the movement once as a trial test.
- *Patient instructions:*
  - "Lift your pelvis and chest together just off the supporting surface, stay there for 10 seconds, and then come down again."
  - "The chest and pelvis should be equally far apart from the supporting surface."
- *Control parameters:*
  - This is an evaluation of the anchoring quality between the trunk and pelvis.
  - Ideally, the longitudinal axes of both segments of the body should form one line.
  - The therapist should observe from the side to assess an imaginary connecting line between the chest and pelvis.
- *Note:* If endurance is being tested, the patient should repeat the movement 10–15 times.

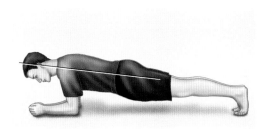

**Fig. 3.30** Ventral bridge.

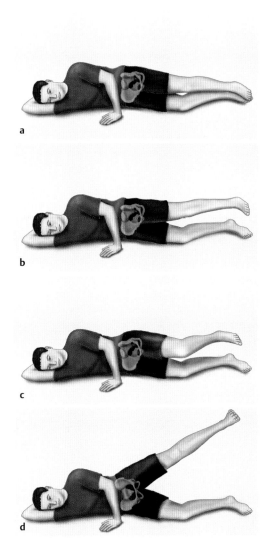

**Fig. 3.31a–d** Abduction test.
**a** Starting position with ideal stabilization of the trunk.
**b** Final position.
**c** Substitution of abduction by bending: dysfunction of the global stabilizers.
**d** Substitution of abduction by sidebending: dysfunction of the global stabilizers.

*The test requires special coordination between the local and global stabilizers. A deviation as soon as the first test phase (without repetitions) is nearly always a sign of weakness of the local muscles. Further training of the local system is needed.*

### Test of the Global Stabilizers in an Open System

Everyday functions also include control of all extremity movements in an open system. This necessitates proximal stabilization and selective distal mobility; the potential amplitudes (mainly in the proximal joints) may be tested to their fullest or at smaller levels.

### Abduction Test (Fig. 3.31a–d)
This test was first described by Janda (1979).

*This test has a high reliability in terms of the quality of movement control of the leg where it joins the trunk.*

- **Action:**
  - Selective control of leg movement in abduction.
  - This test evaluates the global stabilizers on the top side, primarily the gluteus medius muscle, quadratus lumborum muscle, and the oblique muscles.
- **Starting position:**
  - Side-lying position, possibly with a cushion under the waist.
  - The hand of the top arm is placed in front of the abdomen for support.
- **Learning process:**
  - Before performing the test, the patient should understand that it does not test strength, but rather precision.
  - It is best if he or she tries to abduct the leg a few times before beginning the actual test.
- **Patient instructions:**
  - "Slowly raise your top leg upward, hold it for 10 seconds, and then slowly lower it again."
  - "Be sure to perform the movement slowly."
- **Control parameters:**
  - Leg, pelvis, and chest.
  - The therapist should check if the leg moves alone or the back changes position; he or she should also observe the sequence of motion.
  - Ideally, abduction should occur before side-bending of the lumbar spine.
- **Note:** If endurance is being tested, the patient should repeat the movement 10–15 times.

*Frequent deviations are a sign of dominance of the global mobilizers. These include abduction/bending of the hip joint, premature lumbar sidebending, and/or rotation of the pelvis and/or chest.*

## Testing the Global Mobilizers

This test analyzes the extensibility of the muscles and their sensitivity to stretching. The test of the musculature for shortening is based on a standardized procedure (Janda 1979, Kendall 1993) that includes isolation of local changes. Given the principle of continuity, depending on the position of the body, the need for extensibility of the muscle varies. Thus, one must also test the extensibility of the muscle within a pattern of movement that is relevant to the patient.

*If the primary activity of the patient occurs in the sitting position, then it is in this position that the hamstring muscles should be tested.*

### Test for Muscle Shortening in a Function Position (Sitting) (Fig. 3.32a, b)

*Ideally, this test should simulate the working conditions of the patient.*

- *Action:* Extend the lower leg to evaluate the extensibility of the hamstring muscles.
- *Starting position:* Seated with the spinal column in a neutral position.
- *Learning process:* The patient should understand that the test evaluates whether the length of certain muscles (the hamstrings) allows the spine to be held in a safe position.
- *Patient instructions:*
  - "Extend your lower legs as much as possible."
  - "Say right away if you feel any changes."
- *Control parameters:*
  - This test evaluates the amount of knee joint extension as well as the behavior of the pelvis and lumbar spine.
  - Ideally, the patient should be able to perform full extension without any additional movement of the pelvis or lumbar spine.

*If there is any additional movement of the lumbar spine, the therapist should determine whether the hamstring muscles are shortened or whether there is a problem with the stability of the dorsal structures of the lumbar spine. Sensitivity of the sciatic nerve can lead to a misinterpretation of results.*

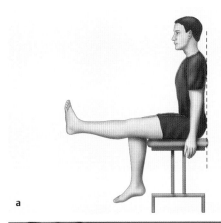

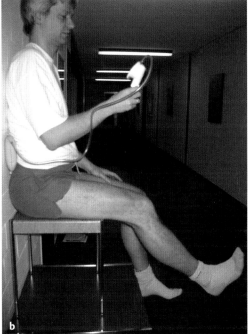

Fig. 3.32a, b  a Active selective stretching test of the hamstring muscles. b Self-test.

## Diagnosis of the Myofascial Chain

The concept of structural continuity of the muscles and the fascia, along with their adaptation to increased strain with connective tissue proliferation, raises the question of whether a certain chain might exacerbate a postural fault. By way of example, the following test evaluates the length of the dorsal myofascial chain:

- *Action:* Evaluation of the behavior of the dorsal chain during elongation (**Fig. 3.33a, b**).
- *Starting position:* Sitting with the legs outstretched in front.

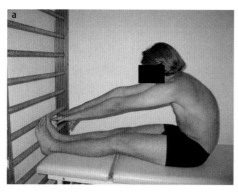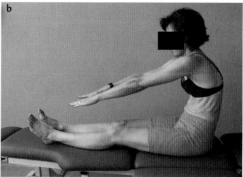

**Fig. 3.33a, b** Diagnosis of the myofascial chain with the legs outstretched in front. The path of least resistance is in the region of the lumbar spine and lower thoracic spine (**a**), only in the lower thoracic spinal region (**b**).

- *Learning process:*
  - The patient should understand that the muscles are connected, without interruption, from head to foot.
  - The test reveals any weakness in the chain. A rope may help with visualization.
- *Patient instructions:*
  - "Try to touch your feet with your hands."
  - "Say right away if you feel any changes."
- *Control parameters:*
  - This test evaluates the behavior of the legs, the pelvis, and the spinal column in relation to hypo- and hypermobile structures.
  - Ideally, there should be a harmonious, arc-like curvature of the spine. The knees should remain extended, and the thighs should be neutral in the hip joints without rotation.
- *Note:* The result should be compared with any postural deviations: if there is a fixed swayback with kyphosis, there will be hypomobility of the lumbar spine and hypermobility of the thoracic spine.

**Clinical Relevance**

In stretching of the lumbar spine extensors, the behavior of the entire chain should be taken into account. It is essential that during the stretch, priority is placed on active fixation of the thoracic spine.

## Adapted Muscle Function Testing

If the test of posture in relation to muscle length supports a hypothesis of lengthening, then muscular strength should be tested with the muscle in its shortest position.

**Modified Test of the Psoas Muscle**
- *Action:* After passively flexing the patient's leg (over 90°), they should actively maintain this position for 15 seconds.
- *Starting position:* Sitting with the spinal column in a neutral position.
- *Learning process:* The patient should understand that muscle strength is being tested with the muscle in a shortened position. They should actively hold the initially passively established flexed position for 10–15 seconds.
- *Patient instructions:*
  - "Keep your leg in the same position after I let go of it."
  - "Keep your trunk as still as possible."
- *Control parameters:*
  - This test evaluates whether the position is held and if the back remains still.
  - The muscle should be able to hold the weight of the leg for the required length of time.

*If the patient can actively hold the position, the therapist should increase the difficulty by applying slight resistance.*

## Sensorimotor Control

Sensorimotor control refers to the involuntary efferent response to an afferent signal in the form of joint stabilization. In terms of the musculature, the signals come from the muscle spindles. By virtue of anticipatory (feed-forward) pre-programming of the muscle, this sensory loop prevents trauma from occurring (see 3.3.3 Functional Classification of the Musculature in the Myofascial System).

The function and/or dysfunction of the musculoskeletal system cannot be divided from the mechanisms modulating the neural system. Peripheral

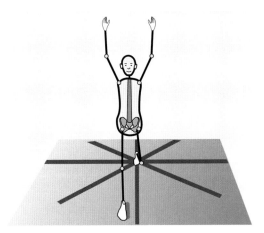

**Fig. 3.34** Lunge.

**Summary**

The assessment of postural and myofascial imbalance includes an evaluation of the interaction between various components of the locomotor system.

In the analysis described here, the components consisting of *posture* and *musculature* enable the use of recurrent observational parameters and a systematic approach to identifying any deviation. For correct diagnosis, and hence individually tailored treatment planning and implementation, proper knowledge of muscular responses and their classification in terms of function is essential.

trauma can often trigger adaptive mechanisms in the CNS (or the reverse), which are evidenced by altered movement programming. Various studies have provided explanatory models for the relationships between articular lesion and the resulting uncoordinated muscle functions.

### Lunge (Fig. 3.34)

> Given its frequent use in everyday motor skills, the lunge position may be considered a functional movement.

- *Action:* The lunge leads to a certain inertia and sudden loading. Responsive stabilizers, in particular, are needed.
- *Starting position:*
  – Standing upright.
  – The patient should stand on the center of an "X" marked on the floor. Their feet should be placed hip-width apart.
- *Learning process:*
  – The patient should understand that the test requires involuntary tensing of the muscles.
  – When they are asked to do so, they should lunge forward, placing their front foot on a line drawn on the floor.
- *Patient instructions:*
  – "When I give the signal, lunge forward."
  – "Try to land with your front foot on the line drawn on the floor."
- *Control parameters:*
  – The patient's trunk should remain in a neutral position.
  – There is axial loading of the front leg and the pelvis should remain horizontal.

### References

Bacha P. Klassifikation der Muskelfunktion. Teil 1. Manuelle Therapie 2003;7:157–167

Bacha P. Muskelsysteme. Teil 2: Von der Muskeldysbalance zur myofaszialen Dysfunktion–Assessment. Manuelle Therapie 2004;8:28–38

Basset CL. Effect of force on skeletal tissues. In: Downey RC, Darling RC, eds. Physiological Basis of Rehabilitative Medicine. Philadelphia: W. B. Saunders; 1971

Bergmark A. Stability of the lumbar spine. A study in mechanical engineering. Acta ortho Scan 1989;60:20–24

Bogduk N. Klinische Anatomie von Lendenwirbelsäule und Sakrum. Rehabilitation und Prävention, Vol 57. Berlin: Springer; 2000

Brumagne S, Cordo P, et al. The role of paraspinal muscle spindles in lumbosacral position sense in individuals with and without low back pain. Spine 2000;25(8): 989–994

Enneking WF, Harrington P. Pathologic changes in scoliosis. J Bone Joint Surg (Am) 1969;51:165

Fortin C, Ehrmann Feldman D, et al. Inter-rater reliability of the evaluation of muscular chains associated with posture alterations in scoliosis. BMC Musculoskelet Disord 2012;13:80

Guimond P. Intricate correlation between body posture, personality trait and incidence of body pain: a cross-referential study report. PLoS ONE 2012;7(5)

Hamilton C. Stabilisierendes System. In: Klein-Vogelbach S, et al. Funktionelle Bewegungslehre. Bewegung lehren und lernen. 5th ed. Berlin: Springer; 2000

Hodges PW, Richardson CA. Inefficient muscular stabilization of the lumbar spine associated with low back pain. A motor control evaluation of transversus abdominis. Spine 1996;22:2640–2650

Janda V. Muskelfunktionsdiagnostik. Leuven: Acco; 1979

Kendall FP, McCreary E, et al. Muscles: Testing and Function. Baltimore: Williams & Wilkins; 1993

Klein-Vogelbach S. Functional Kinetics; Observing, Analysing, and Teaching Human Movement. Berlin: Springer; 1990

Klein-Vogelbach S. Funktionelle Bewegungslehre, Bewegung lehren und lernen. 5. Aufl. Berlin: Springer; 2000

Lephart SM, Fu FH, eds. Proprioception and Neuromuscular Control in Joint Stability. Champaign, IL: Human Kinetics; 2000

Levangie P, Norkin C. Joint Structure and Function: A Comprehensive Analysis. 2nd ed. Philadelphia: Davis; 1992

Luomajoki H. Movement control tests of the low back; evaluation of the difference between patients with low back pain and healthy controls. BMC Musculoskelet Disord 2008;9:170

Nashner LM. Sensory neuromuscular and biomechanical contributions to human balance. Balance: Proceedings of the American Physical Therapy Association Forum. Nashville: American Physical Therapy Association; 1989

Panjabi MM. The stabilizing system of the spine. Part II. Neutral zone and instability hypothesis. J Spinal Disord 1992;5(4):390–396

Posture Committee of the American Academy of Orthopaedic Surgeons. Posture and its Relationship to Orthopaedic Disabilities: A Report of the Posture Committee of the American Academy of Orthopaedic Surgeons. Evanston, IL: American Academy of Orthopaedic Surgeons; 1947

Richardson CA, Juli C, et al. Therapeutic Exercise for Spinal Stabilization in Low Back Pain—Scientific Basis and Clinical Approach. Edinburgh: Churchill Livingstone; 1999

Richardson CA et al. Therapeutic Exercise for Lumbopelvic Stabilisation: A Motor Control Approach to Treatment and Prevention. Oxford: Elsevier; 2004

Sahrmann A. Diagnosis and Treatment of Movement Impairment Syndromes. St. Louis: Mosby; 2002

Sheth P, Yu B, et al. Ankle disk training influences reaction times of selected muscles in a simulated ankle sprain. Am J Sports Med 1997;25(4):538–543

Soysa A, Hiller C, et al. Importance and challenges of measuring intrinsic foot muscle strength. J Foot Ankle Res 2012;5(1):29

Wolff J. Das Gesetz der Transformation der Knochen. Stuttgart: Schattauer Verlag; 1991 (Reprint Dt 1892 edition, Berlin: Hirschwald)

# 4 Pain as the Chief Symptom

# 4 Pain as the Chief Symptom

*Mechthild Doelken*

## 4.1 Theoretical Foundations of Pain as a Chief Symptom

### 4.1.1 Definitions

- Pain is an unpleasant sensory and emotional experience that is associated with actual or potential tissue damage or is described in such terms (Merskey and Bogduk 1994).
- Pain is the perception of a physical event with the following characteristics:
  - Physical perception accompanying stimulation, which causes—or potentially causes—tissue damage (nociceptive perception)
  - Experience of a threat to the body, which is accompanied by nociceptive perception
  - An uncomfortable feeling accompanying nociceptive perception and perception of a threat to the body (modified definition based on Price et al 1999).

This latter new definition avoids the assumption that pain is always associated with a real or potential tissue-damaging event.

Pain is the chief symptom in many orthopedic diseases, and it is what brings the patient to the doctor and then to the physical therapist. The patient's quality of life may be severely impaired as a result of prolonged pain. Most patients expect their doctor or physical therapist to alleviate the pain as quickly as possible. Recent discoveries related to pain make these expectations all the more important.

Rapid pain relief avoids central hypersensitivity. Repeated, persistent pain leads to a change in the central pain synapses, resulting in hypersensitivity. Physiological afferents are thus altered to such a degree that they are perceived as pain. The patient perceives pain, although there is no longer any tissue damage. This is the distinguishing feature of chronic pain.

The perception of pain is subjective and may vary greatly between individual patients. Pain perception and pain processing are closely interwoven. Pain perception is determined by psychosocial factors; pain is influenced by our thoughts and feelings. The neural pathways that transmit information, for example, about the location and intensity of a harmful stimulus, differ from those that transport affective or emotional stimuli. Our response to a harmful stimulus reflects the activities of both systems.

Within orthopedics, physical therapists treat patients with acute and chronic pain.

### Acute Pain

Acute pain may be preceded by tissue damage or by a stimulus that is potentially harmful. This type of pain is useful, as it alerts the organism to danger. The tissue damage is not necessarily always associated with acute trauma, but may also result from strain on the body's structures. Acute pain is caused by tissue-damaging chemical, mechanical, or thermal stimuli. If the stimulation persists, acute symptoms may be prolonged for an unlimited length of time.

> *In long-term pain, what was initially a helpful and useful pain may manifest physically due to deficient adaptive processes of the nervous system. Thus, the pain may persist after it is no longer necessary.*

If there is excessive perception of pain (hypersensitivity), even harmless stimuli (e.g., mechanical) may be transmitted as pain. This useless pain is also referred to as *chronification of pain* or *neuropathic pain*.

### Chronic Pain

There are various definitions of chronic pain. The International Association for the Study of Pain (IASP) defines chronic pain as pain that occurs persistently or intermittently for 6 months (IASP 2013a,b).

Preferably, the definition should also include various aspects related to tissue healing. The term *chronic pain* should be used only for pain persisting for longer than 6 months, which, given normal healing processes, should have disappeared (Linton 1996). In other words, patients with disorders such as chronic polyarthritis would not be included with those who have chronic, unnecessary pain. The disadvantage of this definition, however, is that it assumes prior tissue damage, although this applies to only a minority of patients with chronic pain.

In recent years, the concept of chronic pain has changed. It is no longer the duration of pain, but rather the type of pain that is central to the concept. For many patients, pain no longer reflects nociceptive processes, but rather it develops its "own life."

Psychological aspects are crucial. Pain is not merely an expression of tissue damage, but rather an expression of what it means—positively or negatively—to the patient. Positive experiences serve as positive reinforcements of chronification.

*Examples:*
- Positive:
  - Experience of physical attention (e.g., hands-on therapies)
  - Time off work
- Negative:
  - Social isolation
  - Insomnia

According to Linton (1999), the primary goal of all therapists who deal with musculoskeletal pain is to identify those patients who are at risk of chronification of pain and impairment. He emphasizes the risk of chronification in patients with acute musculoskeletal pain.

Physical therapists should have an understanding of pain that is useful for clinical practice. It is not enough to merely consider pain centers and pain pathways, as well as involved neurons and chemical interactions. Pain needs to be studied in a larger, multilayered and multidimensional context. The social environment surrounding the patient, such as family and work, should be taken into account, as well as his or her conceptualization of their pain and its importance to them. Pain must also be considered in research-oriented, diagnostic terms in order to provide the patient with adequate explanations and prognoses and develop the best possible basis for treatment. The skill of the therapist lies in his or her ability to use multilevel, multidimensional data for treatment (e.g., Gifford's Mature Organism Model [MOM]—see p. 152; Gifford 1998, 2000).

## 4.1.2 Pain Perception

### Dimensions of Pain Perception

Melzack and Wall (1996) have distinguished three dimensions of pain:
- *Sensory discriminative pain dimension:* Perception of the region, intensity, and behavior of the pain.
- *Cognitive evaluation pain dimension:* The attitude of the patient toward pain is influenced by his or her previous experience and knowledge (e.g., if a physical therapy measure has caused pain, next time the patient will signal earlier that pain is being triggered).

- *Affective-motivational pain dimension:* The patient's thoughts about pain and his or her emotional response to it (e.g., anger, anxiety, fear, concern).

All of these dimensions are essential parts of pain experience, and they combine to change physiological outputs and thus ultimately influence the pain behavior of the patient as well. Negative thoughts about an injury or pain can stimulate the autonomic and neuroendocrine system. This, in turn, also has a negative effect on the sensory system. At the same time, the patient uses altered movement patterns that are influenced by unconscious pain-processing mechanisms.

Pain is part of a warning system against damaging stimuli. Various mechanisms are involved in the perception and response to potential stimuli (Wall 1979):
- Flight reflexes.
- Pain perception.
- Behavior, learning, and memory (e.g., "How should I behave the next time so that I avoid hitting my knee?").
- Affective response.
- Autonomous, respiratory, endocrine, and immune responses (e.g., patients with long-term pain have a tendency toward infections).

## The Influence of Psychosocial Factors on Pain Perception

Psychosocial risk factors include the patient's emotions and expectations as well as the interactions between the patient and his or her surroundings (Kendall et al 1997). Job satisfaction, expected compensation, depression, or an extremely caring partner may be very significant for the severity of symptoms and the pain behavior of the patient (Flor et al 1990; Nicholas and Sharp 1999).

The secondary benefit of the patient's pain—of which he or she may or may not be aware—may prevent their symptoms from improving (Kendall et al 1997; Nicholas and Sharp 1999). Long-term symptoms, for which there is no diagnosis, may intensify the patient's insecurity and worries. They may focus their attention on their body and alter their daily life according to the intensity of the pain. An exaggerated alertness to any sensory signal may result. Heightened awareness may be directed toward any potential sources of danger that may contribute to the pain, such as moving. Patients can develop fear-avoidance behavior, causing them to adopt protective positions and restrict their movement. This, in turn, leads to increased perception of pain and a lower level of pain tolerance. In the literature, fear of movement has been discussed as the main feature in the development of chronic musculoskeletal problems (Zusman 1998; Vlaeyen and Linton 2000).

## Cortical Changes in Patients with Chronic Pain

For pain chronification, not only is nociceptive stimulation significant, but also the way in which the brain processes non-nociceptive characteristics of a painful event. Because chronic pain leads to cortical changes, modern treatment strategies target the brain with the goal of altering negative reorganization. This hypothesis was developed by Lorimer Moseley in one of his most recent research projects. Lorimer Moseley is a physical therapist and professor of neuroscience in Australia. In 2012, he and his team received important awards for research on chronic pain.

Chronic pain is associated with reorganization of the primary somatosensory and motor cortex as well as the angular cingulate cortex of the insular region. The correlation between cortical reorganization and the intensity of pain influences prevention and treatment strategies. Tactile discrimination training can improve sensory discrimination. Graded motor imagery is a promising approach for normalizing motor representation. The technique uses a computer program to show visual images of healthy parts of the body in various positions. The patient views the images and in his or her imagination assumes these positions. Similar to graded motor imagery, there is also very good evidence on mirror therapy for the treatment of patients with neuropathic pain affecting the hand after a distal radius fracture; in the acute stage using mirror therapy and in the chronic stage using graded motor imagery (Moseley 2006). Both concepts involve transmitting an image of the healthy hand to the affected hand using a mirror image of the healthy hand; in graded motor imagery, there is the additional use of computer images. The goal of both concepts is to use activation of the premotor and primary motor cortical areas to achieve cortical reorganization, thus interrupting the cycle of chronic pain (Moseley and Flor 2012)

Patients with chronic pain have abnormal processing of tactile impulses. In the summer of 2012, Moseley and his team published the results of their studies on patients with chronic low back pain. Various vibrating stimuli were applied, either in pairs or at different times, and the patients were asked to say when they felt the stimuli occurred simultaneously. The results showed much slower processing of stimuli from the affected region. Patients with chronic low back pain have abnormal spatial representation of vibrating tactile stimuli (Moseley et al 2012).

## 4.1.3   Classification of Pain

Pain may be classified in terms of duration or in terms of physiology. For the classification of pain, different authors have proposed various systems.

## Classification of Pain Duration Based on Waddell (1998)

- Acute pain: Less than 6 weeks
- Subacute pain: 6 to 12 weeks
- Chronic pain: Longer than 3 months

This raises the question as to whether pain has a direct relationship to tissue damage (acute pain) or not (persistence of chronic pain despite healing or, occasionally, without any tissue lesion; Gifford and Butler 1999).

Yet, if there is repeated tissue damage or abnormal wound healing, the pain may be related for longer than the 6-week acute phase with peripheral tissue damage. This is very common in patients with orthopedic problems. Degenerative diseases lower the ability of the body's structures to withstand strain over the long term, and thus there is a constant risk of renewed tissue damage. The documentation of the pain duration should therefore include the pain behavior: is the pain continuous, intermittent (daily), or does it appear in (rare or frequent) episodes (Waddell 1998)?

> Intermittent pain requires an examination of the conditions that trigger the pain (e.g., mechanical influences such as posture and movement).
> Continuous pain is rather more a sign of inflammation or chronification with hypersensitivity of the central nervous system (CNS).

## Physiological Classification

Pain may be divided into three phases:

### First Pain Phase

The pain occurs when it is triggered. Patients usually experience it on the surface of the body as bright and circumscribed; it stops when the stimulus disappears, and it is directly related to impending or actual tissue damage. It is also referred to as *rapid pain* or pain due to A-delta pain impulses because it is primarily carried by A-delta fibers, which transmit pain rapidly. Pain is transmitted to the dorsal horn via alpha-amino-3-hydroxy-5-methyl-4-isoxazole propionic acid (AMPA) receptors. The goal is to avoid immediate injury, which is why pain generally triggers a withdrawal reflex (e.g., if one touches a hot burner on a stove). Its function is to warn and protect; the pain lasts only as long as the stimulus is present.

This first pain pathway is made up of A-delta fibers with a conduction velocity of 30 m/second. It is responsible for first pain and precedes second pain in terms of perception. The fibers of the first pain pathway are thin, myelinated fibers, which respond very quickly to stimuli. Most are located in the skin; they transmit a bright, well-localized, stabbing, cutting pain.

The cell bodies of the first peripheral pain neurons are surrounded by connective tissue. Together with other sensory neurons, they form the spinal ganglion in the dorsal root of the spinal nerve. Their axons end in the dorsal root at the second neuron, whose axons cross in the same spinal cord segment to the opposite side of the spinal cord; then they travel the neothalamic pathway (lateral part of the spinothalamic tract) to the third neuron in the thalamus.

The thalamus is part of the diencephalon. Via the diencephalon, all sensory tracts (except for the olfactory tract) pass to the cerebral cortex, whose axons mainly pass to the sensory area where pain perception occurs.

### Second Pain Phase

Long-term pain occurs during the second pain phase. Presumably, unmyelinated C-fibers are the main ones responsible for the second pain phase. These activate N-methyl-D-aspartate (NMDA) receptors in the dorsal horn. Thus, it is also referred to as *C-pain*, and it occurs at a different time from the beginning of the stimulus. This type of pain is dull and not as well localized. It lasts longer than the traumatic stimulus. This type of pain is usually caused by chemical substances related to tissue damage as well as the inflammation. C-pain ensures the avoidance of stress on the injured tissue; thus, it has a protective function for normal wound healing (Cervero and Laird 1991).

The long-term, spreading pain is most apparent when related to the joints. This is followed by, in order of decreasing intensity, the periarticular tissue, the viscera, the muscles, the deep fascia, and the skin, which triggers this type of pain in the least apparent manner (Melzack and Wall 1996).

This second part of the pain pathway is formed by C-fibers with a conduction velocity of 3 m/second. They are responsible for second pain, because they come after the first pain pathway. C-fibers are thin, unmyelinated fibers, which cause a delayed, dull, diffuse, burning, piercing pain. They are carried by the older paleothalamic pathway (medial portion of the spinothalamic tract and spinoreticular tract).

Phase 1 and 2 pain are useful in terms of protecting the injured tissue (adaptive pain). The afferents of A-delta or C-pain originate in receptors in the body's tissue; hence, this is also referred to as receptor pain. The receptors also include nociceptors (*nociceptive pain*).

Nociceptive pain is mainly related to acute pain, although it can also occur with adaptive chronic pain. This usually occurs when the tissue is in poor condition and is less able to tolerate stress. Diseases involving abnormal tissue biology (e.g., inflammation, rheumatoid arthritis, and degenerative diseases such as osteoarthritis) produce nociceptive pain in musculoskeletal tissues.

### Third Pain Phase

In the third pain phase, pain may transition from the subacute phase to chronic pain.

For several years it has been suggested that, under the influence of a longer-term tissue lesion, the CNS may change various aspects of its function (Mense 1999). Apparently, signals reaching the spinal cord from the injury in the periphery of the body transform the processing of the incoming sensory information. In extreme situations, the patient may still feel pain although the injury has healed (Mense 1999).

This may lead to change in the synapses and lead to hypersensitivity. This is the beginning of the third phase of pain. The pain is no longer useful for protection of the injured tissue (maladaptive pain). The physiological afferents are altered to such a degree that they are perceived as pain. In this phase, acute pain increases due to the mechanisms of peripheral and central sensitization.

### Peripheral Sensitization

After a tissue injury, rapid formation of pro-inflammatory substances sets a series of events in motion, which lead to peripheral sensitization. At the injury site, a "sensitizing soup" forms.

Peripheral sensitization serves to sensitize the normally high-threshold nociceptors so that they discharge in response to stimuli, which normally would be too weak to trigger a response. The sensitized nociceptors also discharge more often, and the dormant nociceptors are "awakened." The latter are only active in inflammation. To modulate the inflammatory response, opioid receptors form. It is their task to decrease the excitability of the cell or inhibit pro-inflammatory neuropeptides. The production of opioids may be increased by physical therapy measures (e.g., gentle massage, careful movement in the pain-free range, lymph drainage). During the subacute phase, this can have a positive effect against chronification.

Persistent chronic pain that endures long after the injury has healed is attributed to negative learning processes in nerve cells in the spinal cord. Radiating pain occurs due to a misinterpretation of nerve signals.

A main feature of learning processes at the level of individual nerve cells is that an external stimulus causes lasting changes in the cell function. Such behavior is termed "plasticity." This concept of neuroplasticity is central to pain research. For some time, plastic changes affecting nerve cells have been discussed as a possible explanation for the chronification of pain (Mense 1999).

### Central Sensitization

The pain afferents synapse in the dorsal horn. The milieu of the dorsal horn consists of "jostling" primary afferent excitatory firings, stimulation, and inhibition of neurons in the spinal cord and descending modulation. Similar to a room full of noisy children, only the loudest signals make it through.

Peripheral sensitization in the "sensitizing soup" reinforces the input from the periphery. This leads to a temporary increase in synaptic strength and the activation of dormant receptive neurons in the dorsal horn. The reinforcement increases the peripheral neurons' receptive fields; some sensations, which are normally harmless, are now interpreted as pain. The result is a more effective voice reaching the brain.

An important aspect in central sensitization is the activation of the glutamate receptor NMDA in the dorsal horn cells of the spinal cord, leading to their increased sensitivity. The hyperactivity is triggered by glutamate, nitrous oxide, and substance P (Ren 1994). NMDA receptors are located on the cell membrane of neurons in the spinal cord and brain cells. Their function is to activate the neurons on which they are located. They play a role in many tasks related to learning and memory, and they help store long-term memory. This explains the development of pain memory in patients with chronic pain.

Central sensitization at the level of the dorsal horn means that touch and vibrations affecting the body's tissue, as well as information from low-threshold sensory A-beta fibers, which normally transmit touch and vibration stimuli, are perceived as pain. During this phase, hands-on physical therapy treatments (e.g., massage, manual therapy) are no longer perceived as pleasant.

Various factors play a role in the development of maladaptive pain, for example, the cognitive evaluation and affective-motivational dimensions of pain perception (p. 144). Injury to the neural structures can also trigger maladaptive pain. Injury of the connective tissue sheaths of the neural structures initially causes phase 1 and 2 pain. Yet, the actual axonal lesion may also provoke impulses in the axon. Thus, the axon triggers impulses at a site where they would otherwise not occur; normally, pain is produced at the receptor or nerve ending.

The axolemma of the peripheral nerves is made for the transmission of pain impulses and not for their production. The axonal impulses enter the CNS and at some point are perceived as pain; this is neuropathic pain. Inflammatory mediators, and in some instances, fibers from the sympathetic nervous system, may cause pathological stimulation of nerve fibers at injured, and thus no longer isolated sites. Healthy nerve fibers do not possess any adrenergic receptors, while damaged nerves may form them. This makes them receptive to sympathetic stimuli, and the sympathetic nervous system can sustain the pain.

**Example:** The situation may be compared to an alarm that is set off by opening a window: in nociceptive receptor pain, the alarm system would be activated by a short circuit in the cables leading to the window.

> The three phases of pain may occur consecutively. The pain may stop after the first phase, or it may transition into phase 2 pain and ultimately, due to sensitization of the central synapses, it may transition into chronic phase 3 pain. Yet, phase 3 pain may also occur without phases 1 and 2.

## 4.1.4   Causes of Pain

- Mechanical tissue damage: Tensile and compressive strains on the body's tissues.
- Thermal stimuli: $> +45°C$.
- Chemical stimuli: For example, potassium ions that are liberated from destroyed cells; lactic acid; substances that arise with decay of tissue or inflammatory reactions (e.g., prostaglandin reduces the nociceptor threshold).
- Psychological condition: The patient's individual psychological state (e.g., stress, grief) can significantly influence the perception and processing of pain (see cognitive evaluation and affective-motivational dimensions of pain perception, p. 144).
- Nociceptors (see section 4.1.5 below) are often found in the body's tissues adjacent to the arterioles, where the efferents of the sympathetic nervous system are also located; due to the release of chemical substances (e.g., noradrenaline) these can change the nociceptor threshold (Gifford 2002, 2003).
- All processes leading to the lowering of the nociceptor threshold cause increased sensitivity of the tissue (peripheral sensitization) and sometimes pain (C-pain). The lowering of the threshold thus serves to protect the body's tissues so that wound healing can proceed undisturbed.

Etiopathogenetic features may be divided into physiological (warning pain if there is noxious stimulation of healthy tissue), pathophysiological (if an organ is diseased), and neuropathic pain (if there is damage of nerve cells/nerve fibers).

## 4.1.5   Nociceptors

Pain can occur in any tissue in the body that contains nociceptors. Nociceptors are the alarm system for pain (signaling the damage) and are found in all tissues except for the cartilage and the brain. They are nerve cells that code and process noxious stimuli. The nociceptive system consists of the peripheral and central systems. When a person is conscious, its activation creates a situation of subjective pain perception.

## Nociceptor Localization and Structure

Nociceptors are located in the following structures (except in cartilage—where only the subchondral layer has nociceptors—and in the brain):
- Bone
- Muscle
- Tendons and tendon sheaths
- Bursae
- Nerves
- Vessels
- Skin and subcutaneous tissue

## Nociceptor Stimulation

Nociceptors are primary afferents with free nerve endings and slow conducting axons. Free nerve endings are thin and unmyelinated. Some of the endings are covered with Schwann cells, or they end directly in the surrounding tissue. Along with receiving stimuli, free nerve endings also release mediators (e.g., substance P and glutamate) from the nerve fiber.

The cell body of a nociceptor is the spinal ganglion. Via axoplasmic transport, substances are transported in the intracellular system from the cell body to the ending and the reverse. The cell body has similar receptor properties to the nerve ending. Nociceptors are distinguished by whether or not they produce mediators. These are neuropeptides such as substance P.

The nociceptors are the body's alarm system, providing information about any tissue damage that occurs. Each time pain is perceived the "initial ignition" is stimulation exceeding the nociceptor threshold. Normally, nociceptors have a high stimulation threshold, that is, they require strong stimuli.

Depending on the organ and structure, the stimulation threshold varies. It depends on which mechanical, thermal, or chemical intensities are dangerous to a given organ or structure. As with all receptors, their activation is caused by a decreased membrane potential. This occurs due to the opening of ionic channels, which are present in large numbers on the nociceptors, and that react to various stimuli. The stimulation threshold of the nociceptors can change greatly; various influences may lower it. Over the course of the sensitization process, the stimulation threshold can be lowered to a non-noxious level.

Along with their afferent sensory function, many nociceptors also have efferent functions that influence tissue processes. The efferent effect is due to the release of neuropeptides from the nerve endings. Neuropeptides stimulate receptors on other cells, causing vasodilation and increased permeability for instance.

In addition, neuropeptides can bring about the degranulation of mast cells. These, in turn, release inflammatory mediators and thus increase the sensitivity of the nociceptors. The release of the mediators from the nerve endings also leads to neurogenic inflammation, which contributes to the overall inflammation.

## Nociceptor Functions

- Triggering pain sensations.
- Influencing motor neurons in the muscles of the trunk, the extremities, the eyes, and the masticatory apparatus.
- Influencing the gamma system of regulation of muscle function.
- Influencing the cardiovascular and respiratory systems.

The term *alarm system* refers to the actual task of these receptors. Although they are often referred to as *pain receptors*, that term does not reflect the entire range of their functions.

## Response Behavior of Nociceptors

### Unimodal and Polymodal Nociceptors

#### Unimodal Nociceptors
- These react only to one quality (mechanical, chemical, thermal) of the irritating stimulus.
- Stimulation occurs if only a single quality of irritation is present.
- They increase their impulse rate in response to the following stimuli:
  - Noxious-mechanical (extreme pressure or tension on the body's tissues, e.g., meniscus damage).
  - Noxious-thermal (e.g., heat over + 45°C, e.g., touching a hot burner on the stove)
  - Noxious-chemical (e.g., irritation due to inflammatory mediators).

#### Polymodal Nociceptors
- These respond to several qualities.
- Stimulation occurs only with combined irritation.

- They increase their impulse rate in response to the following stimuli:
  - Noxious-mechanical + thermal
  - Noxious-mechanical + thermal + chemical.

> *Polymodal receptors are useful because the stimuli that trigger pain vary greatly and can occur in various combinations.*

### Primary Mechano-insensitive (Silent) Nociceptors

These normally do not respond to noxious stimuli. Yet, during an inflammatory process, they are sensitized to respond like polymodal nociceptors. If silent nociceptors are activated by an inflammation, they will respond to mechanical and thermal stimuli. Studies on silent nociceptors have shown that, after their sensitization, they demonstrate a discharge behavior that corresponds to pain perception (Weiss and Schaible 2003).

The sensitization of the nociceptors occurs via inflammatory mediators in the tissue (e.g., prostaglandin, bradykinin, serotonin, histamine).

### Non-nociceptive Neurons

These are not nociceptors, but rather their neurons that transmit pain; they, too, can respond to noxious stimuli.

## Altered Response Behavior of the Nociceptors

The response behavior of the nociceptors can change. For instance, due to increased synthesis and release of inflammatory mediators (histamine, bradykinin, serotonin, prostaglandins), tissue inflammation may lead to nociceptor sensitization in the following manner:
- The stimulation threshold for mechanical and thermal stimuli is lowered so much by the inflammation that a normally harmless stimulus may trigger impulses.
- The impulse frequency of the nociceptors increases.
- In "silent" nociceptors, even mechanical stimulation can trigger impulses.
- If afferent nerve fibers have been damaged they may be activated by transmitters in the sympathetic nervous system (e.g., adrenaline or similar substances), because they build adrenergic receptors.

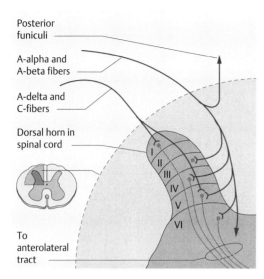

**Fig. 4.1** Structure of the dorsal horn in the spinal column with the Rexed laminae.

### 4.1.6 Transmission of Pain Impulses

The nociceptive process consists of the transmission of nociceptor impulses via the nociceptor axons to the spinal cord, and from there via the brainstem to the cortex. Conscious perception is the subjective perception of pain at higher levels in the brain.

#### Nociceptor Axons

- A-delta fibers: Thin myelinated fibers that respond very rapidly to stimuli and are located primarily in the skin. They trigger a bright, very well-localized, stabbing, cutting pain (primary pain).
- C-fibers: Thin, unmyelinated fibers that have a delayed response and trigger a dull, diffuse, burning, piercing pain (secondary pain).

#### Spinal Level

In the area of segmental connections in the dorsal horn, various phenomena for the modification of afferent input can occur and thus alter the pain. The information about the tissue damage is conducted in a well-localized form (via fast A-delta nerve fibers) and in a less well-localized form (via unmyelinated slow C-fibers) to the first synapse in the dorsal horn of the spinal cord (Wolff 1996).

The afferent fibers end in the spinal cord, in the laminae (layers) of the dorsal horn; these were numbered I–VI by the Swedish scientist Bror Rexed in 1952 (Fruhstorfer 1996; Melzack and Wall 1996).

The A-delta and the C-fibers end in the cell-rich laminae I and II (Rolando's gelatinous substance). Melzack and Wall (1996) suggest that this is also where inhibitory interneurons that block pain transmission are found (**Fig. 4.1**).

A few A-delta fibers end in lamina V. Laminae III and IV contain cells that can respond to low-threshold afferents of the thick A-beta fibers. Lamina VI is where the low-threshold afferents from the muscles and the joints end (Fruhstorfer 1996; Melzack and Wall 1996).

The dorsal horn contains three different types of cells (Melzack and Wall 1996):

- Cells that respond only to the low-threshold afferents from the A-beta fibers are located in laminae III and IV.
- Cells that respond only to high-threshold afferents from the thinner A-delta and C-fibers (specific nociceptive neurons).
- Cells that can respond to both afferents and thus are termed multi-receptive cells or *wide-dynamic-range cells* (WDR cells). They respond with a low discharge rate to non-noxious stimuli and with a high discharge rate to noxious stimuli. The cells have a low stimulation threshold; they also respond to non-noxious stimuli and are thus easily irritated.

Sensitization of the nociceptive neurons and the WDR cells plays a major role in central sensitization. Long-term incoming nociceptive stimuli lead to an increase in the receptors, which respond to nociception and the release of substances such as amino acids, glutamate, prostaglandins, and peptides such as substance P in the dorsal horn region. These substances lead to hyperacidity in the dorsal horn.

One hypothesis on central hypersensitivity is the dying off of inhibitory interneurons in the dorsal horn (dark cells) as well as sprouting of mechanoreceptive afferents in the dorsal horn to fibers of the spinothalamic tract. Both lead to potentiation of pain afferents (Zusman 1998).

The hyperacidity of the dorsal horn leads to death of pain-inhibiting interneurons. Nociceptive-specific neurons are activated. These are interneurons that stimulate the WDR cells and make them sensitive to pain stimuli and thus "open the door" toward the cortex (Butler 2000).

Noxious stimuli in the dorsal horn lead to stimulation of spinal motoneurons and vegetative neurons in the lateral horn. This explains the accompanying motor and vegetative response to pain (increased muscle tone) and vegetative reactions (altered blood circulation and sweating).

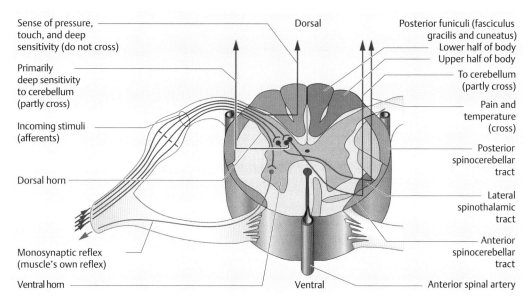

Sense of pressure, touch, and deep sensitivity (do not cross)

Primarily deep sensitivity to cerebellum (partly cross)

Incoming stimuli (afferents)

Dorsal horn

Monosynaptic reflex (muscle's own reflex)

Ventral horn

Dorsal

Ventral

Posterior funiculi (fasciculus gracilis and cuneatus)
Lower half of body
Upper half of body

To cerebellum (partly cross)

Pain and temperature (cross)

Posterior spinocerebellar tract

Lateral spinothalamic tract

Anterior spinocerebellar tract

Anterior spinal artery

**Fig. 4.2** Cross-section of the spinal cord with the conduction pathways.

In the traditional understanding of neurology, the transmission of pain afferents occurs in the anterolateral tract (lateral spinothalamic tract, spinomesencephalic tract, and spinoreticular tract). These tracts contain not only nociceptive fibers, but also non-nociceptive fibers. Other important structures are the dorsolateral portion of the spinothalamic tract and the *Lissauer tract*.

According to Gifford (2000), there are no typical pain pathways. This means that pain may travel in many various ways to the brain (**Fig. 4.2**).

## Central Regulatory Levels

### Brainstem

The reticular formation also plays a role in the transmission of motor, autonomic, and affective functions in response to noxious stimuli. It consists of a network of neurons in the brain stem with various chemical neuron systems and reflex centers; among other things, it is responsible for consciousness.

The neurons that are in relation in the medulla and mesencephalon to the reticular formation, and to the periaqueductal gray matter in the brainstem, seem especially important. They can produce autologous substances with morphine-like effects with an inhibitory effect on the pain stimuli. They are probably produced in the hypophysis (Benedetti 1997). The stimulation of these regions inhibits the transmission of noxious stimuli in the dorsal horn:

- Thalamus: In this important center, the arriving nociceptive stimuli are linked to the sensory, motor, and visceromotor centers. The thalamus region also connects the somatic afferent fibers with the cerebrum; only then is pain perceived. This makes it the "gateway to consciousness." Parts of the nuclear regions in the thalamus are the starting point for the lateral thalamocortical pain processing system, which analyzes somatosensory aspects of pain processing, localization, duration, and intensity.
- Cerebrum (neocortex and limbic system): While the cerebral cortex is primarily responsible for perception, discernment, localization, evaluating, and actively responding to the pain (cognitive component), the limbic system adds to the character of pain (affective and emotional components). The thalamic nuclei receive feedback projections from the somatosensory areas of the cortex.

## Plasticity

Repeated, severe pain can lead to a type of pain memory in the CNS. If new pain impulses are received, previous, similar ones are "recalled" and thus the current stimuli are perceived as more intense (Gifford 1999). Both the supraspinal system (spinal cord, brainstem, thalamus) for pain processing, as well as large portions of the somatosensory cortex, demonstrate plasticity.

## Mechanisms of Plasticity

- De-inhibition processes: Pain inhibition is reduced.
- Long-term potentiation (learning processes): Somatosensory reception fields increase in size with repeated stimulation.
- Sprouting of dendritic and axonal endings.

> *A patient who reports chronic pain is not imagining it. Some therapists may respond with astonishment or disbelief when the patient says he or she feels pain during the physical therapy examination; the symptoms are not clearly attributable to mechanical causes. The complex adaptive processes of the CNS can cause changes in pain processing that are often only partly reversible. Patients will usually have lasting pain symptoms.*

## Gate Control Theory (Melzack and Wall 1996)

Branches of the nerve fibers for pressure and touch (myelinated fibers = A-alpha fibers, A-beta fibers, and the non-nociceptive portion of A-delta fibers) pass to the second pain neurons in the dorsal horn of the spinal cord segment. There they form an inhibitory synapse (afferent, segmental inhibition).

Mechanical stimuli (e.g., massage and transcutaneous electrical nerve stimulation [TENS]) stimulate the above-named fibers and reduce the activity of the pain neurons. The same principle may be applied to nociceptive receptor pain to inhibit pain. In chronic pain, with changes affecting the CNS, there is no effect (or the pain may worsen under certain conditions). In these patients as well, mechanical stimuli are interpreted as pain stimuli.

Diseases that cause demyelination of the thick fibers for pressure and touch (e.g., polyneuropathies) reduce their activity and thus the inhibiting effect on the second pain neurons in the dorsal horn of the spinal cord. This explains the occurrence of spontaneous pain in these diseases.

### 4.1.7    Behavior Strategies at the Level of the Therapist–Patient Relationship

The experience of pain is not only the result of ascending nociceptive processes from peripheral structures. It is also influenced via descending tracts in the CNS. Cortical processes play a role in the integration of sensory and affective aspects of pain. Pain may be the result of processes in neural networks and can therefore occur in the absence of any tissue pathology. Cognitive, emotional, social, cultural, and behavioral aspects are therefore increasingly considered important factors in the experience of pain (Hengeveld 2003).

The new findings have led to the development of new thought models in research and clinical practice. These include biopsychosocial models, which are also relevant to physical therapy.

The most important one is the *Mature Organism Model* (MOM) (Gifford 1998, 2000). This notion describes a person as a biological being with a dynamic and plastic nervous system, in which input and output mechanisms constantly exert an influence. Information is constantly being absorbed from the environment and the body and, depending on physiological, affective, cognitive, and sociocultural influences (input), it is processed. This is expressed in physiological processes (e.g., changed muscle tone and vegetative responses) as well as in a person's behavior (e.g., avoidance of activities, withdrawal) (output). The special feature of this model is that the output of the system also influences the input. The experience of pain thus becomes a dynamic process. Impairment due to pain may occur as a direct result of cognitive, affective, or behavioral factors.

This notion shows that pain patients should not be treated in purely biomedical terms relating to the body's structures. The cognitive processing level is also very important. Pain patients must understand the cause of pain, the ability to withstand stress, and various factors that may influence the pain. This means that physical therapists must have solid clinical knowledge of pain. The output level may also be influenced. This may occur, for example, through body perception strategies or by influencing avoidance behavior by introducing activities and training in a step-by-step process.

Introducing a biopsychosocial perspective into the treatment of pain patients necessitates a deeper conceptualization of certain psychosocial aspects that physical therapists are confronted with on a daily basis. This usually occurs unconsciously (Hengeveld 2000).

For pain patients, treatment goals must be defined not only at the level of impairment (structures and functions), but also at the level of activities and participation (in society). Behavior and experience effects should be taken into consideration during the examination and treatment the same as the movement system.

Physical therapists analyze tissue processes, pain, suffering, and impairment, as well as the patient's experience of disease and behavior from a biopsychosocial perspective, and consider these aspects in treatment (Hengeveld 2000). This is the beginning of a clinical reasoning process that departs from a unidimensional approach where first the pain is relieved, and then the impairment automatically improves. This unidimensional approach is unproductive in pain patients.

The specific physical therapy examination of the body's structures and functions, as well as the patient's activities, followed by targeted treatment, should never be neglected. In addition to treatment techniques that influence receptor pain at the level of the body's structures (e.g., manual therapy, massage, electrotherapy), therapists should develop *coping strategies* with the patient.

Coping refers to the way in which people deal with difficulties in life (Waddell 1998). The physical therapist should help the patient with coping strategies early on so that he or she can use these in various everyday situations to influence their pain and their sense of well-being. In the acute phase, appropriate strategies can counteract the chronification of pain (e.g., movement in pain-free ranges promotes wound healing and the release of pain-inhibiting substances such as opioids).

Many pain patients use passive coping strategies only (e.g., medication, bed rest). These promote chronification (Wittink and Hoskins 1997). The use of merely passive physical therapy measures (e.g., massages) can also support chronification; the attention can encourage the patient's passive coping strategies.

If the patient learns to influence their pain, they may steadily lose their fear of movement. Movement avoidance strategies can be dismantled. These are often already present with acute pain, due to the fear of pain, and they have a negative influence on wound healing.

It can also help alleviate the fear of movement if the patient has knowledge of wound healing and the pathobiological process that occurs in the tissue. Patients need information and education strategies about the regeneration potential (e.g., of intervertebral disks), the influence of these processes, and the various neurophysiological pain mechanisms. The therapist should check whether the patient has absorbed and understood the information.

> Treatment should include an assessment of the patient's ideas about the source of pain and how he or she hopes to deal with it in the future.

The biopsychosocial thought model is new to physical therapy. There is thus a risk of overemphasizing these aspects while overlooking pathobiological processes or failing to perform a thorough manual therapy examination.

Hands-on therapy is a special feature of the physical therapy profession. This should not be forgotten when treating patients with chronic pain. Yet, mere hands-on therapy is also not the best option. A professional therapist–patient relationship is characterized by clinical reasoning strategies that take in the whole picture of the patient and lead to selection of the right treatment at the right time.

## 4.2 Physical Therapy Examination of Patients Whose Chief Symptom is Pain

> To understand the patient's pain situation, a thorough patient history is essential. It is impossible to fully assess and document his or her perception of pain. Pain is not measurable like temperature, weight, or range of motion. It is impossible to quantify it physically.

Another problem is the many factors that influence pain. These are shaped by pain perception and the pain behavior of the patient. Along with the physical symptoms of pain, psychosocial factors must also be considered; these may determine and sustain the process. Both components should be evaluated during the physical therapy assessment of pain in order to develop an adequate treatment approach.

The treatment concepts for acute nociceptive receptor pain mainly contain physical therapy techniques that act on the mechanoreceptors. Many of these are hands-on techniques (e.g., manual therapy, massage). In maladaptive chronic pain, the physical therapist must develop other treatment strategies. Patient management is crucial; hands-off therapies are also often used. For example, patients need to learn to overcome their fear of movement.

A good and thorough examination reassures the patient that he or she is being taken seriously. This is an important first step in building cooperation between the therapist and the patient. Often, pain patients have been assumed to be faking their symptoms, and, especially with chronic pain, the symptoms change frequently. Nor are they explainable on a purely mechanical level, and thus patients often face a lack of understanding as well as frustration on the part of doctors and therapists, because treatment often does not lead to immediate success.

At the end of the initial examination, the physical therapist should use the clinical reasoning process to develop hypotheses concerning the pathobiological processes as well as sources of the movement dysfunction. He or she should also develop additional prognoses and identify any potentially serious conditions (*red flags*).

Hypotheses about the patient's individual experience of disease should also be developed. Psychosocial factors (*yellow flags*) should be included in the patient history. These are related to the emotions and the expectations of the patient as well as interactions between them and their environment (Kendall et al 1997).

*Examples:*
- *Red flags:* Red flags are symptoms that can indicate serious disease. The physical therapist should refer the patient to their treating physician for further diagnostic testing, and the therapist should also contact the doctor directly. If any of the following symptoms are present, extra caution is warranted. These may be signs of a serious spinal disorder:
  - Age at the onset of symptoms < 20 years or > 50 years (note additional diseases)
  - Fever
  - Rapid weight loss
  - Progressive pain that is not due to mechanical causes
  - Significant trauma or a fall
  - Severe night pain (indication of inflammation)
  - Pain that worsens when the patient is lying down
  - Extensive neurological complaints (loss of sensation or strength)
  - History of cancer
  - Thoracic pain without any mechanical cause/change due to mechanical influences.
- *Yellow flags:* These refer to psychosocial factors and additional diseases that have an influence on the pain behavior of the patient and increase the risk of chronification of pain:
  - Fear of consequences
  - Worry about the future
  - Dissatisfaction with work
  - Extremely caring partner
  - Expectation of compensation (e.g., after a car accident)
  - Depression

- Restlessness
- Additional diseases (e.g., diabetes mellitus) that have a negative influence on the neural system and wound healing
- Fear of movement
- Passive coping strategies (e.g., doctor-hopping).

### 4.2.1  Patient History

### Pain Characteristics

#### *Pain Location*

The site of the pain and its origin may be identical, although often this is not the case. Pain may also be felt away from the site of tissue damage. The pattern of pain often involves several structures. Radiating pain often depends on the structure causing it, and the extent may vary:

*Examples:*
- *Compression of the spinal nerve root:* When a spinal nerve root is damaged, the pain may radiate into the corresponding area of skin, but does not always follow a dermal distribution.
- *Hyperalgesia of skin zones due to visceral pain:* Pain fibers from internal organs form synapses at the same switching neurons in the dorsal horn of the spinal cord as the pain fibers from skin areas. If an internal organ is damaged, the patient perceives pain mainly in the skin, because the CNS interprets the cause of pain as trauma from an external source (e.g., with ischemic noxious irritation of the cardiac muscle, the pain often projects into the left arm). The patient feels pain in areas of the skin whose afferents project into the same segments as the primary afferents from the internal organs. These *Head zones* are named after the neurologist who discovered them (Head 1898). In this way, various physical therapy measures, such as connective tissue massage, influence the internal organs via the skin zones.
- *Referred pain:* If there is a dysfunction affecting a spinal facet joint, referred pain may occur in the supply area in the shoulder/arm (cervical spine) or pelvis/leg region (lumbar spine) related to this motion segment.

In a study by Fukui et al (1996) in the region of the cervical spine (**Fig. 4.3**), in symptomatic patients, the facet joint, which was provoking pain, was infiltrated with a contrast agent. Local anesthesia elimi-

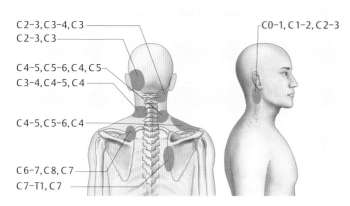

C2–3, C3–4, C3

C2–3, C3

C4–5, C5–6, C4, C5

C3–4, C4–5, C4

C4–5, C5–6, C4

C6–7, C8, C7

C7–T1, C7

C0–1, C1–2, C2–3

**Fig. 4.3** Source of pain in facet joint: pain area based on Fukui et al (1996); C2–C3 = facet joint, C3 = medial branch of the dorsal branch in the corresponding segment.

nated the pain, and the anesthetic was injected again into the facet joint. Among the patients who responded to the procedure, the medial branch of the dorsal root was electrically stimulated. They then marked the site of their pain on a body chart.

Using this procedure, Fukui et al (1996) were able to identify the pattern of radiating pain from the facet joint and dorsal branch separately from one another.

## Pain Quality

- Stabbing and rapid pain that can be precisely localized, if conducted via A-delta fibers (30 m/ second).
- Dull, piercing, and lasting pain that cannot be well-localized, if conducted via C-fibers, 3 m/second).
- Burning pain after myelin damage of the sheath surrounding the peripheral nerves, e.g., in neuropathy.
- Pulsating pain may be a sign of inflammation.
- Hyperalgesia: Increased sensitivity to pain.
- Allodynia: Normally nonpainful touch causes pain.

## Type of Pain

- Neuropathic pain: Pain caused by a lesion or disease of the somatosensory nervous system (Treede et al 2008).
- Physiological nociceptor pain:
  - Superficial pain: Origin of pain in the skin.
  - Deep pain: Origin of pain in the joints, bones, connective tissue, or muscles.
- Visceral pain (pathophysiological nociceptor pain): Origin in the internal organs, but sometimes projected to the surface (see Hyperalgesia of skin zones due to visceral pain, p. 154).

- Psychogenic pain: Origin in the CNS. Not every pain that is felt is caused by nociceptor irritation and transmission via pain pathways.

## Duration of Pain

- Acute: Sudden onset, appeared recently.
- Chronic: Not only is time an essential factor, but also whether the pain is related to tissue damage or not.
- Intermittent: The pain occurs in intervals and periodically decreases.
- Physiological (adaptive): The pain has a purpose, for example, after acute trauma it protects the damaged tissue against strain to aid tissue healing.
- Pathological (maladaptive): The pain no longer has a function. It often occurs as a constant, persistent pain and cannot be influenced mechanically. Although the tissue has long since healed, the pain persists. Many factors play a role in the development of maladaptive pain, for example, the emotional response to the pain. Fear, depression, or anger can lead to an increased release of epinephrine from the adrenal medulla. In the peripheral tissues, this causes the release of neurotransmitters such as prostaglandins, catecholamine, and noradrenaline. The neurotransmitters produce a neurogenic inflammation in the peripheral tissue, which leads to a vicious circle. The neurotransmitters, in turn, cause tissue damage that triggers stimulation of nociceptors in the periphery. Thus, the emotional response of the patient leads to the release of adrenaline. This mechanism can lead to a prolonged cycle of pain that can be self-sustaining (see pp. 143–145).

## Conditions of Onset (24-hour Pain Behavior)

- Usually due to strain
- Mainly at rest, night pain
- Often associated with certain activities

As a part of therapy, chronic pain patients should record their pain behavior in a diary for a certain length of time. Even minimal changes in the pain behavior will thus be evident. The patient should be instructed to make an entry in a table roughly every 2 hours, noting the pain intensity and any accompanying symptoms. The patient should include the date of their physical therapy so the treating physician can also see its influence.

## Accompanying Symptoms

- Changes to the circulation in the hands and sweat gland secretion: This occurs as a result of sympathetic reflexes. After the pain impulses have arrived in the CNS, the impulses are carried away in the descending tracts. These pass to the sympathetic neurons in the lateral horn of the spinal cord, and then on with the spinal nerves to the cutaneous vessels, sweat glands, and smooth muscles of the skin hairs.
- Tonus changes affecting the musculature.
- Muscle atrophy and regional osteoporosis (objectifiable sign of protection): The protection of the painful body part can lead to muscle atrophy and regional osteoporosis.

### 4.2.2   Documentation of Pain History

A *body chart* may be used to document the pain characteristics. The patients should draw the site of the pain. If there are several pain sites, they may number these hierarchically in order to emphasize the primary pain (see 4.2.7 Pain Measurement).

The patient should describe the quality of pain in his or her own words, for example, "I feel like there are ants crawling on my legs" (sign of paresthesia—involvement of neural structures?). Adjective lists are also available, for example, in the McGill Pain Questionnaire (see section 4.2.7). Scales may be suitable for reporting the intensity of pain. The patient may estimate the intensity of pain using, for example, a visual analogue scale (VAS scale; see section 4.2.7).

For developing various hypotheses about the patient's individual experience of disease, the physical therapist should ask specific questions:

- What does the patient know about their problem?
- What does the patient expect from treatment?
- How can the patient influence their pain (whether the patient tends to use passive or active coping strategies; see 4.1.7, Behavior Strategies)?
- How does the patient see their future?
- How is the patient's partner responding to his or her disease?

Especially in pain patients, the patient history is an essential part of the evaluation. The patient history enables the therapist to develop an initial hypothesis; it also provides information about any additional strategies needed for examination and treatment. The physical therapist must learn to listen closely and observe carefully, and to use these skills from the beginning of the greeting phase and when taking the patient history. This will help obtain clues to the patient's experience of their pain and their pain behavior.

### 4.2.3   Movement Behavior

The main question in terms of movement behavior is whether the patient's spontaneous movement behavior agrees with his or her description of the pain behavior.

**Example:** A patient complains of persistent pain in the lumbar spine and buttock region with a score of 9 on the VAS. When getting dressed or undressed, however, there are no signs of protective mechanisms. At first glance, her report and her behavior do not seem to fit together; this is usually seen in patients with chronic pain. Due to the complexity of pain processing and chronification, the patient continues to report her subjective pain as extremely intense. Positive experiences and impressions may make it seem to diminish temporarily (see p. 144).

During the interview and later examination, the therapist should note the patient's gestures and facial expression, as well as his or her responses (e.g., shouting out if touched without pressure). The more acute and intense the pain, the more care must be taken during the examination. At the same time, exaggerated reactions should be filtered out. This is very difficult, especially for novices and physical therapy students. They have not yet stored many clinical patterns and therefore may not detect an exaggerated response.

If the therapist suspects that the patient's response may be exaggerated, *distraction maneuvers* during the examination may be used. These allow

**Table 4.1** Waddell test

| Five categories | Symptoms |
|---|---|
| Tenderness | • Superficial tenderness on the back, also over the area supplied by the dorsal branch<br>• Deep tenderness over a widespread area affecting the entire spine |
| Simulation maneuver | • Compression: Low back pain with application of slight compression on the skull in the standing patient<br>• Trunk rotation: Low back pain with simultaneous extension of the shoulder girdle and pelvis |
| Distraction maneuver | If the SLR is not positive in the sitting position, but was definitely positive when the patient was supine (see example below with patient supine, legs stretched out in front) |
| Neuroanatomy | Sensory disorders that cannot be attributed to a dermatome, and diminished strength that cannot be attributed to a segment |
| Overreaction | Exaggerated responses during the examination, such as pulling a face, groaning, or muscle tension, tremors, collapse, or sweating (note: risk of over-interpretation) |

one to distinguish objective parameters from subjective ones.

**Example:** During the straight leg raise (SLR) test the patient reports pain at 20° bending of the hip joint. However, he can sit with both legs stretched in front of him without any difficulty. In this position, the hip joint is also flexed, and the knee joint is extended. Thus, the neural structures are just as tense as in the SLR test. If the nerve were so irritated that even 20° bending were difficult, then it would be impossible to sit with both legs stretched out in front.

To determine the prognosis for healing and returning to work, various tests have been developed that can provide information about the behavior and cause of the pain. Are the causes organic, or do psychogenic factors dominate? These tests are used by doctors to estimate retirement age for example, and they are also used to diagnose and treat pain patients. They are also suitable for the physical therapy examination if there are signs of an exaggerated pain response without a clear organic cause.

Using the example of back pain, various tests may be used to determine whether it is due to psychogenic causes; this would increase the risk of chronification and reduce the chances of eliminating the pain. During none of the tests should the back be so strained that the pain could worsen due to mechanical reasons. If the patient still reports more intense pain on the VAS, or if he or she has an exaggerated response to pain, this suggests psychogenic pain behavior. Thus, different treatment strategies must be selected than those used for acute mechanical pain (Waddell test, **Table 4.1**).

## Tests for Developing a Prognosis for Back Pain

If two of the following four tests are positive, the chances that the patient will be able to resume work again are lower. Treatment that merely addresses the level of the body's structures and functions has little chance of success:

- *Step test:* The patient should climb up and down stairs (height: 30 cm) for 3 minutes and then report the intensity of his or her pain using the VAS.
- *Arm holding test:* In the supine position, the patient should hold two 3 kg weights with their arms outstretched toward the ceiling. Afterward, they should report the intensity of their pain.
- *Pain scale* (1–10).
- *Waddell sign* (**Table 4.1**): The Waddell test is considered positive if at least three of the five categories apply:
  - There is no clear organic cause underlying the back pain.
  - During the examination and treatment, psychosocial risk factors (yellow flags) must be taken into account.
  - Often, there is fear of pain and the prognosis.

*The individual signs should not be over-interpreted. The test does not rule out the possibility of organic factors.*

*During the test, one should not make a psychological diagnosis.*

## Effect of Nociceptive Signal on the Sequence of Movement

Every disorder signaled by the nociceptors leads to a reflexive change in the sequence of movement. It occurs already before the nociception is perceived by the patient. There is a change in muscle tone, and any muscle whose activity worsens the problem becomes hypotonic. Those muscles that may protect the problem site against further damage, for instance, by maintaining the joint in a certain position, become hypertonic. The cause of the problem is initially irrelevant for this neurovegetative reflex mechanism for the protection of the area around a lesion.

### 4.2.4    Symptoms of Altered Tonicity Affecting the Musculature

### Hypotonic Muscles

- Tenderness of the muscle increases when it contracts.
- Contraction pain.
- Painful muscle fatigue.
- Fascicular twitching when the muscle is tired.

### Hypertonic Muscles

- Tenderness of the muscle increases when it stretches.
- Stretching pain.
- Painfully stiff muscles.
- Cogwheel rigidity during passive stretching, that is, muscle gives way in jerks as it stretches.

Both muscle groups are less able to withstand stress, fatigue very quickly, and have significantly diminished strength. Such muscular symptoms are often first noticed by the patient when there is a problem affecting the locomotor system.

**Example:** A patient with beginning hip joint arthritis feels increasing stiffness in the muscle surrounding the hip, especially after getting up in the morning. After walking around for about 15 minutes, he feels as if his legs are tired and lame. Although he does not yet feel any typical joint pain, people have mentioned his "side-to-side" gait to him and say that it has worsened in recent weeks. He had not yet noticed that he had developed a limp as a type of protection in response to the problem.

## Fear of Movement is Common Among Patients with Pain

The fear of pain can lead to avoidance strategies. Patients avoid any movement that, in their experience, has a negative influence on their pain. This is a reasonable strategy during the acute phase, when pain functions as a warning signal. Given their reduced ability to withstand strain, the affected structures need rest until wound healing is complete. This does not mean, however, that they should not move at all. It is the physical therapist's responsibility to inform the patient about wound healing and regeneration of the body's structures, and to work together with him or her on protective movement behavior for the injured parts of the body. This will help the patient regain trust in movement functions.

---

**Case Study 1**
A patient with an acute herniated disk in the lumbar spine experienced extreme pain exacerbation after getting up quickly from the supine position. The pain shot like lightning into his right leg. Since then, he hardly trusts himself to move, because he is afraid it will happen again. He holds his spine very stiffly when walking and has a protective position with loss of lumbar lordosis and sidebending to the opposite side.
In nonweight-bearing starting positions, the physical therapist works on movements of the lumbar spine that do not involve lifting weight against gravity. At the moment, only bending and sidebending (toward the pain-free side) are possible without increasing the pain. The patient only feels confident performing the movements after the therapist has explained the conditions involved in disk healing. He learns that movement is essential in the acute phase as well, using self-exercises.
He also learns how to get up from lying on his back by rolling first onto his side. When doing so, he experiences that this is less painful than his previous strategy. As a result of the self-exercises, his previously very tense muscles (due to the protective posture) relax, and he feels increasingly better. The economic way he is able to get up also increases his independence. His confidence in these movements grows. Under the guidance of the physical therapist, he gradually feels confident performing more movements, and he varies his positions as he becomes familiar with various nonweight-bearing positions and postures.

---

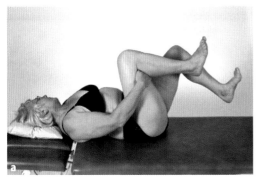 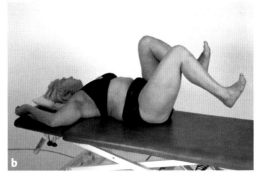

**Fig. 4.4a, b** Self-exercises for reactive abdominal muscle activation in the supine position.
**a** Easier version, supporting the leg with the hand. **b** Increasing the difficulty.

*During the examination, the therapist should observe the spontaneous movement behavior of the patient. The therapist should avoid being obvious about it, however, because if the patient feels "watched" he or she will probably stop moving spontaneously and choose different strategies than they would in everyday life.*

## Analyzing Pain-triggering Movements with the Patient

Pain-provoking activities and sequences of movements should be analyzed together with the patient. These provide them with important information. The patient should actively participate in the analysis. After the patient has received information on the triggering of pain and the reduced ability of the structure to withstand stress, the therapist should share his or her thoughts about why a certain movement sequence worsens the pain.

### Case Study 2

A patient has a painful lumbar spine when she raises her outstretched leg in the supine position, for example when standing up. Her abdomen protrudes strongly, and she has diastasis recti.

The therapist explains the functional relationships (i.e., lacking ventral connection, tension from the iliopsoas muscles worsens hyperlordosis). When she performs the movements again, the patient experiences these relationships through perception of the distances of the abdomen as well as the supporting surface under the lumbar spine.

Together, the therapist and the patient should develop strategies for avoiding pain. The patient learns that before getting up she should first roll onto her side after flexing the hip and knee joints to shorten the lever for the lumbar spine.

She is also given self-exercises for reactive abdominal activation with a leg weight (**Fig. 4.4a, b**). While lying on her back, she holds her legs with maximum hip and knee joint bending against her stomach so she feels the contact between the lumbar spine and the table. From this position, she learns to slowly bring one leg down to the table, without losing contact between the lumbar spine and the table. The movement amplitude can gradually be increased.

## Avoidance Strategies and Fear Promote the Chronification of Pain

Over time, the extreme fear of movement, and the resulting avoidance strategies, strains the body's structures. This is the start of a vicious cycle. The body's structures need to move to live, and lacking movement promotes their degeneration.

The steadily decreasing ability to withstand strain lowers the stress threshold; constant triggering of irritation promotes new pain processes. As a result of the diminished movement ability, the patient increasingly loses their independence in everyday life, and they are less able to participate in social life. Depression and pain chronification can result.

### 4.2.5 Nociceptive Receptor Pain from the Structures of the Locomotor System

Pain may be triggered by the following structures in the locomotor system:

## Joints

In terms of the joints, one should distinguish between degenerative and inflammatory causes of pain. The following articular structures may cause nociception:
- Subchondral layers of the articular surface
- Periosteum
- Ligaments
- Joint capsule
- Synovial membrane
- Bursae

### Degenerative Joint Pain

*Causes*
- Result of trauma
- Being in damp conditions for a long period of time

*Localization*
Joint or spinal pain that radiates into the related soft-tissue structures (muscles, tendons, ligaments).

*Pain Quality*
- Dull and piercing, usually deeper
- Acute and sharp with impingement (menisci or joint mouse)

*Onset of Pain*
- Morning, start-up pain
- Increased pain with stress
- Rapid fatigue
- Later, also night pain or pain at rest

*Specific Examination*
- Joint swelling (in active osteoarthritis), assuming nonweight-bearing positions or postures, and possibly limping.
- During palpation, the joints respond with local tenderness, and in the surrounding muscle changes in muscle tone may be palpated.
- When testing movement, pain with movement or restricted motion are present, although not all directions of movement are equally limited (capsular pattern).
- Because of the pain, the patient's strength rapidly diminishes, and the muscle tone changes and

becomes hypertonic or hypotonic. There is contraction or stretching pain of the muscle.

> The impairment of everyday activities depends on the stage of osteoarthritis.

*Pain Provocation*
- If there is involvement of the subchondral region, the joint responds with pain on compression. The therapist should apply compression perpendicularly to the treatment plane.
- In patients who only experience pain with stress, compression is applied using the force of weight.

**Example:** Single-leg standing stresses the hip joint. The therapist should ask the patient to rise onto his or her toes and drop down again onto their heel. The resulting force places stress on the weight-bearing portion of the hip joint. It may reproduce the pain that patient reports related to walking.

### Inflammatory Joint Pain

*Causes*
- Inflammatory bone disease and tumors
- Joint effusion

*Localization*
- Articular or spinal pain with diffuse radiating pain into the surrounding area
- Local periosteal pain with bone processes

*Pain Quality*
There is massive, sharp, pulsating, piercing, inflammatory pain.

*Onset of Pain*
- Extreme, persistent pain
- Pain at rest, and especially at night, worsening in the early morning hours

*Specific Examination*
- Massive swelling and loss of joint contours are seen. Patients assume nonweight-bearing positions and postures, and they report feeling very unwell. They fatigue quickly, and often they are feverish.
- Palpation reveals excessive warmth and severe local tenderness about the inflamed joint.
- The patient's autonomy is extremely restricted, because the painful joint cannot tolerate any strain or movement.
- When testing movement there is extremely painful limitation in all directions. Inflammatory

changes in the region of the joint capsule worsen the pain if the capsule is placed under tension (e.g., due to traction).

- There is a significant loss of strength as a result of pain. All of the surrounding muscles become hypotonic; any movement exacerbates the pain.
- The constant pain disturbs the patient's sleep at night.
- Patients often appear sad or sometimes even angry at the persistent pain.

### Pain Provocation

The joint responds to pressure (compression) and tension (traction, hanging weights) with severe pain.

## Ligaments

### Source

Especially in hypermobile joints, stretching, compressive, and tensile forces strain the ligamentous structures, given the altered rotational axes.

### Localization

At the insertion sites of the tendons and ligaments, there is local receptor pain, often radiating into the related musculature.

### Pain Quality

- Diffuse, dull, pulling, piercing pain.
- When the spine is involved, patients often report a feeling of "giving way."

### Onset of Pain

The pain steadily worsens if the patient stays in one position for a prolonged period of time.

### Specific Examination

- Joint malposition (e.g., genu recurvatum—knee joints are hyperextended when standing or walking, axis deviations at the knee joints with increased valgus position, increased lumbar lordosis). Patients with pain in the lumbar spine often stand with their legs far apart.
- Poor constitutional factors may worsen the altered position of the joints and increase the provocation of the ligament pain (e.g., extra abdominal weight can increase lordosis).
- Trophic conditions of the skin are changed.
- There are doughy-looking transverse striations about the spinal column. The folds are indented; there is hardening of the skin and subcutaneous tissue. In hypermobile spinal segments, the skin is thicker with large pores. Upon palpation, there is extreme reddening of hyperalgesic zones.

- Patients avoid being in one-sided positions for longer periods of time (e.g., standing in one spot for a long period of time).
- Passive movements about the hypermobile joints and translational joint play are greater.

### Pain Provocation

- If the ligaments are placed under tension during the stability tests, they respond after about 30 seconds with pain radiating into the related musculature.
- Palpation reveals local tenderness at the insertion site or over the actual ligament.
- If there is long-standing pressure, the pain radiates.

## Gliding Structures (Bursae, Tendon Sheaths)

### Causes

- Rheumatic or metabolic diseases (e.g., primary chronic polyarthritis [PCP], gout)
- Hormonal or vitamin imbalance (e.g., with major hormonal changes, menopause, vitamin E deficiency)
- Single or repeated microtrauma

### Localization

Locally, over the bursae and tendon sheaths.

### Pain Quality

The pain has a pulling, tearing quality.

### Onset of pain

Pain often occurs following a strain injury or after repeatedly performing the same task.

### Specific Examination

- Local swelling in the bursa region.
- On palpation, the bursae are suddenly palpable due to swelling; pain worsens with pressure application. Movement produces crepitation about the tendon sheaths.
- Motion is painful and usually limited in certain directions (e.g., in subacromial bursitis, shoulder abduction is most severely limited).
- There is less pain with movement, as long as the joint is in a nonweight-bearing position (e.g., in subacromial bursitis, abduction is less painful if tension is applied to the humerus, as this frees up the subacromial space).

### Pain Provocation

- Pain affecting the bursae may be provoked by compression.

**Example:** Pain affecting the subacromial bursa may be provoked by upward movement of the head of the humerus. Compression applied via the humerus in the direction of the acromion can trigger pain.

- During palpation, the tendon sheaths respond with pain to local pressure or tensile forces.

**Example:** Pain affecting the tendon sheaths for the finger flexors may be provoked during passive dorsal finger extension. Elbow extension increases the effect.

## Muscular Causes of Pain

### Causes

- Reflexive changes to muscle tone in order to protect a lesion (e.g., in degenerated or blocked joints)
- Stress or strain, often due to static conditions and constitutional deviations
- After trauma (e.g., muscle tear)

### Localization

- Local pain affecting the muscle; pain increases with contraction or stretching. The muscle often exhibits an increased tendency to cramp when it contracts. There is a significantly increased sensitivity to stretching.
- Pain affects all aspects of muscle synergy, that is, in all muscles forming a functional unit. This leads to *chain reactions.*

### Pain Quality

- Diffuse, dull, piercing pain.
- Bright and sharp about the trigger points (local circumscribed areas of muscle hardening).
- Activated trigger points demonstrate radiating pain into one of their typical reference areas.
- Latent trigger points respond to pressure with dull, local pain.

### Onset of Pain

- Start-up pain after longer-term immobilization (e.g., morning pain) or staying in one position for a prolonged period of time.
- Pain worsens if the muscle contracts or stretches.
- Ischemic pain with static contraction.

### Specific Examination

- If the pain persists for a longer period of time, muscle atrophy, or more pronounced muscle contours with extreme hardening of the muscle may be found.
- During movement testing, there is altered movement quality. Resistance may be increased, and often there is cogwheel rigidity. Motion may be restricted.
- Active movement (especially eccentric muscle activity) triggers pain.
- Passive movements are painless. At the end of the movement, there is increased sensitivity to stretching.
- The affected muscles are tender. Tenderness may increase with contraction or stretching of the muscle. Local hardening of the muscle responds to pressure with radiating pain and active trigger points.

### Pain Provocation

- Palpation of the muscle belly, the musculotendinous junction, and the tenoperiosteal junction, causes pain. In the region of the muscle belly, there are often active trigger points that respond to pressure with radiating pain.
- Static contraction from the middle position and dynamic concentric and eccentric contraction trigger pain. Strength is diminished.
- Muscle selection test: Often several muscles in a single muscle group have the same function. The affected muscle may be identified by testing the individual muscles.
- The following questions should first be answered:
  - What are the individual muscles that make up the group?
  - How do they differ in terms of course and function? Do other muscles in the group have secondary functions?
  - Which antagonistic functions may be used for differentiation?

**Example:** Muscle selection in the region of the hand extensors (**Fig. 4.5a, b**)
Active wrist extension against resistance is painful throughout the entire group of muscles. Point tenderness is found over the belly of the muscle and its origin on the lateral epicondyle. The extensor carpi radialis brevis muscle and the extensor digitorum both originate on the epicondyle and are active during wrist extension. They may be distinguished from one another due to the additional function of the extensor digitorum muscle (finger extension).

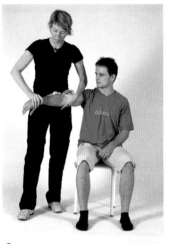
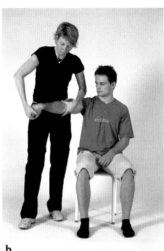

**Fig. 4.5a, b** Pain provocation test of the hand extensors.
**a** Extensor carpi radialis muscle.
**b** Extensor digitorum muscle.

a

b

When testing the extensor carpi radialis brevis muscle, the extensor digitorum may be inhibited by having the patient grasp an object.

The evaluation of the extensor digitorum muscle tests finger extension against resistance, while the patient presses his or her palm against the table. This causes reciprocal inhibition due to the activity of the antagonists of the extensor carpi radialis brevis muscle.

- Static resistance from a "pre-stretched" position: With tension from the middle position, the muscle will not respond to mild irritation. The provocation may be greatly increased using a "pre-stretched" position. First, static tensing is used to test the muscle. If the patient fails to respond, the provocation may be increased to its maximum, with dynamic eccentric and concentric contraction against resistance, from a "pre-stretched" position.

> *Muscle selection is used here the same as for testing from the middle position.*

### Examples:
- The starting position for testing the extensor carpi radialis brevis muscle is volar bending with elbow extension and forearm pronation; the fingers should remain relaxed. From this position, the patient actively performs dorsal extension, keeping the fingers relaxed.
- The starting position for testing the extensor digitorum muscle is finger bending and volar bending, along with simultaneous elbow extension and pronation. From here, the patient actively performs finger extension.

## Nerves

### Causes
Pain is triggered by direct irritation of nerve pathways:
- Mechanical irritation due to pressure on the nerve root in patients with intervertebral disk herniation.
- Pressure applied to the peripheral nerve in compression syndrome (e.g., carpal tunnel syndrome = compression of the median nerve, for example, due to swelling of the tendon sheaths in the carpal tunnel).
- Applying pressure to the nerve increases the tension and exacerbates the pain. Gliding of the nerve may be impaired.

### Localization
- Local or projected pain in the area supplied by the nerve or the nerve root
- Sharply demarcated

### Pain Quality
- Bright, stabbing, cutting, sharp, tingling, or shooting pain; pulsating pain is often seen in involvement of the autonomous nervous system.
- In nerve root compression, sudden, shooting pain occurs in the respective innervation area.

### Onset of Pain
- In nerve root compression (radicular pain), the pain occurs in weight-bearing positions. Pain can radiate into the dermatome. Movement that constricts the intervertebral foramen often provokes the pain (e.g., extension and rotation).

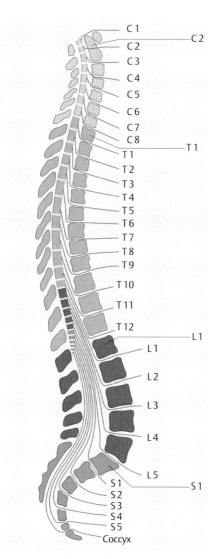

**Fig. 4.6** The relationships between the motion segments and the spinal cord segments along with the exit sites of the spinal nerves.

- Highly acute pain can also occur in non-weight-bearing positions.
- Any motion, including coughing, abdominal pressure, or sneezing may worsen the pain.
- In peripheral nerve compression, pain occurs in its sensory innervation area. There may be steady pain, which worsens with increased tension on the nerve or if pressure is applied to the site of constriction.

***Specific Neurological Examination***
- In radicular compression, the affected area may be held in a nonweight-bearing position; peripheral

compression may be accompanied by muscle atrophy.
- Involvement of the autonomic nervous system often involves swelling of the extremities. As a result of altered blood circulation, the skin is often a bluish color, and sometimes it may be taut or have a shiny appearance.
- Active and passive movements trigger pain. If the irritation is severe, the pain continues after the movement.
- The sensitivity of the nervous system to movement and pressure may be tested using neural tension (e.g., straight leg raise), described in Chapter 2.1.6.
- The neurological examination may reveal reflex and sensory disturbances (hyperesthesia, hyperalgesia, paresthesia) in the dermatome or in the area of the peripheral nerve. There may be motor deficits affecting the segment-indicating muscles or muscles supplied by the peripheral nerve. Abnormal secretion of sweat occurs only with peripheral nerve lesions.

***Basic Principles of the Neurological Examination***
Damage to the peripheral nerve pathway is also seen in orthopedic patients. The cause is usually compression, for example, disk prolapse, spinal canal stenosis, or peripheral compression neuropathies.

This portion of the examination involves various tests that distinguish individual peripheral disturbances. Damage to the peripheral nerve pathway can affect the following:
- Spinal nerve/spinal root (nerve root)
- Peripheral nerve

Depending on the height of the lesion, various symptoms can dominate; these may be identified during the neurological examination. To understand the different symptoms, a brief look at neuroanatomy is helpful.

### 4.2.6    Neuroanatomy of the Peripheral and Spinal Nerves

The number of the spinal cord segments corresponds to the exiting spinal nerves (**Fig. 4.6**). In the region of the cervical spine, eight segments may be distinguished (C1–C8), given that eight spinal nerves exit here. The first spinal nerve arises between the occiput and the atlas. In the cervical spine, the spinal nerve is thus referred to by the vertebra above which it exits:

- The spinal nerves T1–T12 exit from the thoracic spine; these are named after the vertebra below which they exit.
- The spinal nerves L1–L5 exit from the lumbar spine and are also named after the vertebra below which they exit.
- The spinal nerves S1–S5 exit the sacral canal via the intervertebral foramina.

The discrepancy between the spinal cord segment in relation to the motion segment from which the spinal nerve exits increases from cranial to caudal. In the cervical spine, the spinal cord and the motion segment are at the same height.

The difference starts in the thoracic spine. At the level of the motion segment TI–T6, it is two spinal cord segments; and at the level of T7–T9, it is three spinal cord segments. The region of T9–T10 contains the lumbar spinal cord segments, and at T11–L1 are the sacral spinal cord segments. The spinal cord ends at L1–L2, and below this the spinal nerves travel in the spinal canal as the cauda equina.

The peripheral motor nerve fibers leave the spinal cord through the ventral root. In each segment, a certain number of nerve fibers join and thus form the motor portion of the spinal nerve.

The peripheral sensory nerve fibers enter the spinal cord via the dorsal root. Their cell bodies are in the spinal ganglion, which is found outside of the CNS. They are responsible for impulse conduction of sensory information (e.g., from the skin, muscles, tendons, and joint capsules).

The general principle still holds that all *sensory* fibers (including nociceptive ones) reach the spinal cord via the dorsal root, while all *motor* fibers leave via the ventral root. The notion of a strict division appears to be increasingly questionable based on the results of clinical studies.

According to Coggeshall (1973), 30% of the fibers in the ventral root are unmyelinated, and a large number of them at all levels of the spinal nerve are nociceptive in nature. This is an important neuroanatomical finding in terms of our understanding of the symptoms related to ventral root compression. These are by no means merely motor symptoms, but are also nociceptive in nature.

Clinical findings have supported the involvement of the ventral root in the conduction of nocisensory impulses (Winkel et al 1985). Before exiting the spinal column, the spinal nerve unites before traversing the intervertebral foramen to become the spinal root. The spinal root exits the intervertebral foramen—surrounded by a "sleeve" called the dura mater (the "hard skin" of the spinal cord)—distal to the spinal ganglion and continues into the epineurium (outermost layer of a peripheral nerve).

Compared with a peripheral nerve, a spinal nerve has a much more sensitive structure. The nerve fibers are parallel, rather than wavy as they are in peripheral nerves. This makes the spinal nerve much more vulnerable to outside pressure or tension and more susceptible to injury.

Each spinal nerve branches off outside the intervertebral foramen into a dorsal branch and a ventral branch. Both contain somatomotor and somatosensory fibers. The spinal nerve also contains autonomic fibers (afferent and efferent), for example for the innervation of blood vessels of the locomotor system. Compression would thus also change the circulation in the segmental area.

The meningeal branch (recurrent nerve) contains somatic afferent fibers and autonomic afferent and efferent fibers. If there is damage of the spinal nerve root, the anterior (motor) roots, or the dorsal (sensory) roots, or both may be affected. If there is compression of the anterior roots of T2–L2, sympathetic fibers may also be compressed. Above T2 (arm region) and below L2 (leg region), there are more sympathetic fibers only distal to the spinal nerve roots. Thus, in these regions, damage to the nerve root does not cause sympathetic nerve symptoms. This important difference is relevant for the differential diagnosis of damage of the roots and peripheral nerves.

## Innervation Areas of the Various Portions of the Spinal Nerves

### Dorsal Branch

This is a monosegmental (limited to one segment) nerve. It provides *sensory* innervation to the joint capsule of the intervertebral joints (spinal joints). Several branches from various dorsal branches innervate a single spinal joint; innervation is not monosegmental. Thus, pain from a single intervertebral joint radiates over several segments.

In terms of *motor* innervation, it supplies the autochthonous back muscles and provides *sensory* innervation to the dermatome (area of skin supplied by the segment) in the dorsal region. The skin and zones of subcutaneous tissue that receive sensory and autonomic innervation from the dorsal branches of the spinal nerves extend from the crown of the head over the occiput, and then continue paramedian to the midline (about a hand-width) into the region of the sacral hiatus. The area ends in a diamond shape, the lower sides of which run diagonally over the gluteal region while the distal sides are roughly marked by the anal fold.

### Meningeal Branch (Sinuvertebral Nerve or Recurrent Nerve)

The meningeal branch primarily contains autonomic afferent fibers (e.g., nocisensory fibers) and postganglionic fibers from the sympathetic trunk. The branch runs monosegmentally back through the intervertebral foramen into the spinal cord. It sends collateral branches into the spinal canal, which bridge various segments caudally and cranially. It innervates the following tissues:

- Posterior longitudinal ligament
- Annulus fibrosus of the intervertebral disk
- Vertebral body and arch
- Anterior portion of the dura mater
- Ventral root

> *Symptoms associated with compression of the dura mater (e.g., due to disk protrusion) thus never affect merely a single segment, but rather spread over multiple segments, often bilaterally.*

### Ventral Branch

The ventral branches of the cervical, lumbar, and sacral spinal nerves blend to form plexuses (cervical plexus, brachial plexus, lumbar and sacral plexuses). This ultimately gives rise to the peripheral nerves, which receive fibers from several spinal nerves.

The ventral branch supplies motor, sensory, and sympathetic innervation to the anterior regions of the body (trunk) and the extremities. Compression triggers the classic radicular symptoms with pain radiation and weakened sensation in the respective dermatome (area of skin that receives sensory impulses from a spinal cord segment via its posterior sensory root) as well as weakening or malfunction of the segment-indicating muscles.

The skin, muscles, and joints always receive peripheral innervation through the blending of the peripheral nerves in the plexus from several segments of the spinal cord. Clinical studies have shown that certain muscles are characteristic for a certain segment (*segment-indicating muscles*). Malfunction of the segment-indicating muscles provides a clue as to the affected segment.

**Example:** The extensor hallucis longus muscle is innervated monosegmentally from L5. Compression of the L5 root leads to paresis/weakening of the muscle, so that active extension of the great toe is no longer possible or is significantly limited. In the thoracic

region, the ventral branches run monosegmentally. Here they are known as intercostal nerves.

Only after exiting the intervertebral foramen does the spinal nerve divide into a dorsal and a ventral branch. The meningeal nerve originates before the division. Compression of the spinal nerve (e.g., due to a herniated disk) always occurs before the division. Thus, there are mixed findings in all three portions of the spinal nerve.

If a peripheral nerve is damaged, the symptoms do not occur in the dermatomes, but rather in the sensory skin area of the peripheral nerve. This area is different from the dermatome. A peripheral nerve receives sensory fibers from various spinal cord segments. This important difference helps to distinguish damage at the root level from damage at the nerve level.

### The Neurological Examination

> *The neurological examination allows for an assessment of the level of the affected segments and any peripheral nerve damage.*

- *Testing sensation of the dermatomes* (**Fig. 4.7a, b**): Hyposensitivity (e.g., numbness) indicates a loss of function and is suggestive of nerve root damage. Hypersensitivity indicates a gain in function. It can be present with neuropathic pain, however it can also be present with nociceptive pain due to lowering of the nociceptive threshold in the corresponding dorsal horn complex:
  - In allodynia, touch causes pain. This sensory alteration may be related to the dermatome in case of nerve lesions, however it may also occur as a generalized pain feature in non-neuropathic pain disorders.
  - If peripheral nerve damage is suspected, sensation in the corresponding peripheral area of the skin should be examined (**Fig. 4.8**).
- *Testing the strength of the segment-indicating muscles:* If there is a deficit, lax peripheral paralysis occurs along with muscle atrophy, possible muscle fasciculation (twitching of the muscle without movement), and hypotonicity of the affected muscle. In a peripheral lesion, there may be weakness of all muscles that are innervated by this nerve.
- *Reflex testing:* If the ventral root of a motor nerve is affected, the reflexes are weakened. If there is a peripheral lesion, there is loss or weakening of the reflex.
- *Testing sympathetic deficits:* Sympathetic deficits only occur with nerve root compression in the

thoracic spine and do not occur in the cervical or lumbar spines. They can be present with a peripheral lesion.

## Sympathetic Deficits

- Diminished secretion from the cutaneous sweat glands, resulting in dry skin.
- The smooth muscle of the hairs on the skin cannot be provoked by pinching the skin, that is, this does not cause goose bumps with the hair standing on end (piloreaction).
- A deficit affecting the smooth musculature in the skin prevents vascular constriction, and thus vasodilation results.

A distinction should be made between the responses of the sympathetic nervous system during the onset of pain and the role of the sympathetic nervous system in producing pain. In general, pain is always accompanied by autonomic components such as circulatory changes, sweating, temperature changes in the painful area, as well as heart rate and blood pressure changes.

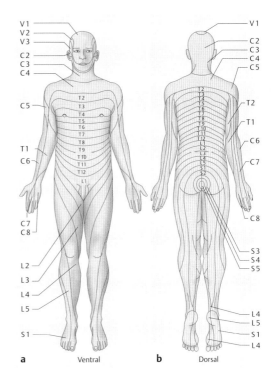

**a** Ventral  **b** Dorsal

**Fig. 4.7a, b** Dermatomes.
**a** From ventral. **b** From dorsal.

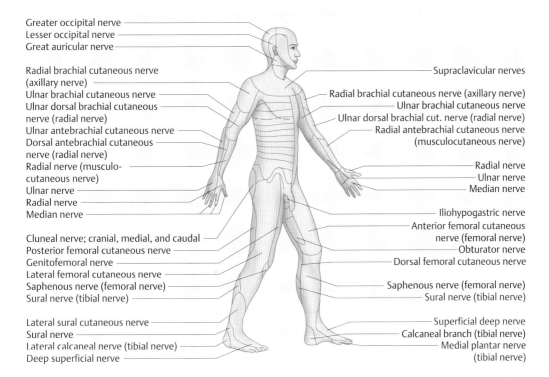

Greater occipital nerve
Lesser occipital nerve
Great auricular nerve

Radial brachial cutaneous nerve
(axillary nerve)
Ulnar brachial cutaneous nerve
Ulnar dorsal brachial cutaneous
nerve (radial nerve)
Ulnar antebrachial cutaneous nerve
Dorsal antebrachial cutaneous
nerve (radial nerve)
Radial nerve (musculo-
cutaneous nerve)
Ulnar nerve
Radial nerve
Median nerve

Cluneal nerve; cranial, medial, and caudal
Posterior femoral cutaneous nerve
Genitofemoral nerve
Lateral femoral cutaneous nerve
Saphenous nerve (femoral nerve)
Sural nerve (tibial nerve)

Lateral sural cutaneous nerve
Sural nerve
Lateral calcaneal nerve (tibial nerve)
Deep superficial nerve

Supraclavicular nerves
Radial brachial cutaneous nerve (axillary nerve)
Ulnar brachial cutaneous nerve
Ulnar dorsal brachial cut. nerve (radial nerve)
Radial antebrachial cutaneous nerve
(musculocutaneous nerve)

Radial nerve
Ulnar nerve
Median nerve

Iliohypogastric nerve
Anterior femoral cutaneous
nerve (femoral nerve)
Obturator nerve
Dorsal femoral cutaneous nerve

Saphenous nerve (femoral nerve)
Sural nerve (tibial nerve)

Superficial deep nerve
Calcaneal branch (tibial nerve)
Medial plantar nerve
(tibial nerve)

**Fig. 4.8** Sensory innervation zones of the peripheral nerves.

The sympathetic origin site may also influence the pain. If mechanical irritation is applied there, this can decrease the sympathetic activity (Sato and Schmidt 1973).

■ *Decreasing sympathetic activity can reduce the pain.*

- Sympathetic innervation of the head and neck: C8–T2
- Sympathetic innervation of the arms: T3–T7 (T9)
- Sympathetic innervation of pelvis and legs: T10–12

The efferent sympathetic nervous system may also be involved in producing pain. Complex regional pain syndrome (CRPS) occurs after trauma affecting the extremities or injuries involving the nervous system. A distinction is made in CRPS between type 1 and type 2 (formerly known as causalgia). In addition to the often spontaneously evoked pain, these diseases are characterized by changes to the skin circulation, sweating, and trophic alterations affecting the skin, the subcutaneous layers, and the bone. Severe edema in the initial months and hyperalgesia (touch causes severe pain) are typical. In addition, complex motor disturbances such as paresis, tremors, and dystonia can occur (Stanton-Hicks et al 1995; Baron et al 1996).

If the nervous system is involved in causing the pain, the following examinations may be performed.

### Pain Provocation Tests of Neural Structures

Neural provocation tests are considered positive when the patient's symptoms are reproduced. The entire nerve is placed under increasing tension or pressure in order to test its sensitivity to the mechanical stimulation. If the nerve is sensitized, the mechanical provocation will cause pain.

**Example:** Pain provocation test
- *Compression test:* If irritation of the cervical roots is suspected:
  - Spurling test: The cervical spine is flexed laterally and rotated to the same side. Additional extension narrows the intervertebral foramina to their smallest size. The weight of the head alone is adequate to produce the effect. No pressure should be added. The therapist should now observe whether the position of the head reproduces or worsens the pain: if there is nerve sensitivity, the patient will experience a sudden, shooting pain in his arm. Pain that slowly migrates distally, or local pain in the cervical

spine, suggests compression pain affecting the vertebral joint due to maximum convergence.

**Examples:** Tension tests
- *For irritation of the L4–S1 roots (sciatic nerve):*
  - Lasègue test with Bragard sign (straight leg raise, SLR): The patient is lying on his back with his leg extended at the knee. The therapist passively flexes his leg in the hip joint. A reproduction of the patient's pain during hip bending is considered pathological.
    To rule out muscle stretching pain affecting the hamstrings, or neural pain, the Bragard test may be performed. The leg should be extended in the hip joint until the pain subsides. Additional dorsal extension places tension on the tibial nerve. If the pain is reproduced, the Lasègue and Bragard tests are positive.

*One should always perform the tests with a comparison of sides. Shooting pain with minimal hip bending indicates acute symptoms. The Bragard test is mainly useful for the upper region of bending for differential diagnosis.*

- Crossed Lasègue test (SLR): The test is performed in the same manner as the Lasègue test. The test is positive if pain occurs in the opposite leg when moving the unaffected leg.

*This is often a sign of a severely herniated disk in the lumbosacral region.*

- *Irritation of the L2–L4 roots (femoral nerve):*
  - Reverse Lasègue test (prone knee bend, PKB): With the patient lying prone, the leg is passively extended in the hip joint and flexed at the knee, causing tension on the femoral nerve (L2–L4). Shooting pain in the groin and/or ventral thigh is pathological.
    The cause of pain may also be arthritis of the iliosacral joint or the hip joint. If so, there is a different pain quality. By adding neck bending, the nervous system is tensed more via the dura and can thus be differentiated from joints and muscle.

### Sensitivity Testing

The following criteria are evaluated as part of neural sensitivity testing:
- Which perceptions are changed?
  - Superficial sensitivity: Pain and temperature; pressure and touch.

– Deep sensitivity: Position, movement, and vibration perception.
- Localization of the sensory disturbance:
  – Dermatome-bound (e.g., disk herniation).
  – Sensory skin area about a peripheral nerve (e.g., positional-related lesion of the peroneal nerve).
  – Stocking-like area on the leg or glove-like area on the arm may be indications of polyneuropathy.

If various sensory qualities are absent, this may provide clues as to the height of the lesion.

### Superficial Sensitivity
Superficial sensitivity is conducted by two main pathways: one for pain and temperature and one for pressure and touch. Most of the receptors are located near the surface of the body. Muscles, tendons, joint capsules, and bones contain pain and pressure receptors only:

#### Pathway for Pain and Temperature
The nerve fibers cross in the anterior region of the spinal cord, immediately after entering over the dorsal root, to the opposite side. Thus, in central lesions in the spinal cord, pain and temperature deficits occur on the opposite side:
- *Testing pain perception:* Pain perception may be tested on the basis of skin irritation (e.g., pinching). It may be stronger or weaker. The test should always be performed with a comparison of sides.
- *Testing temperature perception:* The response to cold or thermal stimuli is tested with a comparison of sides.

#### Pathway for Pressure and Touch
After entering via the dorsal root, the nerve fibers pass on the ipsilateral side in the posterior column of the spinal cord to the brain stem. There they cross to the opposite side to the sensory area of the cerebral cortex. Thus, if there is a central lesion affecting the spinal cord, pressure and touch deficits occur on the same side as the lesion:
- *Testing pressure and touch perception:* The examiner should touch the skin with a cotton swab, fingertips, or brush to administer sensory stimuli. The patient should report the sensory qualities; this should be done on both sides.

*A feeling of "ants crawling," burning, tingling, or a sensation similar to an electric shock, are typical symptoms in patients with neuropathic pain. They can be accompanied by hypersensitivity to mechanical or thermal stimulation.*

*Hypoqualities occur when there is compression of a neural structure. These are often described by patients as "woolly" feeling.*

### Deep Sensitivity
The cerebellum is the coordinating center for motor activity. All of the information from the proprioceptors located in the joints, tendons, and muscles is processed here, resulting in the perception of position and movement.

Deep sensitivity may be tested by evaluating the sense of position (imitating position and movement sensation) as well as by vibration behavior:
- *Testing positional sense:* The examiner places the affected extremity in a certain position. Keeping his or her eyes closed, the patient should imitate the position on the opposite side.
- *Testing movement sense:* The examiner places a joint (e.g., the great toe joint) in a certain position. With his or her eyes closed, the patient should state the position of the joint. The therapist and patient should first agree on the terms the patient should use in their description. For the movement direction, the orientation in space and in relation to the body should be tested (e.g., the great toe moves toward the nose). The test should be performed several times.
- *Testing vibration sense (part of the physician's neurology examination):* This test identifies early sensory symptoms in deep sensory disturbances. A tuning fork is struck and placed on an area of the arm or leg that is not covered by soft tissue. The patient then says whether or when they stop sensing the vibrations of the tuning fork. The measurement scale is 8/8–1/8. A value lower than 6/8 is considered pathological.

## Testing Reflexes

Using a reflex hammer, the relaxed tendon is quickly tapped. The muscle contracts briefly due to the stretch stimulus applied to the tendon:
- Reflexes should always be tested with a comparison of sides, given that only a discrepancy is considered pathological.
- The reflex test should be performed several times.
- If the reflex is too weak, the patient may help increase it. The reflex may be reinforced by acti-

vating other muscle groups (e.g., by clenching the teeth).

- Example of documentation of reflex level: 0 = absent; 1 = diminished; ▪2 = normal; ▪3 = increased; 4 = clonus; BRT = broad reflex trigger zone.

**Examples: Reflexes**

> *Three important reflexes are described, by way of example, in the following.*

- Biceps tendon reflex (BTR), biceps brachii muscle; C5–C6; musculocutaneous nerve: The patient's forearm is positioned in a neutral pronation/supination position. The examiner places his index finger on the biceps tendon at the elbow. Using a reflex hammer, he taps his fingers, causing the biceps brachii muscle to contract.
- Patellar tendon reflex (PTR), quadriceps femoris muscle; L2–L4; femoral nerve: With slight knee bending, striking the patellar tendon with the reflex hammer causes the quadriceps femoris to contract.
- Achilles tendon reflex (ATR) triceps surae muscle; S1–S2; tibial nerve: Striking the Achilles tendon causes plantar bending of the foot.

### Testing Muscle Strength in Patients with Motor Lesions

Test the strength of the segment-indicating muscles of the lumbar spine and cervical spine.

## 4.2.7   Pain Measurement (Algesimetry)

Pain cannot be quantified using objective measurement techniques; there is no method or apparatus that allows one to assess perceived pain as a parameter.

For the physical therapist, pain measurement first and foremost serves to control treatment progress during therapy. The procedures are simpler than those used in diagnosing the pain process. For diagnosis, objective and subjective measuring techniques are used. Objective algesimetry uses procedures that measure the physiological responses of the patient to noxious stimuli. They are not based on the subjective pain perception of the patient. The evaluation is accomplished by comparing parameters for different stimulus intensities as well as norm data. Noxious stimuli include mechanical, thermal, chemical, and electrical stimuli. Various devices may be used to apply specific stimuli (e.g.,

pressure stimuli) to the body's structures. The patients report pain intensities that are then compared with norm data. The administration of these standardized stimuli serves for the examination of pain perception as well as accompanying physiological responses (e.g., hyperemia, sweating).

In the field of physical therapy, clinical algesimetry is very important. It deals with subjective pain perception and the level of impairment in the patient's everyday life as well as the identification of pain behavior.

Various methods are available for determining these qualities.

### Pain Localization with Pain Drawing

Pain locations may be documented using pain drawings (Pain Disability Index, pp. 173, 174). The drawings should initially be evaluated independently of the cause of pain. One should see whether the patient can precisely outline the painful region and whether the pain is deep or superficial. This may be suggestive of the cause. For instance, chronic pain often is diffuse, poorly bounded, and very widespread, while acute receptor pain is often more well-localized.

> *The assessment of pain location is important for treatment, because it shows whether the localization has changed as a result of therapy. Yet, the quantification of these results is just as difficult as the estimation of pain character.*

### Assessing Pain Character with Adjective Lists

The character of the pain may provide clues to the differential diagnosis. Various proposed qualitative descriptions have attempted to evaluate the different components of pain (e.g., sensory or affective), yet they are less suitable for an immediate assessment of the progress of treatment (Pain Disability Index, pp. 173, 174).

The McGill Pain Questionnaire (MPQ) was presented in 1975 by Melzack. The questionnaire consists of several sections, including lists of adjectives that describe pain in terms of increasing intensity. According to Melzack (1975), these may be divided into somatosensory/discriminative (e.g., hot, burning, fiery, scalding), affective/emotional (e.g., annoying, tortuous, excruciating), and evaluative blocks (e.g., circumscribed, radiating, disseminating). Various German surveys are also available, although these have not yet been as well evaluated as the

**Fig. 4.9** Visual analogue scale.

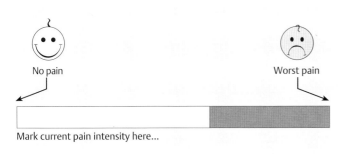

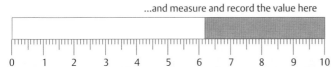

English versions (Weiss and Schaible in Scherfer 2003).

## Assessing Pain Intensity using Unidimensional Scales

The assessment of pain perception is accomplished using various scales that patients may use to estimate their pain intensity. These scales may also be used to monitor the progress of treatment during therapy.

### Visual Analogue Scale (VAS; Fig. 4.9)

The most well-known of these scales is the visual analogue scale (VAS). The VAS is a simple, but very useful means of documenting a treatment result succinctly and precisely. The VAS meets all of the requirements for a standardized test, including feasibility.

Various studies on the psychometric properties of the VAS have shown that this clinical "measurement instrument" is exceedingly reliable and valid (Schreiber and Winkelmann 1997). For surveying pain, the VAS is generally clear and easily understood by patients, although it does require their constructive cooperation. In clinical practice, the VAS may be used to estimate the immediate effects of treatment (baseline values and treatment outcome) as well as for monitoring the progress of treatment series. It may be used with patients with acute or chronic pain.

The VAS consists of a single line (usually 10 cm long). The starting point is *no pain*, at one end, and at the opposite end is *maximum pain imaginable*. No other pain descriptors are provided. The patient marks the severity of his or her pain on the scale, between the two points. This distance of the marking from the starting point may be measured in millimeters. In this manner, a numerical value is obtained that may be analyzed in terms of reporting and comparison.

Various instruments have been developed with different designs. Most of these are slide-rule devices for easy use in clinical practice. These may also be used by children from about age 6. They have different "smilies" on them, which makes them easy to use by children and patients who do not understand numerical scales.

The scale should be positioned in the same manner as if a person were to write on a piece of paper, that is, it should be horizontal and be read from left to right. A direct comparison has shown that horizontally placed pain intensity scales tend to elicit lower values than vertically positioned scales (Schreiber and Winkelmann 1997).

Between the beginning and endpoint, the horizontal line should contain no markings and should be at least 10 cm long. The word choice used on the scale is crucial, because it influences the patient's assessment. With terms such as *unbearable pain* or *strongest imaginable pain*, the entry is more toward the right; for ones such as *considerable pain*, it is more to the left.

### Tips for Using the VAS in Clinical Practice

*The information provided by the VAS depends on how one asks about the pain. Various questions may be used to query the patient's current pain status or other aspects related to the duration of pain.*

**Examples:** Questions
- Current status: How is your current pain?
- Twenty-four-hour behavior: How was your pain in the last 24 hours?
- One week: How was your pain in the last week?
- Related to pain maximum and minimum:
  - What was your most severe pain in ... (duration)?
  - What was your most mild pain in ... (duration)?
- Relation to pain region: How was your pain in ... (region–relation to pain drawing)?
- Relation to impaired function: Activities of daily living (ADL): How much does your pain limit certain functions (walking, job, housework, contact with other people, sleeping, enjoyment of life)?

The visual analogue scale should be used before starting treatment and the results recorded. This will enable an immediate comparison of pain intensity after individual treatment sessions. Immediately after therapy, the results should be analyzed with care, however. Pain perception at that point is strongly influenced by the psychological situation of therapy; a strong stimulus may temporarily increase pain. It is advisable, for the purpose of documenting the treatment success, to register the results of the VAS before treatment.

In particular, older patients, and those with pain in many regions of the body, are often unable to respond to a summary pain questionnaire or to use a slide-rule. The therapist should patiently tell them how to perform the test and provide clear instructions. It is advisable to test using a different categorical scale as well, such as a numerical rating scale.

In order to properly assess the results, the therapist should have knowledge of the influences of additional therapies (e.g., pain relievers, acupuncture), and ask about these in the patient history. An altered living situation or habits should also be taken into account.

Features of the VAS should be taken into consideration. Certain variants may lead to grave measurement errors. To document the progress of treatment, the same form of VAS scale should be used each time.

Additional unidimensional scales for evaluating pain intensity are the following:

## Numerical Rating Scale (NRS)

The patient is given a series of numbers (from 0–10 or 0–100) and asked to rate the severity of his or her pain within the given range.

## Verbal Rating Scale (VRS)

The pain is evaluated using adjectives that are arranged in terms of increasing intensity. The patient chooses the adjective that best describes his or her momentary pain intensity from the adjectives provided.

> Verbal rating scales are often more readily understood than numerical ones, but they are less suitable for documenting treatment progress and statistical analyses.

## Assessments

Along with standardized tests (e.g., scales), assessments (evaluation, rating, estimation) may be used to measure pain. These allow the patient to express his or her perception and experience in the form of a self-assessment or evaluation. Tests that have been positively assessed in terms of their quality criteria are scientifically sound instruments. Often they allow for a documentation of the progress and success of treatment just as well as objective measurements of visible changes (e.g., measurements of altered mobility).

### The Definition of an Assessment

The term "assessment" generally refers to procedures that attempt to measure something that evades direct observation or that cannot be quantified using simpler methods (Biefang et al 1999; Hasenbein and Wallesch 2003).

The advantage of these procedures is that they offer patients the possibility to provide their own assessment and document their evaluation or treatment. Thus, both the patient and the therapist can describe how the health impairment or the course of therapy or rehabilitation are affecting daily life and thus their impact on the level of activities and participation.

The use of standardized tests and assessments—especially self-assessment instruments—thus leads not only to a scientific basis and assessment of physical therapy, it also helps the field to be perceived as a whole by patients, to develop a professional identity, mold it, and present it to the public.

Assessment procedures aim to measure complex constructs. These are abstract terms that must be specifically formulated in order to render visible something that is not directly observable for scientific discussions as well as make it tangible in everyday clinical practice (Dornholdt 2000). Compared with *mobility of the joints*, the terms *patient satisfac-*

tion, *health-related quality of life with chronic pain*, and *impairment of daily life* are more abstract terms that elude a simple operational definition.

The *Pain Disability Index* (PDI) is one example of a self-assessment tool for patients whose chief symptom is pain. The PDI gives patients with chronic pain the opportunity to describe the impairment they experience in daily life as a result of their pain (Dillmann et al 1994). There are seven basic categories that make up the index on *pain-related limitations in daily life*. The abstract construct is divided into sub-points and criteria, taking all major aspects into account:

- Family and household duties
- Recuperation
- Social activities
- Job
- Sexual life
- Self-care
- Elementary vital activities

Using a numerical rating scale of 0–10, patients report the degree of their impairment in various areas due to pain. In addition to point values (scores) for the individual items, the PDI calculates a summary score for all items. It is designed in such a manner that patients can fill it out in only a few minutes, outside normal treatment times.

In addition to the above-named items, it also includes information on assessing pain intensity, localization, influence, and the patient's knowledge of the cause of pain. To assess the quality of pain, a list of verbs is available; the patient reports whether the descriptor applies to the quality of his or her pain or not.

The original version of the PDI was developed by the Pain Research Group (Department of Neurology, University of Wisconsin, Madison Medical School). **Fig. 4.10** shows an English translation of the German-language pain questionnaire on the website of the Mainz Pain Center.

The PDI may be used to describe the pain related to various diseases. These assessments are primarily used for patients with chronic pain, although they may also be used to estimate the risk of chronic pain. They are used both for diagnosis of pain as well as in physical therapy.

Specific instruments have also been developed for certain diseases. In regard to the locomotor system, the German survey "Funktionsfragebogen Hannover" (FFbH) for self-assessment of functional capacity in patients with back pain (FFbH-R) or osteoarthritis (FFbH-OA; **Fig. 4.11**) is available (Raspe and Kohlmann 1989; Raspe et al 1996).

## Summary

Examining patients with pain is a major challenge for doctors and physical therapists. For chronic pain patients, treatment often requires cooperation with professionals in other fields of medicine (e.g., psychotherapists).

The patient's emotional state may be severely altered. The more acute and intense the pain, the more careful and gentle the procedure must be. The pain dictates the rhythm of the patient's life. Patients with chronic pain, in particular, structure their day around their pain. They often no longer have control over the pain or feel responsible for influencing it. They go from one doctor to the next, from one therapist to the next, hoping for help (passive coping strategy). The patient must relearn to assume responsibility for influencing his or her pain. This requires various steps in the examination and treatment.

Solid, comprehensive examination: The patient needs to feel that they are believed and are being taken seriously with their pain, given that many patients will have been thought to be faking it. Maladaptive pain may also be explained functionally and physiologically (see pain processing and characteristics of pain).

In addition to a thorough history of the pain, the examination of mobility and movement behavior is also important; it should not be neglected, even if there is suspicion of pain without an organic cause (psychogenic pain). When asking about the individual symptoms, the therapist should specifically ask about any changes in the patient's symptoms rather than about an increase in pain. The latter would restrict the perception of the patient and cause them to focus only on the pain. Specific simulation maneuvers help determine whether the pain has an organic origin (e.g., Waddell sign). Questions help determine the specific individual experience of disease and the pain behavior of the patient (note yellow flags).

Specific pain provocation tests for individual structures confirm the source of pain in patients with nociceptive receptor pain (organic source).

Given that pain cannot be objectively measured, it is always a subjective feeling. For the documentation of pain, body charts, scales for estimating the intensity of pain, and pain questionnaires may be used. Clear documentation is considered evidence of the effectiveness of treatment.

**(1) Marital status:**

| | | |
|---|---|---|
| 1 ☐ Single | | 3 ☐ Widowed |
| 2 ☐ Married | | 4 ☐ Divorced/separated |

Date: ___  Time: ___
Surname: ___  First name: ___
Date of birth: ___  Sex: ☐ Male ☐ Female

**(2) Educational level** (please state the number of years you were in training/school/vocational training/college)

Years  4 5 6 7 8 9 10 11 12 13 14 15 16 17 18 19 20

Degree: ___

**(3)** Current occupation (please explain your title; if you are unemployed, please state your previous occupation): ___

**(4)** Partner's occupation: ___

**(5)** What is your current occupation?

| | |
|---|---|
| 1 ☐ Full-time work, outside the home | 4 ☐ Retired |
| 2 ☐ Part-time work, outside the home | 5 ☐ Not employed |
| 3 ☐ Housewife/House husband | 6 ☐ Other |

**(6)** How long has it been since you were diagnosed?  ☐ Months

**(7)** Did you ever have pain related to your current disease?
1 ☐ Yes   2 ☐ No   3 ☐ Not sure

**(8)** At the time of the initial diagnosis, was pain one of the symptoms?
1 ☐ Yes   2 ☐ No   3 ☐ Not sure

**(9)** Were you operated on in the past month?
1 ☐ Yes   2 ☐ No

**(10)** Most people have pain from time to time (e.g., headache, toothache, sprained joints). Did you have **another type of pain in the past week**, other than such everyday types of pain?
1 ☐ Yes   2 ☐ No

Today:  1 ☐ Yes   2 ☐ No

If you answered yes to the last two questions, please continue with the survey. If you answered both questions with no, please stop here. Thank you.

**(11)** Please shade in the areas on the following diagrams where you have pain. Place an "x" on the site with the worst pain.

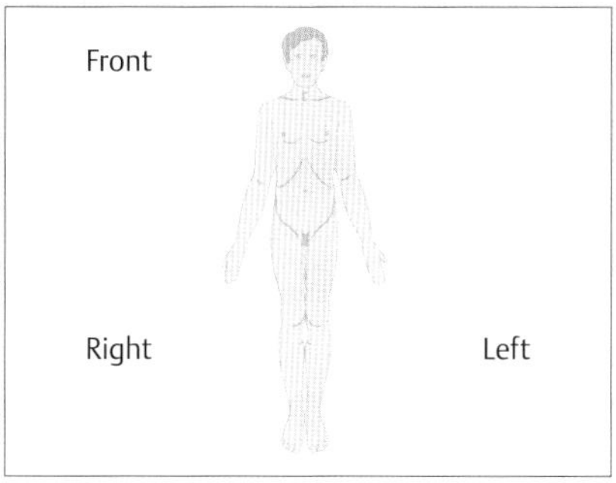

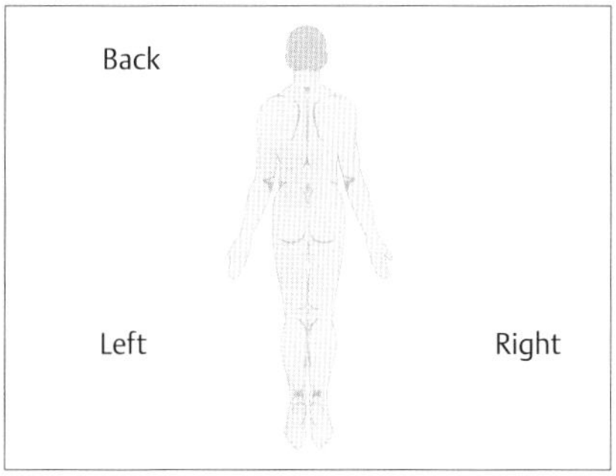

**Fig. 4.10** Pain questionnaire.

Continued ▷

**12**  Circle the number that best describes your worst pain in the past week:

| 0 | 1 | 2 | 3 | 4 | 5 | 6 | 7 | 8 | 9 | 10 |
|---|---|---|---|---|---|---|---|---|---|---|
| No pain | | | | | | | | Worst possible pain imaginable | | |

**13**  Circle the number that best describes your lowest pain level in the past week:

| 0 | 1 | 2 | 3 | 4 | 5 | 6 | 7 | 8 | 9 | 10 |
|---|---|---|---|---|---|---|---|---|---|---|
| No pain | | | | | | | | Worst possible pain imaginable | | |

**14**  Circle the number that best describes your average pain in the past week:

| 0 | 1 | 2 | 3 | 4 | 5 | 6 | 7 | 8 | 9 | 10 |
|---|---|---|---|---|---|---|---|---|---|---|
| No pain | | | | | | | | Worst possible pain imaginable | | |

**15**  Circle the number that best describes your pain at this moment:

| 0 | 1 | 2 | 3 | 4 | 5 | 6 | 7 | 8 | 9 | 10 |
|---|---|---|---|---|---|---|---|---|---|---|
| No pain | | | | | | | | Worst possible pain imaginable | | |

**16**  Which things and activities relieve your pain (e.g., heat, medications, rest)?

**17**  Which things and activities exacerbate your pain (e.g., walking, standing, lifting)?

**18**  Which treatments or medications do you receive to manage your pain?

**19**  Take a moment to recall the past week. How much pain relief did treatment or medication provide you? Please circle the percentage that best describes your level of pain relief.

| 0 | 10 | 20 | 30 | 40 | 50 | 60 | 70 | 80 | 90 | 100% |
|---|----|----|----|----|----|----|----|----|----|------|
| No relief | | | | | | | | | Compete relief | |

**20**  If you take pain medication: how many hours does it take until your pain recurs?

| 1 | | Pain medications are of no help | 5 | | 4 hours |
|---|--|--------------------------------|---|--|---------|
| 2 | | 1 hour | 6 | | 5–12 hours |
| 3 | | 2 hours | 7 | | More than 12 hours |
| 4 | | 3 hours | 8 | | I do not take any pain relievers |

**21**  What do you believe is the cause of your pain? Please mark the answer that best applies.

1. Due to therapy (e.g., drugs, surgery, radiation, prosthesis)  1 ☐ **Yes** 2 ☐ **No**
2. Primary diseases (this is the disease that is being treated and evaluated at present) 1 ☐ **Yes** 2 ☐ **No**
3. Medical cause that is unrelated to primary disease (e.g., arthritis)  1 ☐ **Yes** 2 ☐ **No**

**Fig. 4.10** Pain questionnaire. (Continued)

Continued ▷

**22** Pain perception: Please state whether each of the following words applies to your pain.

| | None | 0 | 1 | 2 | 3 | Extreme |
|---|---|---|---|---|---|---|
| Dull, pressure | None | 0 | 1 | 2 | 3 | Extreme |
| Throbbing, pulsatory | None | 0 | 1 | 2 | 3 | Extreme |
| Burning, hot | None | 0 | 1 | 2 | 3 | Extreme |
| Electric-shock–like, shooting | None | 0 | 1 | 2 | 3 | Extreme |
| Stinging, piercing | None | 0 | 1 | 2 | 3 | Extreme |
| Cramp-like, colic-like | None | 0 | 1 | 2 | 3 | Extreme |
| Pulling, tearing | None | 0 | 1 | 2 | 3 | Extreme |
| Pain upon slight touch | None | 0 | 1 | 2 | 3 | Extreme |
| Unbearable | None | 0 | 1 | 2 | 3 | Extreme |
| Exhausting, fatiguing | None | 0 | 1 | 2 | 3 | Extreme |
| Terrible | None | 0 | 1 | 2 | 3 | Extreme |

**22** Circle the number that describes how much impairment your pain caused in the past week.

**General activity**

**A**
| 0 | 1 | 2 | 3 | 4 | 5 | 6 | 7 | 8 | 9 | 10 |
|---|---|---|---|---|---|---|---|---|---|---|
| No impairment | | | | | | | | | Worst impairment | |

**Mood**

**B**
| 0 | 1 | 2 | 3 | 4 | 5 | 6 | 7 | 8 | 9 | 10 |
|---|---|---|---|---|---|---|---|---|---|---|
| No impairment | | | | | | | | | Worst impairment | |

**Walking ability**

**C**
| 0 | 1 | 2 | 3 | 4 | 5 | 6 | 7 | 8 | 9 | 10 |
|---|---|---|---|---|---|---|---|---|---|---|
| No impairment | | | | | | | | | Worst impairment | |

**Normal work (outside and household), capacity**

**D**
| 0 | 1 | 2 | 3 | 4 | 5 | 6 | 7 | 8 | 9 | 10 |
|---|---|---|---|---|---|---|---|---|---|---|
| No impairment | | | | | | | | | Worst impairment | |

**Relationships with other people**

**E**
| 0 | 1 | 2 | 3 | 4 | 5 | 6 | 7 | 8 | 9 | 10 |
|---|---|---|---|---|---|---|---|---|---|---|
| No impairment | | | | | | | | | Worst impairment | |

**Sleep**

**F**
| 0 | 1 | 2 | 3 | 4 | 5 | 6 | 7 | 8 | 9 | 10 |
|---|---|---|---|---|---|---|---|---|---|---|
| No impairment | | | | | | | | | Worst impairment | |

**Enjoyment of life**

**G**
| 0 | 1 | 2 | 3 | 4 | 5 | 6 | 7 | 8 | 9 | 10 |
|---|---|---|---|---|---|---|---|---|---|---|
| No impairment | | | | | | | | | Worst impairment | |

**Fig. 4.10** Pain questionnaire. (Continued)

**The following questions ask about activities in everyday life.**
**We would like to know how well you can perform the following activities.**
**Please answer each question in terms of your current (last 7 days) situation.**

| You have **three** possible responses: |
| --- |

| | | |
| --- | --- | --- |
| 1 | **Yes** | i.e., you can perform the activity without any difficulty |
| 2 | **Yes**, with difficulty | i.e., you have difficulty performing the activity (e.g., weakness, stiffness, it takes longer or you need to support yourself) |
| 3 | **No**, or only with help from someone else | i.e., you cannot perform this activity at all unless another person helps you |

|  | Yes | Yes, but with difficulty | No, or only with help |
| --- | --- | --- | --- |
| Can you walk on a level surface (e.g., footpath) for 1 hour? | 1 | 2 | 3 |
| Can you walk outside on uneven surfaces (e.g., in the woods or on a dirt path) for 1 hour? | 1 | 2 | 3 |
| Can you go **up** the stairs from one floor to the next? | 1 | 2 | 3 |
| Can you go **down** the stairs from one floor to the next? | 1 | 2 | 3 |
| Can you run quickly for 100 meters (not walking), such as to catch the bus? | 1 | 2 | 3 |
| Can you stand for 30 minutes without taking a break (e.g., waiting in line)? | 1 | 2 | 3 |
| Can you get into and out of a car? | 1 | 2 | 3 |
| Can you use public transportation (bus, train, etc.)? | 1 | 2 | 3 |
| Can you bend down from standing to pick up a small object (e.g., coin or piece of paper) off the floor? | 1 | 2 | 3 |
| Can you bend down from sitting and lift a small object (e.g., coin) next to your chair? | 1 | 2 | 3 |
| Can you pick up a heavy object off the floor and place it on a table (e.g., crate of bottled water)? | 1 | 2 | 3 |
| Can you lift a heavy object (e.g., bucket of water or suitcase) and carry it 10 m? | 1 | 2 | 3 |
| Can you get up out of a chair of normal height? | 1 | 2 | 3 |
| Can you put on and take off your stockings or socks? | 1 | 2 | 3 |
| Can you get into and out of the bathtub? | 1 | 2 | 3 |
| Can you wash yourself from head to foot and dry yourself off? | 1 | 2 | 3 |
| Can you use a normal toilet (normal height, no handrails)? | 1 | 2 | 3 |
| Can you get up out of a normal (height) bed? | 1 | 2 | 3 |

**Fig. 4.11** Functional questionnaire for patients with osteoarthritis.

# References

Baron R, Blumberg H et al. Clinical characteristics of patients with CRPS type I and type II in Germany with special emphasis on vasomotor function. In: Jänig W, Stanton-Hicks M, eds. Reflex Sympathetic Dystrophy—A Reappraisal. Progress in Pain Research and Management, Vol. 6. Seattle: IASP; 1996:25–48

Benedetti F. Cholecystokinin type A and type B receptors and their modulation of opioid analgesia. Physiology 1997;12(6):263–268

Biefang S, Potthoff P, et al. Assesmentverfahren für die Rehabilitation. Göttingen: Hogrefe; 1999

Butler DS. The sensitive nervous system. Adelaide: Noigroup Publications; 2000

Cervero F, Laird JMA. One pain or many pains? A new look at pain mechanisms. News Physiol Sci 1991;6:268–273

Coggeshall RE, Coulter JD, et al. Unmyelinated fibers in the ventral root. Brain Res 1973;57(1):229–233

Dillmann U, Nilges P, et al. Assessing disability in chronic pain patients. [Behinderungseinschätzung bei chronischen Schmerzpatienten] Schmerz 1994;8(2):100–110

Dornholdt E. Physical Therapy Research. Principles and Applications. Philadelphia, London, Toronto: W. B. Saunders; 2000

Flor H. Psychobiologie des Schmerzes. Empirische Untersuchungen zur Psychophysiologie, Diagnostik und Therapie chronischer Schmerzsyndrome der Skelettmuskulatur. Bern: Huber 1991

Fruhstorfer H. Somatoviszerale Sensibilität. In: Klinke R, Silbernagl S, eds. Lehrbuch der Physiologie. Stuttgart: Thieme; 1996

Fukui S, Ohseto K, et al. Referred pain distribution of the cervical zygapophyseal joints and cervical dorsal rami. Pain 1996;68(1):79–83

Gifford  L. The mature organism model. Topical Issues in Pain 1. , Science and management, fear avoidance beliefs and behavior. CNS Press, Falmouth, 1988; 45–56

Gifford L. Schmerzphysiologie. In: Van den Berg F (Hrsg.) Angewandte Physiologie 2, Organsysteme verstehen und beeinflussen. Stuttgart: Thieme; 2000; 467–518

Gifford  L. Perspektiven zum biopsychosozialen Modell. Manuelle Therapie 2002;

Gifford L. Perspektiven zum biopsychosozialen Modell. Teil 3: Patientenbeispiel—Anwendung des Einkaufskorb-Ansatzes und der abgestuften Exposition 2003;1:21–31

Gifford L, Butler D. Die Eingliederung der Schmerzwissenschaften in die klinische Praxis. ÖVMP-Zeitschrift 1999;1:1–7

Hasenbein U., Wallesch C-W, Räbiger J. Ärztliche Compliance mit Leitlinien. Ein Überblick vor dem Hintergrund der Einführung von Disease-Management-Programmen. Gesundheitsökonomie und Qualitätsmanagement 2003; 8: 363–375

Head H. Die Sensibilitätsstörungen der Haut bei Viszeralerkrankungen. Berlin: Hirschwald; 1898

Hengeveld E. Psychosocial issues in physiotherapy: manual therapists' perspectives and observations [thesis]. London: University of East London, Dept. of Health Sciences; 2000

Hengeveld E. Compliance und Verhaltensänderung in Manueller Therapie. Manuelle Therapie 2003;3:122–132

International Association for the Study of Pain (IASP). IASP Curriculum outline on pain for occupational therapy. Available at: http://www.iasp-pain.org/Content/NavigationMenu/GeneralResourceLinks/Curricula/Occupational_Therapy/default. Accessed December 16, 2013; 2013a

International Association for the Study of Pain (IASP). IASP curriculum outline on pain for physical therapy. Available at: http://www.iasp-pain.org/Content/NavigationMenu/GeneralResourceLinks/Curricula/Therapy/default.htm. Accessed December 16, 2013; 2013b

Kendall NAS, Linton SJ, et al. Guide to assessing psychosocial yellow flags in acute low back pain: risk factors for long-term disability and work loss. Accident and Rehabilitation and Compensation Insurance Corporation of New Zealand and the National Health Committee. Wellington, New Zealand: Ministry of Health; 1997a

Linton SJ. Early intervention for the secondary prevention of chronic musculoskeletal pain. In: Campbell JN, ed. Pain 1996—An Updated Review. Seattle: IASP Press; 1996: 305–311

Linton SJ. Cognitive-behavioral intervention for the secondary prevention of chronic musculoskeletal pain. In: Max M, ed. Pain 1999—An Updated Review. Seattle: IASP Press; 1999:535–544

Melzack R. The McGill Pain Questionnaire: major properties and scoring methods. Pain 1975;1(3):277–299

Melzack R, Wall PH. The Challenge of Pain. New York: Basic Books; 1996

Mense P. Neurobiologische Grundlagen von Muskelschmerz. Schmerz 1999;1:3–17

Merskey B, Bogduk N, eds. Classification of Chronic Pain—IASP Task Force on Taxonomy. Seattle: IASP Press; 1994

Moseley GL. Graded motor imagery for pathologic pain. A randomized controlled trial. Neurology 2006;67(12): 2129–2134

Moseley GL, Flor H. Targeting cortical representations in the treatment of chronic pain: a review. Neurorehabil Neural Repair 2012;26(6):646–652

Moseley GL, Gallagher L, et al. Neglect-like tactile dysfunction in chronic back pain. Neurology 2012;79(4):327–332

Nicholas M, Sharp TJ. A collaborative approach to managing chronic pain. Modern Medicine of Australia 1999;10:26–33

Price DD, Milling LS, et al. An analysis of factors that contribute to the magnitude of placebo analgesia in an experimental paradigm. Pain 1999;83(2):147–156

PT-Zeitschrift für Physiotherapeuten_65, Springer2013/3

Raspe & Kohlmann 1989: Funktionsfragebogen Rücken (FFb-H-R) heruntergeladen auf der Homepage des Schmerzzentrums Mainz

Raspe & Kohlmann. Hannover Functional Questionnaire in ambulatory diagnosis of functional disability caused by backache. Rehabilitation (Stuttgart) 1996; 35(1): I–VIII

Ren 1994. In: Mense S. Neuroplastizität und chronischer Schmerz. Beilage zum Script NOI – Mobilisation des Nervensystems, Level II; 1995

Sato A, Schmidt RF. Somatosympathetic reflexes: afferent fibers, central pathways, discharge characteristics. Physiol Rev 1973;53(4):916–947

Schaible H.-G, Weiss T. Physiologie des Schmerzes und der Nozizeption. In: Van den Berg F (Hrsg.) Organsyteme verstehen und beeinflussen. Angewandte Physiologie, Band 2, Stuttgart: Thieme; 2003

Scherfer E. Standardisierte Tests und Assessments: Bindeglied zwischen Forschung, Praxis, Qualitätssicherung und einer ganzheitlichen Perspektive. Z Physiother 2003; 55(7):1178–1184

Schreiber TU, Winkelmann C. Die Visuelle Analogskala (VAS) zur Schmerzmessung in der Physiotherapie. Krankengymnastik 1997;49(11):1856–1865

Stanton-Hicks M, Jänig W, et al. Reflex sympathetic dystrophy; changing concepts and taxonomy. Pain 1995;63(1): 127–133

Treede R-D, Jensen TS, et al. Neuropathic pain. Redefinition and a grading system for clinical and research purposes. Neurology 2008;70: 1630-1635

van den Berg F. Angewandte Physiologie. Band 2: Organsysteme verstehen und beeinflussen. Stuttgart. Thieme; 2000

van den Berg F. Angewandte Physiologie. Band 3: Therapie, Training, Tests. Stuttgart: Thieme; 2001

Vlaeyen JWS, Linton SJ. Fear-avoidance and its consequences in chronic musculoskeletal pain: a state of the art. Pain 2000;85(3):317–332

Waddell G. The Back Pain Revolution. Edinburgh: Churchill Livingstone; 1998

Wall PD. On the relation of injury to pain. The John J. Bonica Lecture. Pain 1979;6(3):253–264

Winkel D, Vleeming A, et al. Nichtoperative Orthopädie der Weichteile und des Bewegungsapparates. Band 1: Anatomie in Vivo. Stuttgart: G. Fischer; 1985

Wittink H, Hocking T. Chronic Pain Management for Physical Therapists. Oxford: Butterworth-Heinemann; 1997

Wolff HD. Neurophysiologische Aspekte des Bewegungssystems. 3rd ed. Berlin: Springer; 1996

Zusman M. Structure-oriented beliefs and disability due to back pain. Aust J Physiother 1998;44(1):13–20

# 5 Examining Cardiopulmonary Functions

# 5 Examining Cardiopulmonary Functions

## 5.1 Respiration—Examining the Pulmonary System

*Petra Kirchner*

### 5.1.1 Useful Information on Breathing

Preliminary and accompanying examinations are an important part of disease-specific and individual respiratory therapy. Physical therapists guide their treatment based on its success or failure (during treatment as well as with repeated examinations). The following criteria may be used:

- Changed breathing type/breathing pattern
- Patient's description of ease or difficulty of breathing
- Audible breathing noises
- Cyanosis

> Breathing patterns (breathing types) in unhealthy patients can only be evaluated in terms of how they compare with normal breathing patterns or normal variants in healthy adults or children.

**Marked Deviations in Breathing Patterns in a Healthy Person**

- Increased respiratory frequency at rest
- Strong use of inspiratory and expiratory accessory breathing muscles
- More thoracic and less abdominal respiratory motion
- Frequent yawning

Doctors and physical therapists often describe these deviations as incorrect or false breathing. The term should be avoided, however, as what patients demonstrate is required breathing (Ehrenberg 1983).

> Required breathing is the current respiratory potential of a patient. In other words, it describes a typical, disease-related respiratory pattern or one created by the patient's personality.

### Required Breathing in Patients with Restrictions

The type of required breathing in a patient with a *moderate to severely restrictive ventilatory disorder* is characterized by a high respiratory rate (24–40 breaths/minute) and the feeling of respiratory distress during minimal physical exertion.

**Explanation:** Due to the increased respiratory work as a result of increased elastic resistance, the patient breathes small respiratory volumes. The body accepts the increase in dead space ventilation. Thus, much of the inhaled air is not included in the gas exchange. To avoid hypoventilation, it is therefore necessary, both at rest and during exertion, to have a higher respiration rate per minute than a healthy person. The patient compensates by increasing his or her respiratory rate.

Diseases leading to restriction include:

- Pulmonary fibrosis
- Lung tumors
- Postoperative condition after lung resection
- Extensive pleural peel

> Restriction may be irreversible (e.g., in the above-named disorders) or reversible (e.g., in pneumonia or with pleural effusion, which may resolve completely).

### Required Breathing in Patients with Obstructions

Required breathing in a patient with an *obstructive ventilation disorder* is marked by increased respiratory work, that is, the strong use of accessory respiratory muscles of inspiration when inhaling, and then during expiration, the use of the abdominals at rest or with physical exertion. In addition, patients with dyspnea exhibit typical breathing noises, paradoxical movements of the lower ribs (diaphragm thoracic wall antagonism), and more thoracic than abdominal respiratory movements.

**Explanation:** To overcome the increased resistance in his or her narrowed (obstructed) airways, the patient must create much larger intra-alveolar pressure differences for inspiration and expiration than a healthy person would. This requires increased use of the respiratory muscles. The effect of obstruction is stronger during expiration than inspiration. The lungs are overinflated and the diaphragm, which is flattened during inspiration, is barely moveable, which explains the minimal abdominal respiratory movements. Given the permanent inhalation position of the thorax, the intercostal muscles lose their contractibility.

**Obstructive Lung Diseases**
- Bronchial asthma
- *COPD* (chronic obstructive bronchitis and/or obstructive pulmonary emphysema or *chronic obstructive pulmonary disease*)

## Breathing Patterns in Patients with Changes to the Thoracic Skeleton and Motor Deficits Affecting the Respiratory Muscles

Respiratory patterns in patients with changes affecting the thorax (e.g., severe thoracic scoliosis) or motor deficits involving the respiratory muscles (e.g., phrenic nerve paralysis) present with asymmetrical thoracic respiratory movements, paradoxical respiratory movements, such as inspiratory retractions of entire portions of the ribs, the intercostal spaces, or the abdomen, limited rib mobility, and, in severe instances, all signs of restricted breathing.

## Breathing Patterns after Surgical Intervention

- Flat and frequent breaths
- Lacking or strongly diminished coughing ability
- Thoracic respiratory movements mainly with upper abdominal interventions
- Thoracic respiratory movements on the nonoperated side, usually after a lateral thoracotomy

## Expressive Breathing

*Expressive breathing* describes breathing types that are an expression of increased mental tension, due to anxiety, pain, or psychological agitation, or in patients with nervous breathing syndrome. The breathing pattern consists of the following:
- Increased respiratory frequency, which may drop when the patient relaxes
- Predominantly thoracic respiratory movements
- Frequent yawning
- Feeling of not being able to breathe deeply
- Lagging of one side with pain

## Combined Type

Various breathing patterns may be present at the same time in a combined form. To select suitable treatment techniques, and to evaluate the chances of success, a distinction should be made between breathing forms due to *pathophysiology* or *psyche*.

The systematic examination is therefore an important part of breathing treatment in physical therapy.

### 5.1.2   Sample Examination Scheme

The following section provides a *sample examination scheme* for adult patients. The applicable statements should be underlined or marked or written in the space provided. The comprehensive examination can also be modified, depending on the clinic (acute and rehabilitation clinics) or physical therapy practice. What and how much needs to be examined ultimately depends on the level of knowledge of the reader.

Similar to the examinations of other systems, the following is an important prerequisite for the breathing examination:

> *During the initial patient contact, as well as during all later treatments, the physical therapist should sit—if possible—at the beginning of treatment next to the bed or treatment bench, or on a chair across from the patient. In this manner, the physical therapist takes the patient's history or his or her report on their current situation (e.g., if the symptoms have changed). Taking the history hastily or hurriedly can considerably disrupt breathing.*

## Documenting the Results of the Respiratory Examination Using the Sample Examination Scheme

### Patient Data

- Name:
- Age:
- Diagnosis (diagnoses):
- Surgical intervention:
- Section/Station/Room/Unit:
- Physical therapist:
- Date of examination and re-examination:

### Information on the Current Situation

**Relevant Secondary Diagnoses/Findings**
(Own notes based on patient self-report or medical records)

It is especially important to note whether the patient has cor pulmonale and/or osteoporosis.

**Current or Previous Occupation**
(Own notes based on patient self-report or medical records)

**Family, Domestic Situation**
Living alone, cohabiting, children at home, apartment/house, institution, homeless

**Physical Activity**
Normal physical activity in everyday life and occupation, participation in sports (name type)

**Subjective Limitations in Everyday Life**
- None, significant, considerable
- When getting dressed or undressed, personal hygiene, keeping house, climbing stairs, shopping, work

**Physician Instructions for Permissible Physical Activity**
- Strict bed-rest
- Partial bed-rest (sitting on edge of bed, chair, walking in room, in hallway)
- Bed-rest no longer necessary (stair-climbing, moving about hospital grounds, clinic-based group gymnastics)
- No restrictions

**Oxygen-dependency/Ventilation**
- .........$O_2$L/min at rest, under exertion/therapy
- Long-term oxygen therapy
- Ventilation: Controlled, active-assistive, removed from on:.........

**Aids**
- Walking aids:
  - Wheelchair
  - Orthesis/prosthesis
- Compression dressings
- Use of respiratory devices/aids: PEP (positive expiratory pressure) systems, flutter device, RC-Cornet, Acapella, "SMI Atemtrainer," IPPB (intermittent positive pressure breathing), threshold, inhalator

**Measures by Members of the Treatment Team in Other Fields**
Sports therapists, masseurs, speech therapists, occupational therapists, psychologists, social workers, nurses

**Outline of Physician's Findings (Medical Records or Doctor's Report)**
*Results from:*
- Auscultation
- Percussion
- Chest radiograph
- Lung function

- Blood-gas analysis
- Spiroergometry
- Allergy test
- Laboratory results
- Ultrasound
- Endoscopic examinations
- Staging/grading (oncology)
- Karnofsky index (oncology)
- Other, including CT/MRI, nuclear medicine examinations

**Physician Therapy (Medical Records or Doctor's Report)**
*Drug Therapy*
- Substances for lungs/airways:
  - Medication for preventing attacks
  - Bronchodilators
  - Anti-inflammatory drugs
  - Mucolytic agents
  - Antibiotics
  - Specific immunotherapy (desensitization)
- Substances for heart/blood pressure:
  - Nitrates
  - Beta blockers
  - ACE inhibitors
  - Diuretics
  - Other
- Cytostatic therapy
- Other medications (relevant to PT)

*Operative/Invasive Therapy*
- Lobectomy, pneumotomy, volume reduction, lung transplantation, bronchus stent, Bülau drain
- Other

*Radiotherapy*

*Respiratory equipment therapy*
- Inhalation (with.........)
- Home respiratory care

*Rehabilitation, asthma education program, lung sports group, re-education planned/already registered.*

## Patient History

**Disease Onset/Course**
(Own notes based on patient self-report or medical records)

**Accompanying Diseases/Operations**
(Own notes based on patient self-report or medical records)

### Allergies
(Based on patient self-report or medical records)
- Animal hair
- Grass/bee pollen
- House dust mites
- Foodstuffs
- Other

### Symptoms/Self-help
*Dyspnea (Table 5.1)*
- At rest, during physical exertion (specify), orthopnea
- Daytime, at night, alternating
- Gradual onset or attacks
- Related to agitation, anxiety
- Known trigger?
- Self-help for dyspnea due to obstruction:
  – Prompt inhalation of emergency medication, body positions that facilitate breathing, pursed-lip breathing, yawning inhalation, grasping a skin fold in the lower rib region during inspiration, focus on physical processes such as respiratory movements, relaxation techniques
  – PEP systems (mask, mouthpiece)
  – Other
- Self-help for secretion elimination:
  – Flutter device, RC-Cornet, Acapella, modified autogenous drain
  – Other

**Table 5.1** Dyspnea scale (0 = no respiratory distress, 10 = worst respiratory distress; mark the corresponding level with an "X")

| Level | Dyspnea at rest | Level | Dyspnea during exertion (specify form of exertion) |
|-------|-----------------|-------|-----------------------------------------------------|
| 1 | | 1 | |
| 2 | | 2 | |
| 3 | | 3 | |
| 4 | | 4 | |
| 5 | | 5 | |
| 6 | | 6 | |
| 7 | | 7 | |
| 8 | | 8 | |
| 9 | | 9 | |
| 10 | | 10 | |

- Self-help for suppressing (unproductive) dry cough:
  – Distraction, more shallow breathing, drink something
  – Other

*Cough*
- Days, weeks, months, sporadic
- Attacks, cough-free intervals, cough syncope
- At rest, when moving
- Daytime, at night, when waking (bronchial toilet), when lying down
- Triggers: smoke, cold air, dust, changing position, mental strain, medications
- Productive cough, unproductive cough, ineffective cough impulse

*Sputum*
- Hypercrinia, abnormal endocrine secretion, hemoptysis, mucostasis
- Clear, white, yellow-green/purulent, bloody
- Thin, glassy, viscous, foamy
- Small amount, mouthful expectoration

*Pain in chest region*
- Breathing-dependent, independent of breathing, at rest, during physical exertion, with certain movements
- Shooting, clearly bordered, radiating, stabbing, burning, dull

*Other symptoms*
(Own notes based on patient self-report or medical records)

### Risk Factors
- Nicotine abuse, occupational exposure and.........
- Coronary heart disease:
  – Genetic disposition, hyperlipidemia, hypertension, diabetes mellitus, obesity, inadequate activity

### Living Situation
Ground floor, elevator, stairs

### Pets, Hobbies
(Own notes based on patient self-report)

### Psychological Situation/Emotional Attitude, Behavior/Willingness to Talk/Ability to Relax
- Psychological situation: Stable, unstable, alternating
- Emotional attitude/behavior: Well-balanced, realistic, calm, aggressive, hectic, depressive, teary,

complaining, unassertive, fearful, cynical, sarcastic, monosyllabic, listless
- Willingness to talk: Open, communicative, reticent
- Ability to relax: Possible, good, difficult, impossible

**Motivation, Compliance, Understanding of Therapy**
- Motivation: High, low, fluctuating
- Compliance: Good, poor, fluctuating
- Understanding of therapy: Yes, no, intellectual problems

## General Examination

**Strength/Height/Nutritional Status/Weight/Constitution**
- Strength: Normal, reduced, strongly reduced/cachexia
- Height: Normal, tall, short
- Nutritional status/weight: Normal, overweight, underweight, weight strongly fluctuating
- Constitution: Leptosome, athlete, pyknotic, mixed type

**Consciousness**
- Clear, alert, spatial and temporal orientation are good, responsive, languorous, clouding of consciousness, spatial and temporal orientation are not good, lethargic, somnolent, comatose, fluctuating level of consciousness and orientation
- Altered due to medication

**Face/Facial Expression**
- Relaxed, attentive, tense, vacant, contorted, expressionless
- Altered due to medication, for example, Cushing disease

**Skin Tone and Characteristics, Cyanosis, and other Visible Abnormalities**
*Skin tone / skin type*
Normal, pale, marmorated, Mediterranean, darker, colored

*Skin characteristics*
Normal, dry, exsiccated, moist, warm, cool, scaly, paper-like skin, ulcers, "cortisone skin"

*Cyanosis*
- Acute cyanosis: Lips, tip of the nose, earlobes, nail bed
- Chronic cyanosis: Blue-red face, tongue

*Other visible abnormalities*
- Hourglass nails, clubbed fingers
- Emphysema types: Pink puffer, blue bloater
- Emphysema cushion
- Shortened distance between larynx/sternum
- Jugular vein obstruction
- More prominent veins on legs/arms; varicose veins
- Cutaneous, mediastinal emphysema
- Other

**Edema/Effusion**
- Legs: Ankles, lower legs, thighs: Unilateral, bilateral, pitting
- Abdomen: Ascites
- Lungs: Pulmonary edema, pleural effusion

**Temperature**
Hypothermia, normal, subfebrile, highly febrile

**Individual Movement Sequences and Transitions**
Harmonious, coordinated, flowing, uncoordinated, strained

## Respiratory Pattern

**Breathing Rate**
Resting rate:.........; with exercise:......... (specify type of exertion)

**Airways**
At rest, with exercise (specify type of exertion):
- Inhale through the nose, mouth
- Exhale through the mouth, nose
- Exhale through "pursed lips"
- Inhale with "alar breathing"
- Breathing through a stoma following a tracheotomy

**Respiratory Movements**
(Are possible and/or predominate)
At rest, with exercise (specify type of exertion), specify starting position:
- Thoracic—ventral/sternal, cranial, lateral, dorsal
- Abdominal—ventral, lateral, lumbodorsal, caudal
- Symmetrical
- Asymmetrical/lagging of ribs
- Paradoxical breathing: Diaphragm thoracic wall antagonism (Hoover sign)

**Breathing Rhythm**
Normal, prolonged exhalation, absent end-expiratory pause, more frequent yawning, hiccups, alternating flat and deep breaths

## Respiratory Musculature
Inspiratory and expiratory evaluation of strength: Own notes (e.g., possible, difficult, impossible, present, not present) (**Table 5.2**)
- Overall evaluation: Inspiratory power/expiratory power: Normal strength, weaker, strongly diminished
- Results of the examination of respiratory muscle strength in the pulmonary function laboratory:.........

**Table 5.2** Inspiratory and expiratory evaluation of strength

| | |
|---|---|
| Several deep breaths | |
| Rapid, flat breathing | |
| Paradoxical breathing movement: respiratory alternans | |
| Sniffing, snuffling, nasal stenosis | |
| Deep breathing in prone position | |
| Breathing against resistance (therapist's hands) | |
| Voice | |
| Speaking, singing, blowing, whistling | |
| Coughing impulse | |

## Use of Accessory Respiratory Muscles
At rest and with exercise (specify type of exertion; **Table 5.3**)

**Table 5.3** Accessory respiratory muscle use at rest and with exercise

| Muscle | Tone right/left | Shortening right/left |
|---|---|---|
| Scalene muscles | | |
| Sternocleidomastoid | | |
| Trapezius | | |
| Levator scapulae | | |
| Pectoralis major | | |
| Latissimus dorsi | | |
| Abdominal muscles | | |
| Other | | |

## Rib Position
Diagonal, horizontal, wide intercostal spaces

## Voice, Manner of Speaking, Speech
- Voice: Normal, hoarse, soft
- Manner of speaking: Normal, atonal, fading, short, cut off, compressed, monotonous, rapidly and tumbling out
- Throat-clearing
- Interrupted by coughing
- Other abnormalities: Lost for words
- Limited understanding of speech because of.........

## Breathing Sounds
- Inspiratory and expiratory stridor, rattling (audible without stethoscope)
- Results of own auscultation.........

## Breath Odor
- None
- Odor: Purulent, acetone, urine

## Body Position

### Preferred Starting Position of the Patient
Flat on the back, slightly raised headrest, lateral decubitus, beach chair position, sitting

### Positions that Ease Breathing in Patients with Obstruction/Respiratory Distress
Seated comfortably with forearms on thighs (also modified version), seated on table/treatment bench with arms supported, seated and leaning on arms outstretched behind for support, pilot's posture, or in an armchair with arms supported by cushions, standing with torso bent forward and hands on thighs for support, standing using arms for support against the table, standing using arms for support against the pelvic bones, standing with forearms resting on a railing
- Other

### Cardiac Chair Position

### Starting Positions to Avoid or that Cause Discomfort
Flat on the back, left lateral decubitus, prone, head lowered

## Tissue Tension—Upper Body

### Musculature (General)
- Hypotonicity, normal tonicity, hypertonicity
- Atrophy

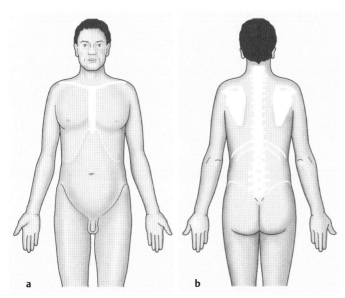

**Fig. 5.1a, b** Body chart for drawing lung and bronchial zones.
**a** Ventral.
**b** Dorsal.

a

b

**Connective Tissue**

Generalized tension, normal tonicity, hypotonicity, hypertonicity

Lung and bronchial zones, draw on body chart (**Fig. 5.1a, b**):

+ = Slight
++ = Clear
+++ = Very clear
Silent/dead zone = draw a circle around it

**Scars**
Type, location

## Locomotor System

**Posture**
Upright, slouched, alternating, expression of mental situation

**Thorax Shape and Mobility**
*Shape of upper body*
Normal, barrel chest, enlarged sagittal diameter, kyphosis, scoliosis, changes due to osteoporosis

*Mobility of thoracic spine and ribs*
See **Table 5.4**.

**Table 5.4**  Mobility of thoracic spine and ribs

| Thoracic spine—active and passive | Notes |
|---|---|
| Bending | |
| Extension | |
| Sidebending | |
| Rotation | |
| *Ribs and costovertebral joints* | |
| First rib | |
| Second to sixth ribs | |
| Seventh and 12th ribs | |
| Costotransverse joints | |
| Costovertebral joints | |

**Thoracic Circumference (Breathing Measurements: Table 5.5), Mobility, Strength, Expandability, Increased Tension**

*(To evaluate peripheral muscle strength, possibly use an orthopedic questionnaire.)*

- Extremity joints and musculature (iliopsoas muscle)
- Spinal column, trunk musculature (quadratus lumborum muscle and rectus abdominis muscle)
- Pelvic floor musculature

**Table 5.5** Thoracic circumference

| Measurement site | Maximum inspiration | Maximum expiration | Difference |
|---|---|---|---|
| Axilla | | | |
| Tip of sternum | | | |
| Five cm below tip of sternum | | | |
| Navel | | | |

**Other Abnormalities of the Locomotor System and Movement Control**

For example, coordination ability

## Cardiopulmonary Performance and Exercise Testing

**Heart Rate/Pulse**

At rest.........; during exertion......... (specify type of exertion); regeneration (after 3 minutes) .........
Rhythmic, arrhythmic

**Blood Pressure**

Respiratory rate (RR) at rest.........; and during exertion based on physician's orders......... (specify type of exertion)

**Pulsoxymetry**

At rest.........; during exertion......... (specify type of exertion)

**Possible Physical Therapy Exertion Tests (Table 5.6)**

- Not possible due to disease severity
- Walking on a level surface, any tempo (give hallway length and time)
- Walking on a level surface at a tempo of 60, 80, 100, 120 steps per minute; report time
- Climbing stairs, any tempo (number of stairs and time)
- Climbing stairs one step per second
- Six-minute walking test (special documentation required)
- Other

## Goals

- Patient's expectations of physical therapy
- Treatment goal(s) of the physical therapist

**Table 5.6** Documentation of walking on a level surface and climbing stairs

| Type of stress | RF | Pulse | RR (if prescribed) | Respiratory distress (number on scale) | Strenuousness (number on Borg scale) | Pallor (P) Redness (R) | Sweating + ++ +++ | Changed movement sequence | Changed behavior and speech | Discontinue |
|---|---|---|---|---|---|---|---|---|---|---|
| Before stress test | | | | | | | | | | |
| Immediately after stress test | | | | | | | | | | |
| 3–5 min after stress test | | | | | | | | | | |

Note: RF = respiratory frequency; RR = respiratory rate.

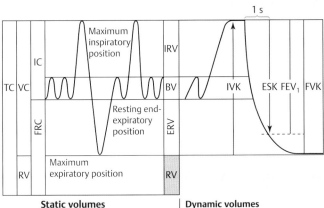

**Fig. 5.2** Lung volumes.

| Static volumes | Dynamic volumes |
|---|---|
| **Static volumes** Static volume consists of the partial volumes making up the total capacity. Spirometry measures static volumes, which allows for an evaluation of restrictive lung disease | **Dynamic volumes** Dynamic volumes require forced expiratory breathing maneuvers and provide standard variables for diagnosing airway obstruction |

### 5.1.3 Examination Steps

#### Current Situation

As part of the medical history, information about the patient's previous or current job is especially important for the doctor. Many occupational disorders are pulmonary diseases, which may limit the ability of the patient to remain on the job. The physical therapist should consider how behaviors that are related to the patient's occupation may be altered (e.g., use pursed-lip breathing during lifting and carrying, emotional effects such as early retirement or disability, as well as potential allergies).

> *Knowledge of any relevant secondary diagnoses is essential for treatment.*

*Examples:*
- In patients with severe osteoporosis, end-range and combined spinal movements must be avoided as should any jarring or compression of the thorax.
- Severe cardiac insufficiency limits the amount of strain the patient can take.

#### *Physician Examinations*

> *Physical therapists should have knowledge of the most important and common doctor's examinations. The therapist should be able to take their results into account during treatment.*

#### *Measuring Pulmonary Function*
The measurement of pulmonary function is important for more than mere diagnosis. It may also be used to evaluate the effects of treatment and the course of disease. Physical therapists should understand the indicators reported by the pulmonary functioning laboratory, in order to appropriately treat the patient's current respiratory situation (**Fig. 5.2**).

#### Measuring Static Lung Volumes
- *Inhalation volumes (IV)* or *breathing volumes (BV)*: The inhaled/exhaled volume per breath:
  - *Middle breathing position:* Position of breath volume as a part of the total lung capacity during normal respiration. It may be more in the direction of inspiration or expiration.
  - *Resting end-expiratory position:* Normal expiratory position, between the elastic tension of the lung inward and the elastic tension of the thorax outward.
- *Inspiratory reserve volume (IRV):* The additional inhalable volume of air after normal inspiration.

- *Expiratory reserve volume (ERV):* Volume that can still be exhaled after normal expiration from the resting end-expiratory position.
- *Residual volume (RV):* Remaining air volume in the lung after maximum expiration.
- *Inspiration capacity (IC):* After normal expiration, the inhalable air volume.
- *Functional residual capacity (FRC):* In the resting end-expiratory position, the volume of air that remains in the lung after normal exhalation.
- *Total capacity (TC):* After maximum inspiration, the volume of air in the lung.
- *Vital capacity (VC):* After maximum inspiration, the volume of air that can be expelled using the greatest amount of force.

> With regard to dynamic volume, it is important to know the forced expiration volume in 1 second (FEV1, Tiffeneau test). This is the volume of air that, after maximum inspiration, can be exhaled with forced expiration in the first second.

### Peak Flow

Peak flow is the maximum expiratory flow rate that is achieved by forced expiration after maximum inspiration. It is a rough measure for obstruction, primarily of the large airways. Normal values depend on sex, age, and size; they are available in the tables accompanying the devices.

> This measurement is especially useful in asthmatics to identify the degree of obstruction. In COPD patients, a drop in the value may indicate that the infection is beginning to worsen.

Measurements of peak flow using a *peak flow meter* may be used to identify an obstruction or worsening of one. Recording values in a diary can help adjust the medication dosage. This important "early warning system" is taught in patient education seminars at which physical therapists are also present.

### Spirometry

Pulmonary function allows for an objectification of characteristic findings and can be reproduced at any time. Classic spirometry enables a direct measurement of respiratory volumes, although its use depends on the cooperation of the patient. The units are inexpensive and are the simplest method a physician has for pulmonary function testing in the private practice setting.

### Body Plethysmography

Body plethysmography (whole-body plethysmography) is a highly sensitive method for determining airway resistance and intrathoracic gas volumes. It does not require active effort by the patient. At present, it is the most comprehensive method of measuring pulmonary function.

### Bronchospasmolytic Test

The bronchospasmolytic test assesses whether a bronchial obstruction is primarily due to bronchoconstriction and whether treatment with bronchospasmolytics is successful.

### Blood Gas Analysis (BGA)/Pulsoxymetry

A blood gas analysis measures oxygen partial pressure, carbon dioxide partial pressure, and other parameters such as the pH level and oxygen saturation in arterial blood. The arterial oxygen value is measured based on an analysis of arterial blood gas (blood is taken directly from an artery or from the earlobe). Oxygen saturation may be simply determined by transcutaneous measurement at the fingertip using a pulsoxymeter.

> The BGA measures oxygen partial pressure in arterial blood. Pulsoxymetry measures oxygen saturation in arterial blood.

In certain pulmonary diseases (e.g., cystic fibrosis, emphysema, fibrosis), the respiratory volume per minute can decrease so strongly that the body is no longer supplied with oxygen, resulting in hypoxemia. This may be determined based on blood gas analysis and, in a simpler way, using *pulsoxymetry* (oxygen saturation measurement without taking blood). If necessary, the patient may be hospitalized and given oxygen or sent later for long-term oxygen therapy. The treatment time with oxygen in long-term therapy is at least 16 hours daily.

Physical therapists often remove the oxygen nasal cannula, arguing that it impairs nasal breathing. This is not so. Patients with hypoxemia should receive oxygen especially during physical therapy treatment.

> When treating at-risk patients at an acute clinic, the physical therapist should ask the treating physician whether the patient can leave his or her room without oxygen.

### Auscultation

Auscultation (from the Latin "to listen") may be used to hear sounds that are produced during respiration or cardiac or gastrointestinal tract activity. When listening to the lung using a stethoscope, respiratory sounds may be interpreted qualitatively and quantitatively.

Normal breathing sounds are soft and quiet. Inspiration should transition into expiration without any interruption. Expiration is only audible at the beginning of the exhalation. Normal breathing sounds in an adult, arising in the bronchioles and alveoli, are referred to as *vesicular breathing* (lung periphery). In children, vesicular breathing is intensified (puerile breathing), and in older people it is weaker.

Breath sounds heard over the trachea are louder and coarser than those heard during normal breathing. Those heard over the lung periphery indicate *bronchial breathing*; on inspiration as well as expiration, there is a pause between the two phases. Greater sound conduction occurs as a result of hardening of lung tissue due to fluid (pulmonary edema) or inflammation (pneumonia).

If the bronchial tubes are displaced in a certain segment of the lung (in atelectasis), or if there is no longer air-filled lung tissue (in pneumothorax), breathing sounds may be quieter or even absent.

**Pathological Noises**
- Dry (continuous) noises (e.g., rhonchus, whistling, or humming) are caused by obstructions that block the flow of air. This may occur—for instance, in asthma or COPD—when mucus clogs and narrows the bronchial tubes. The sounds primarily occur during expiration.
- Moist, coarse rattling sounds (discontinuous noises) when air passes through fluid-filled central airways, for instance, in bronchiectasis, bronchitis, and mucus retention.
- Fine rattling sounds are suggestive of fluid obstruction in the peripheral airways; or there may be crackling sounds with opening of the airways (pulmonary edema, pneumonia, fibrosis).
- Pleural friction rub is perceived as a creaking sound. The inflamed pleural surfaces rub against one another, as in pleuritis sicca.

*Performing auscultation (Fig. 5.3):*
- Disinfect stethoscope.
- Clothing should be removed from the patient's upper body—to avoid anomalies due to clothing or jewelry.
- Ask the patient to cough briefly.
- The patient should inhale and exhale deeply several times through the mouth (caution: risk of hyperventilation).
- Auscultation is performed dorsal to the apex of the lung and down to its base, and then ventral to the apex of the lung. In patients who are weak and can take only a few deep breaths, the base of the lung is the preferred site for auscultation.

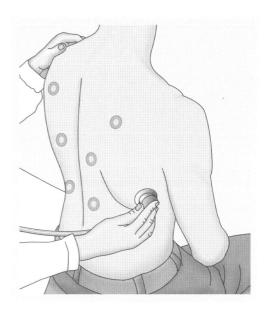

**Fig. 5.3** Auscultation technique—dorsal/lateral.

- Each point is listened to for a complete respiratory cycle, comparing sides.

Physical therapists who work exclusively or primarily with patients with airway symptoms, as well as those working in intensive care, should perform auscultation themselves in order to evaluate treatment success (e.g., elimination of mucus retention). Whether this examination must be learned by students of physical therapy should be critically discussed.

*Percussion*
Percussion is when the physician taps on the patient's chest during the physical examination to evaluate the underlying structures. An air–tissue (e.g., size of the heart, position of the diaphragm) or air–fluid boundary may be evaluated (e.g., infiltrates). The penetration depth of percussion is about 3 cm. A *normal* sound is distinguished from *hypersonorous resonance* over an area of increased air (e.g., emphysema) or *dull resonance* over areas with less air (e.g., in pneumonia, pleural effusion).

*Radiograph of Thoracic Organs*
A radiograph shows changes in patients with atelectasis, emphysema, infiltrates, pleural effusion, and pneumothorax. It is therefore important for the physical therapist to note such diseases in the patient's medical record.

### Spiroergometry

Spiroergometry may be used to analyze physical capacity and also allows for an evaluation of respiratory efficiency and fitness level. In this complex analysis of cardiopulmonary function, the patient exercises at a given level on a cycle ergometer or treadmill. A blood gas analysis (under exertion) is performed, an ECG lead is positioned, and respiratory volume is measured through a face mask over the nose and mouth, as are oxygen intake and carbon dioxide elimination.

### Allergy Diagnosis

Allergy diagnosis begins with a thorough interview using an allergy questionnaire. This is followed by patch testing and, if necessary, blood tests.

### Patch Tests

- *Rub test* (e.g., with animal hair): In a severe allergy, a wheal will develop within a few minutes.
- *Skin-prick test:* A drop of solution containing the allergen is placed on the skin, which is then scratched with a thin needle. If an allergic response occurs, the allergen causes local inflammation in the layer of skin it has entered along with redness and welts.
- *Intracutaneous test:* The solution containing the allergen is injected directly under the skin.
- *Blood test:* Detection of allergen-specific antibodies (IgE antibodies) in blood.
- *Specific provocation tests:* The suspected allergens are placed directly on the nasal mucosa or inhaled.

### Bronchoscopy

This endoscopic examination enables direct inspection of the bronchial tree using flexible or rigid instruments.

A diagnostic bronchoscopy may be performed if there is suspicion of a tumor, pulmonary fibrosis, uncertain hemoptysis, or antibiotic-resistant pneumonia. Depending on the presumptive diagnosis, a *biopsy* may be taken from the mucous membranes, lymph nodes, or peripheral lung tissue. Bacteria, cells, and proteins from the alveoli are obtained using bronchoalveolar lavage.

In terms of treatment, a bronchoscope may be used to remove foreign bodies and secretions; hemostasis can be achieved, and tumor tissue can be removed.

### Karnofsky Index

The Karnofsky index is used to evaluate the patient's overall health:

- 100%: Normal activity, no symptoms

- 90%: Normal activity, mild signs of illness
- 80%: Normal activity, with strain
- 70%: No normal activity, but the patient can take care of him or herself
- 60%: Occasionally needs help
- 50%: Needs considerable help and medical care
- 40%: Constantly needs specialized help and care
- 30%: Significant impairment, hospitalization indicated
- 20%: Severely ill, active supportive therapy needed
- 10%: Dying

> Knowledge of the index is essential to formulating realistic goals for physical therapy.

### Grading/Staging

When working in oncological units, physical therapists should have sound knowledge of grading and staging.

### Grading

The tissue is histologically examined along with an evaluation of tumor differentiation (e.g., G2 = moderately differentiated tumor). Along with the degree of differentiation of a tumor, its spread may also be assessed using ultrasound, radiographs, CT, and bone scintigraphy.

### Staging

Staging is based on the TNM classification. This internationally recognized staging scheme for malignant tumors uses standardized criteria to evaluate tumor size (T), the number of infected lymph nodes (N = nodules), and metastases (M).

## Medication Therapy

Knowledge of medication use is also very important for physical therapists. The medication used to treat patients with pulmonary and airway diseases may be divided into two groups:

- *Controllers:* Protective, basic therapy, which may also be used daily even when the patient is well. These include inhaled corticosteroids, long-acting beta-2-sympathomimetic agents, disodium cromoglycate, and nedocromil, as well as oral steroids.
- *Relievers:* Helpers, which, if needed, may be used for symptomatic treatment of airway obstruction and dyspnea. These include short-acting bronchial-dilating inhaled medications, e.g., beta-2-sympathomimetic agents, and anticholinergics.

### Preventive (Anti-allergy) and Anti-inflammatory Medications

These include cromoglicic acid, disodium salt, and nedocromil sodium. These substances are available in a spray for prophylactic use. They form a protective film around sensitized mast cells, thereby preventing the release of inflammatory substances. These medications are primarily used against allergic asthma.

### Antibody Therapy (Anti-IgE)

The antibody omalizumab inhibits the binding of IgE to mast cells. This prevents histamine release from the mast cell. Subcutaneous administration is appropriate for patients with severe allergic asthma that is present year round.

### Anti-inflammatory Drugs

The most important anti-inflammatory drugs are *corticosteroids* (cortisone). Cortisol is an essential hormone that is produced by the adrenal glands (ca. 30 mg daily). Cortisol production and the release of cortisol into the bloodstream are controlled by complex mechanisms. Cortisol acts by entering the body's cells and alters their metabolic activity. It thus helps the body during stressful situations (e.g., overcoming an infection or in stressful situations); it changes the metabolism of fat, protein, sugar, and alters the salt and water balance.

Corticosteroids have been used as a drug since 1948. Their primary actions are to reduce inflammation and mucosal swelling. Many patients are afraid or concerned, given misinformation in the discussion on the effects and side-effects of the drug. The adverse effects related to long-term oral corticosteroid use, which vary according to duration and dosage, are serious and are relevant to the physical therapy examination and treatment. Effects can lead to a clinical appearance of *Cushing syndrome* (**Fig. 5.4**) in conjunction with the following signs:

- Osteoporosis
- Skin changes (atrophy, acne, furuncles, ulcers, stretch marks, changes affecting hair-bearing skin)
- Weight gain due to increased appetite
- Loss of muscle strength
- Fuller face, adrenocortical obesity
- Ocular changes (gray or green cataracts)
- Hypertension
- Diabetes mellitus
- Increased risk of thrombosis
- Psychological changes (euphoric mood; rarely, depressive mood)

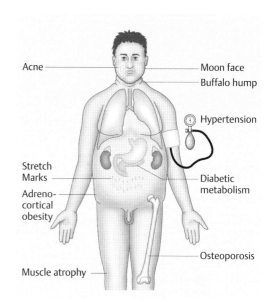

Acne — Moon face
— Buffalo hump
— Hypertension
Stretch Marks —
Adreno-cortical obesity —
— Diabetic metabolism
— Osteoporosis
Muscle atrophy —

**Fig. 5.4** Symptoms of Cushing syndrome.

> Long-term corticosteroid use should not be abruptly stopped or without first consulting the treating physician. During long-term therapy, the body's cortisol production becomes "dormant" and thus stopping treatment can have serious consequences.

An excellent option for avoiding "oral" side-effects is the use of inhalation therapy, which allows the drug to reach the target site in the lung directly (**Fig. 5.5**). Side-effects, such as hoarseness or oral thrush, can be minimized by cleansing the mouth and using an inhaler aid (spacer device).

> Corticosteroid inhalation does not help in an emergency. Instead, patients should inhale short-acting beta-2-sympathomimetic agents.
> The physical therapist should speak with the patient to find out if he or she knows what medication to take in an emergency.

### Leukotriene Antagonists

A relatively new substance group are leukotriene antagonists. These drugs inhibit the effect of leukotrienes, a group of mediators involved in asthma that are released by inflammatory cells. Leukotrienes are involved in various processes, such as mucus production, mucosal swelling, and bronchospasm.

Inhibition of leukotrienes blocks such processes. Yet, given that other mediators also contribute, mere leukotriene inhibition is often inadequate. For long-term therapy, other anti-inflammatory drugs are advised.

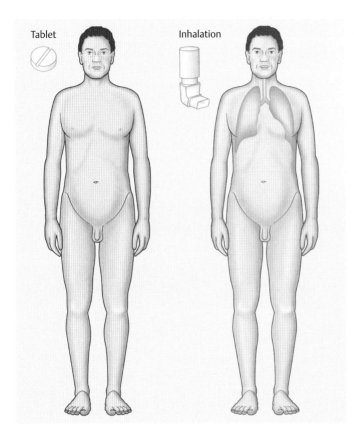

**Fig. 5.5** Pathway from intake to target site.

### Bronchodilators

Bronchodilators include betamimetics, anticholinergics, and theophylline. These drugs reverse the bronchospasm, widen the airways, and prevent overinflation of the lung.

### Betamimetics

Betamimetics are related to adrenaline, one of the body's own hormones. These drugs are able to widen the airways; hence they are also known as beta-adrenergics. Short-acting betamimetics (sprays) rapidly widen the airways and are thus suitable for emergency use in patients with acute respiratory distress. Long-acting betamimetics may be inhaled on a regular basis for prevention.

The retarded drug (tablet) allows for delayed release of the active ingredients over a period of many hours; it is therefore unsuitable for use in an emergency.

> *Side-effects of betamimetics, which may be noted during physical therapy examination and treatment, include shaky hands, restlessness, tachycardia, nausea, and headache.*

### Anticholinergics

Anticholinergics also cause bronchiodilation. In addition, they reduce the formation of mucus. They do not take action as quickly as betamimetics.

> *This substance group has minimal side-effects.*

### Theophylline

The level of bronchiodilation produced by this derivative of caffeine is weaker than that of betamimetics and anticholinergics. Due to various other effects on breathing and the cardiovascular system, it enhances the body's response to stress.

> *The side-effects are similar to drinking too much coffee: nausea, heart palpitations, tremors, restlessness, arrhythmia, sleep disorders, or even seizures.*

### Expectorants

Some patients benefit from the use of expectorants, which dilute the mucus (acetylcysteine) or increase mucus secretion (ambroxol). During antibiotic treatment, the bronchial mucus becomes thicker, and therefore may be difficult to cough up. Thus, the antibiotic does not reach the pathogen in sufficient amounts. For this reason, expectorants are often prescribed during antibiotic treatment. Increasing fluid intake also helps patients cough up mucus if they have a fluid deficiency.

### Antibiotics

Given their complexity, we will not go into detail on treatment with antibiotics or substances that destroy cells (*cytostasis*), which may be prescribed to reduce cortisone use. However, the side-effects of cytostatic therapy are certainly relevant to physical therapy treatment, and the reader is advised to study them carefully.

### Cardiovascular Medications

Among the cardiovascular drugs that are relevant to physical therapy are *beta blockers.*

> *During the physical therapy examination and treatment, blood pressure and heart rate are lowered. In patients taking beta blockers, the heart rate will not increase adequately during exertion. There is thus a risk of strain if the physical therapist does not have sufficient knowledge of these drugs. In addition, beta blockers promote bronchial obstruction and may therefore exacerbate asthma.*

## Specific Immunotherapy (Desensitization)

Specific immunotherapy ("to make less sensitive") in allergic asthma is used if there is a shorter history of allergic disease (less than 5 years) and if the relationship to the allergy trigger is clear (e.g., asthma occurring after exposure to grass pollen).

The basic principle underlying desensitization consists of repeated exposure to increasing amounts of the relevant allergen. The allergens are first given subcutaneously in minute dosages and later in increasing concentrations. The low levels of allergen do not cause an allergic asthma response, but rather they decrease the formation of allergy-related immune substances in the blood.

Because, to a certain extent, the procedure resembles active immunization (vaccination), the term *specific immunotherapy* is preferred.

Desensitization can now also be performed as sublingual treatment (placing the allergen under the tongue).

## Radiation Therapy

Despite technical improvements in radiation treatment, damage to healthy tissue is still not completely preventable.

> *Radiation treatment can lead to acute skin symptoms consisting of redness, scaling, and pigmentation changes. The physical therapist should mark the areas of the skin that were exposed to radiation. No heat or cold should be applied to these areas, and massage or rubbing of the skin should be avoided.*

## Patient History

The patient's main symptoms consist of *dyspnea, anxiety, coughing, sputum,* and pain in the chest region.

## Dyspnea

Dyspnea means difficulty breathing, along with the subjective feeling of respiratory distress. It can range from the perception of greater difficulty breathing (e.g., with physical strain) to discomfort.

Types of respiratory distress may be distinguished by pathogenetic cause (cardiac, pneumological, circulatory, central). The patient should be asked about the onset, frequency, duration, and characteristics of his or her respiratory distress. Sudden shortness of breath, occurring within minutes or hours, may be a sign of an acute asthma attack, pulmonary edema, or pulmonary embolism. Subacute onset, over a period of days, weeks, or months, tends to suggest chronic heart insufficiency, anemia, or bronchial carcinoma.

Dyspnea that develops over the course of several years (insidious) tends to be due to pulmonary emphysema or pulmonary hypertension.

> *Dyspnea is the most common and most important symptom of pulmonary disease.*

### Orthopnea

Strong resting dyspnea that forces the patient to maintain an upright posture or sit up, and necessitates the use of the accessory respiratory muscles, is known as orthopnea.

### Dyspnea Scale

On the scale for dyspnea, "0" indicates no respiratory distress and "10" is the most serious respiratory distress possible. This may be used for resting dyspnea and dyspnea on exertion. This method is a simplified form that may be used in acute care or physical therapy. For rehabilitation clinics and special pneumological facilities, more specific assessment criteria are recommended.

## Anxiety

Patients who suffer from anxiety or significant psychological distress may describe their breathing as follows:

- Feeling of not being able to breathe deeply/fully enough
- More rapid breathing at rest
- Feeling of not being able to exhale enough
- Needing to sigh frequently
- Feeling of suffocation

## Coughing

Coughing is a reflex that is triggered by irritation of the cough receptors in the larynx, trachea, and the large bronchiae. After a deep inhalation, the glottis closes, and the muscles of the chest wall, abdomen, and back cause increased intrathoracic and intra-abdominal pressure. Afterward, the glottis opens suddenly and the air flows out at great speed. During a major coughing episode, the velocity of air may be nearly as great as the speed of sound.

▌ *Coughing is the most effective form of elimination of secretions.*

Coughing is the common symptom for all pulmonary and a few extrapulmonary diseases and is a common complaint. Coughing can contribute to the spread of infectious diseases.

As a protective mechanism (e.g., against choking), coughing ends after or one two coughs. A persistent cough warrants physician consultation, as this does not occur in healthy individuals.

▌ *Persistent coughing is always pathological. Occasionally, compulsive coughing may be due to psychological causes.*

During the examination, the physical therapist should ask when the cough occurs, the frequency of coughing, triggers/exacerbating factors, and the character of the cough. Sometimes, coughing is so routine that the patient is no longer aware of his or her symptom. In rare instances, a coughing fit may lead to syncope or rib fracture (cough fracture).

## Sputum

The presence of sputum (expectorated bronchial secretions) may be a sign of an inflammation and/or nicotine abuse.

## Hypercrinia

Hypercrinia is the overproduction of secretions (e.g., in bronchitis or cystic fibrosis). It is usually difficult for the patient to quantify the amount of sputum, either due to incorrectly estimating the amount or because the mucus is often swallowed. The greatest amount of sputum is coughed up by patients with cystic fibrosis or bronchiectasis (mouthful expectoration, up to 2 L). Its appearance may provide a clue as to the responsible disease:

### Examples:

- White in patients with chronic irritation of the airways
- Foamy (white or rose-colored) in patients with pulmonary edema
- Yellow or green (pus = purulent) in infections if leukocytes are mixed in, or in patients with asthma if there are eosinophilic granulocytes

▌ *Sputum may be thin, stringy, viscous, or glassy.*

### Dyscrinia

Dyscrinia refers to the pathologically changed consistency (viscosity) of mucus (e.g., in asthma).

### Hemoptysis

Depending on the amount of blood the patient coughs up, the sputum may be discolored (hemoptysis). Even pure blood from the lung, or a large amount of blood from the respiratory passages, may be coughed up (hemoptysis: "bloody cough").

Hemoptysis may be harmless (banal inflammation of the tracheobronchial system) or it may be an indication of serious disease (bronchial carcinoma, pulmonary embolism, tuberculosis). Along with blood, there are also other particles (e.g., bits of tissue) in the sputum (e.g., in lung abscess), which have an odor that may be sweet, unpleasant, or putrid.

### Mucostasis

In mucostasis, the mucus remains stagnant in the bronchial system.

## Pain in the Chest Region

A patient may have chest pain that is independent or dependent on breathing. Due to lacking sensory innervation of the lung (and thus it does not cause pain), the pain comes from the pleura (e.g., pleuritis) or thoracic wall.

**Causes of Chest Pain, Depending on Clinical Appearance**

- Sharp, stabbing pain, worsened by respiratory movements, well-localized (arising from the pleura)
- Dull pain, related to a feeling of constriction or pressure, cannot be precisely localized, retrosternal and parasternal also radiating into the left arm with fourth/fifth fingers, not dependent on breathing, triggered and exacerbated during exertion (angina pectoris)
- Well-localized, worsens with thoracic movements, depending on breathing, usually can be reproduced by external pressure (pain of thoracic wall due to muscular causes or rib fracture)
- Well-localized, within segmental borders, superficial, worsens with movement (arising from the spinal column)

## Psychological Situation and Emotional Attitude

The psychological situation and emotional attitude of the patient may be altered due to his or her current diagnosis, family problems, worries about the future, or their pain. The physical therapist should be sensitive to the patient's situation.

## General Findings

### Strength

For a patient with pulmonary and respiratory diseases, strength, and possibly training to build muscle, are important. The decreasing pulmonary functioning exacerbates the patient's dyspnea. His or her lifestyle is increasingly geared toward "avoiding dyspnea," which leads to a downward spiral. As a result of reduced cardiopulmonary activity, the disease progresses, and the patient becomes even less active.

### Body Weight

Significant excess weight impairs the movement of the diaphragm and changes the position of the lumbar vertebrae. Heavier people also need more oxygen during exercise than do people with normal weight. The effects on bronchial diseases are especially negative due to already abnormal ventilation. When there is significant "ventral weight" the rib cage is drawn downward in an expiratory position and the mass must be lifted again with every inhalation.

The causes of *pulmonary cachexia* (emaciation), for instance, in patients with severe COPD, can vary. One possibility is that greater respiratory effort causes patients to consume more energy; they also eat and drink less due to respiratory distress. Chronic inflammations can also lead to cachexia as can consuming diseases (carcinoma). Cytostatic agents may cause side-effects (nausea) that worsen the situation.

Rapid weight gain may be a sign of fluid accumulation due to uncompensated cardiac or renal insufficiency.

## State of Awareness

The patient's state of awareness may be altered or impaired due to residual effects of medication (also postoperatively) or oxygen deficiency. Cerebral sclerosis and dementia should also be considered.

## Skin Color

> *In patients with respiratory or lung diseases, one should also evaluate the color of the skin.*

### Cyanosis

Cyanosis refers to blue discoloration of the skin, mucous membranes, and lips. Pathogenetically, one may distinguish between *central* and *peripheral cyanosis*.

**Central Cyanosis**

This refers to insufficient oxygenation of the blood. It occurs, for instance, in pulmonary diseases with abnormal gas exchange or cardiac defects with a shunt between the arterial and venous system. There are diminished $pO_2$ levels: respiratory partial insufficiency ($pO_2$ diminished, $pCO_2$ normal), or respiratory global insufficiency ($pO_2$ diminished, $pCO_2$ elevated). The cause may be an obstructive or restrictive ventilatory defect and/or a diffusion disorder.

**Peripheral Cyanosis**

Slowed flow velocity in the capillaries may be due to vasoconstriction as a result of cold, or reduced cardiac output, or shock with increased oxygen consumption in peripheral blood.

In clinical terms, a distinction is made between central and peripheral cyanosis. In central cyanosis, the whole body is cyanotic, and in peripheral cyanosis, only the periphery (acral regions: fingers, tips of nose, lips, toes) is cyanotic. Rubbing the earlobe

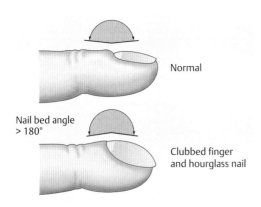

**Fig. 5.6** Clubbed fingers and hourglass nails.

increases peripheral blood flow velocity; peripheral cyanosis will disappear, but central cyanosis will not.

### Visible Abnormalities

Other visble abnormalities that may be present in patients with pulmonary disease are *clubbed fingers* and *hourglass nails.* This pulmonary osteoarthropathy is due to hypoxic damage:

- Due to pulmonary causes, for example, due to pulmonary emphysema, bronchiectasis, pulmonary fibrosis, carcinoma
- Cardiac causes, for example, due to a cardiac defect
- Abdominal causes, for example, due to liver cirrhosis

The precise pathophysiological mechanism is unknown. There have been occasional reports of idiopathic/familial occurrence without any pathological findings (synonym: digiti hippocratici, *clubbed fingers*; **Fig. 5.6**).

- *Nicotine spots* and *stains* on the fingernails and fingers are indicative of nicotine abuse.
- *Cutaneous or mediastinal emphysema* means the penetration of air into the interstitial connective tissue of the mediastinum. This may occur due to injury of the trachea, bronchia, esophagus (e.g., during endoscopy or idiopathically as in spontaneous pneumothorax).

> *For palpation, it is important to know that this collection of air may present as a subcutaneous swelling that makes a crackling noise under pressure ("crunch of snow").*

- *Emphysematous overinflation* is evident when the apex of the lung is visible, protruding above the clavicle.
- In addition to *barrel chest* in a person with emphysema, there is *diminished distance* between the sternum and larynx.
- Disrupted flow in the jugular vein (*jugular vein obstruction*) suggests insufficiency of the right half of the heart (cor pulmonale).
- *Pink puffer* and *blue bloater* are findings in COPD that may be visible upon inspection (**Fig. 5.7**).
  - Pink puffer (panlobular emphysema): Generally occurs in asthenic people with severe dyspnea on exertion, which later progresses into resting dyspnea. The patient's habitus is marked by excessive ventilatory effort (*fighters*); patients tend to have pale rosy skin coloration.
  - Blue bloater (centrilobular emphysema): The main symptoms are chronic bronchitis with coughing, sputum production, and cyanosis. The patient's habitus is usually stout to obese.

## Respiration Patterns (Formerly: Forms of Respiration)

The pattern of respiration is the way in which breathing, or the necessary minute volume, is achieved. The following parameters are involved.

### Respiration Rate

The rate of respiration is the number of breaths per minute. A single breath consists of *inhalation, exhalation,* and an *end-expiratory pause.*

An error in breathing rate measurement may occur if the patient feels watched, which usually causes them to breathe more rapidly.

> *Trick: Inform the patient that you are going to take their pulse. Next, observe their respiratory movements for 60 seconds. This also allows you to simultaneously obtain the "resting pulse."*

#### Eupnea
In adults, this type of breathing occurs without conscious effort. Eupnea is defined as regular successive, equally deep breaths (8–16 breaths per minute with about 500 mL per breath).

#### Normal Values
- Premature infants: 50 to 60 breaths per minute at 1 kg of body weight
- Newborns: 30 to 40 breaths per minute at 3 kg of body weight

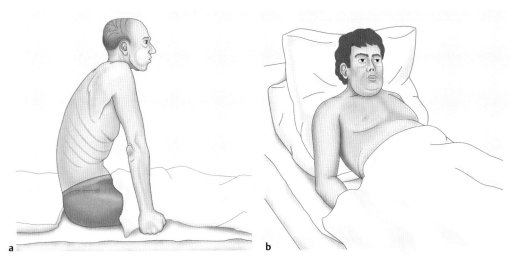

**Fig. 5.7a, b** COPD.
**a** Pink puffer. **b** Blue bloater.

- Small children (1 year old): About 35 breaths per minute
- Children (10 years of age): About 22 breaths per minute

### Deviations in Respiratory Rate

#### Bradypnea
Such patients have—in comparison with normal individuals—a reduced breathing rate under similar conditions. This does *not* necessarily indicate diminished ventilation and bradypnea should be understood in the same sense as bradycardia.

The condition is caused by pressure on the respiratory center (e.g., with head injuries, brain tumors, or inflammation) or chemical influences (e.g., poisoning, sleeping drugs, pain medication, or coma).

| *Bradypnea occurs physiologically during sleep and in athletes.*

#### Tachypnea
Tachypnea refers to an increased respiratory rate compared with a normal person under similar circumstances. The term does *not* refer to hyperventilation and should be understood in the same sense as tachycardia.

Tachypnea is caused by restrictive lung disease (e.g., loss of gas exchange surface compensated for by an increased breathing rate), an increased need for oxygen due to physical exertion, or fever and a diminished hemoglobin count.

### Respiratory Passages

When resting, respiration should occur through the nose, the beginning of the respiratory system. This allows the incoming air to be cleansed, moistened, and warmed. Because more air must be inhaled during physical exertion, there is greater resistance and breathing must also occur through the mouth.

Patients with respiratory distress or severe polyposis also inhale through the mouth, which, however, does not have the air-conditioning effects of nasal breathing. Harmful substances in the air, or cold or dry air, may thus produce bronchial symptoms (e.g., coughing and mucus production). In patients with previous damage and bronchial hyper-reactivity, this situation is exacerbated and the symptoms are more severe.

| *When treating patients with obstruction of the airways, it should be recalled that nasal exhalation produces a natural stenosis.*

#### Nasal Alar Breathing
In nasal alar breathing, there is extreme movement of the ala of the nose, for instance, in conjunction with respiratory distress. This is also a symptom of bacterial pneumonia.

#### Hiccups
Hiccups (*singultus*) occur when there is a sharp inflow of air into the respiratory passages as a result of involuntary contraction of the diaphragm (irritation of the phrenic nerve). This causes the typical

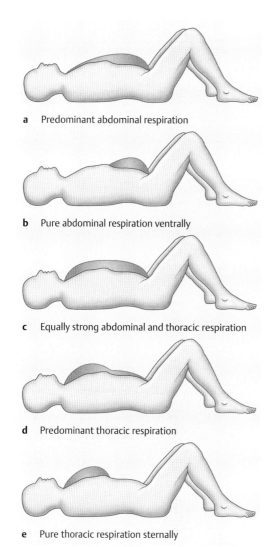

**a**   Predominant abdominal respiration

**b**   Pure abdominal respiration ventrally

**c**   Equally strong abdominal and thoracic respiration

**d**   Predominant thoracic respiration

**e**   Pure thoracic respiration sternally

**Fig. 5.8a–e** Respiratory movements.

hiccup sound. Hiccups can also occur after abdominal surgery in patients with peritonitis, pleurisy, and central nervous disorders.

### Pursed-lip Breathing
Automatic use of pursed-lip breathing, at rest or under stress, may be seen in patients with COPD.

### Tracheotomy/Laryngectomy
Following a tracheotomy (incision of the trachea) or laryngectomy (complete removal of the larynx), the patient must breathe through a *tracheostomy tube*. In patients who have undergone a laryngectomy, the respiratory passages begin at the tracheostomy tube. In patients who have undergone a tracheotomy, the

larynx is not removed. Certain problems can occur in patients as a result of the loss of the larynx/glottis and nasal breathing:

- Absence of the larynx results in:
  - Loss of speaking ability.
  - Lacking vocal cords (or glottis closure), which makes it difficult to cough or clear the throat and there is a high risk of aspiration and infection.
- Loss of nasal breathing results in:
  - Loss of ability to smell.
  - Inability to and blow one's nose, high risk of scalding when consuming hot foods/beverages.
  - Loss of the air-conditioning effect of nasal breathing with potential harm to the respiratory passages due to inhalation of cold and dry air; mucostasis becomes a significant problem.
  - Runny nose without having a cold.

## Respiratory Movements

The movement caused by the muscles used for inspiration (primarily the intercostal muscles and diaphragm) enlarges the thoracic cavity "all the way around." For the purposes of respiratory therapy examination, a distinction is made between thoracic and abdominal respiratory movements.

### Respiratory Movements of the Thorax
The movements of the ribs occur cranially, ventrally and sternally, laterally, and dorsally. The expansion of the "upper" thoracic cavity is more sagittal while expansion of the "lower" portion is more transverse. The diaphragm is involved in the movement of the lower ribs. When it contracts, they are elevated and moved outwardly.

### Respiratory Movements of the Abdomen
Respiratory movements of the abdomen are caused by contraction of the diaphragm during inspiration and its pressure on the abdominal wall and pelvic floor muscles. Intra-abdominal pressure increases and the abdominal organs, which, from a mechanical standpoint, are comparable to a noncompressible fluid-filled sack, are pushed ventrally, laterally, caudally, and lumbodorsally.

The therapist assesses which movements are possible or dominant (**Fig. 5.8a–e**). It should be recalled that in the standing patient, the high level of postural muscle tension, as well as an altered lumbar lordosis, may alter respiratory movements. The respiratory movements should be inspected and palpated from different "angles."

Physical therapists who are also trained as osteopaths can also palpate the diaphragm in the sitting or supine patient in order to obtain the following information:

- Elasticity and resistance of the diaphragm
- Pain
- Locally diminished movement (adhesions)
- Deviations (direction of the movement)
- Defensive tension

### Paradoxical Breathing

Paradoxical breathing involves the inward movement of the lower ribs during inspiration. This can occur if the thorax is fixed in the inspiratory position (pulmonary emphysema), the diaphragm is flattened, and contraction draws the lower ribs inward (*antagonism of diaphragm and thoracic wall or Hoover sign*). The Hoover sign is a cardinal sign of advanced obstructive pulmonary disease. The inward movement may also be an expression of weakness/fatigue or paralysis of the intercostal muscles.

*Respiratory alternans* refers to alternating between almost purely thoracic respiratory movement and purely abdominal respiratory movement. This is an unequivocal sign of respiratory muscle fatigue. The alternating contractions allow the fatigued muscles to recover during the phase in which they are not in use.

In their composition, the muscles of respiration correspond embryologically, morphologically, and functionally to voluntary skeletal muscle. They are composed of the muscle fiber types I, IIa, and IIb. Thus, they can be trained for strength and stamina just as any other skeletal muscle in their concentric (inhalation) and eccentric (slow exhalation) contraction power. Excessive strain causes fatigue and thus respiratory insufficiency. The strength of the respiratory musculature can be measured, for example, in terms of inspiratory pressure:

- PIMAX (maximum inspiratory pressure in kPa)
- P0.1 (inspiratory pressure 0.1 seconds after beginning inspiration in kPa)

### Ventilatory Insufficiency

Patients with ventilatory insufficiency have inadequate ventilation of the lung due to respiratory pump inadequacy (pump insufficiency).

### Examples:

- Neuromuscular disease (poliomyelitis, amyotrophic lateral sclerosis, myopathies), which leads to diminished inspiratory strength as a result of damage to the nerves and/or respiratory muscles.

- Severe thoracic deformities due to scoliosis, or an overinflated thorax due to pulmonary emphysema. Due to constant hyperextension or shortening, the respiratory muscles have a significant loss in contraction ability (lacking conversion of strength into pressure).
- With increased elastic resistance, for example, in pulmonary fibrosis or with increased resistance in the respiratory passages (chronic obstructive pulmonary diseases). Even at rest, there is strain on the respiratory muscles, which must compensate for defective respiratory mechanics.

> All of these diseases strongly limit the function of the respiratory muscles. Inadequate ventilation leads to increased activity and thus strain and exhaustion.

Signs of ventilatory insufficiency include various subjective symptoms (morning headache, sleep disorders, adynamia during the day) as well as clinical findings (e.g., paradoxical respiratory movements; short, flat, frequent breathing; short phonation duration; soft, weak voice) and altered pulmonary function parameters (e.g., increase in $pCO_2$ with concomitant reduction of $pO_2$: respiratory insufficiency).

### Respiratory Musculature

A precise physical therapy evaluation of respiratory muscle strength is difficult and often only possible indirectly. One may *observe* whether there are normal breathing movements and whether deeper breathing is possible (e.g., ask the patient to smell something: concentric contraction of the muscles of inspiration) or whether there is paradoxical breathing or respiratory alternans.

During *tactile evaluation*, the therapist should place his or her fingers in the intercostal spaces and determine the quality and quantity of inhalation and exhalation—also using adequate resistance. He or she should also test whether the patient can overcome resistance (the therapist should place his or her hands on the patient's abdomen and lower ribs and apply dosed resistance) or whether the patient must resort to thoracic respiratory movements. Changes in the starting position should be taken into account.

> The activity of the diaphragm is easier when the upper body is upright (due to gravity) and is more difficult when the patient is reclining.

Lying prone is also very strenuous for the diaphragm, and inspiration is often accomplished with much huffing. Due to nasal stenosis, sniffing and snuffling during inspiration may be used to test the function of the diaphragm as well as its strength, elasticity, and activity.

| *In patients with a weak diaphragm, rapid successive puff-type inhalations are barely or not at all possible.*

Speaking, singing, blowing, and whistling require stopping the outward airflow, which means slowly releasing the air for long phonation duration (tone or breath support). The muscles used for inhalation perform an eccentric contraction, and thus act with "braking power" against a rapidly collapsing thorax (Bänsch 1989, 1992).

### Rib Position

If the thorax is in an inspiratory position (e.g., in COPD), the position of the ribs changes. The ribs are horizontal, and the intercostal spaces are widened.

### Respiratory Noises

In addition to breathing sounds that can only be heard with auscultation (pp. 192–193), physical therapists can also simply listen with their ears. If there is an obstruction, inspiratory and expiratory stridor will be heard; pulmonary edema is accompanied by a rattling sound, even without the aid of a stethoscope.

### Breath Odor

Unpleasant smelling breath (foetor ex ore/halitosis) has not yet been considered in the respiratory examination. The breath of a healthy person has virtually no odor. For physical therapists, it is important to be aware that an unpleasant odor (e.g., ichorous) may accompany an upper airway infection, especially bronchiectasis, pulmonary abscess, or a pulmonary tumor. A foul-smelling or sweet odor (pus) is characteristic of a bacterial infection such as bronchitis or pneumonia.

| *In patients with uremia, the breath and skin smell like urea.*
| *If a patient with diabetes mellitus smells like acetone, this is a sign of impending coma. A physician should be consulted immediately.*

## Voice and Speaking Manner

When a patient with respiratory symptoms comes in for physical therapy, the therapist should evaluate any visible signs of cyanosis and the use of accessory muscles of respiration in the neck. He or she should also evaluate acoustic clues, such as the patient's voice and manner of speaking. The patient's voice may be hoarse (due to inhalation corticosteroids or recurrent paresis, e.g., in bronchial cancer), and his or her sentences may be shorter, cut off, or spoken in a compressed fashion (e.g., in dyspnea and airway obstruction).

Speaking softly may indicate a weakness affecting the respiratory muscles; it is also possible that the patient was recently removed from ventilatory support. Patients with a very nasal speaking voice may have paranasal sinus problems. A soft, monotonous voice also reflects the patient's emotional mental state.

## Body Position

### Obstructive Airway Disease

Patients with obstructive airway disease assume positions of the body that make breathing easier when they have respiratory distress or difficulty breathing after physical exertion (e.g., sitting with the forearms on the thighs or resting the arms on a table). Some of these positions may also be used for treatment.

### Cardiac Chair Position

In the cardiac chair position, the patient's legs are lower than the heart. This reduces strain on the heart by slowing venous backflow (in patients with cardiac insufficiency).

## Tissue Tension—Upper Body

### Connective Tissue Zones

Teirich-Leube (1990, modified after Schuh 1986) has described the connective tissue zones for the lungs and bronchial system as such: in bronchitis, the connective tissue zones are in segments C3–C8 and T1–T9.

- Particularly high tension and irritability are found on the *dorsal side:*
  - Tissue between the shoulder blades, in chronic disorders in the region of the entire thoracic spine and cervical spine as well as the upper lumbar spine
  - Tissue over the neck and shoulders
  - Tissue along the lower margin of the thorax and the borders of the latissimus dorsi muscle

- *Ventral side:*
  - Tissue over the sternum and costal cartilage of T2–T6
  - Tissue in the region of the jugular fossa and the origins of the sternocleidomastoid muscles and well as their posterior borders
  - Tissue below the clavicle on the anterior portion of the deltoid muscles
  - Tissue in the region of the lower margins of the thorax

In asthma, the connective tissue zones are more extensive, often extending caudally to T12 and L1. The following tissue segments are especially tense:

- Paravertebral as far as the sacrum
- In the region of the anterior superior iliac spine as far as the groin
- Bilaterally on the border of the latissimus dorsi and into the axilla
- Bilaterally on the lower border of the thorax and over the intercostal spaces T7–T10

> Given the size of the zones described here, this cannot be determined visually. The physical therapist must rely fully on tactile perception.

## Kibler Fold Test

Tissue tension in the upper body region and dermatomes may also be evaluated via the Kibler fold test (skin rolling test) and connective tissue massage assessment.

> Both examinations cause extreme autonomic irritation.

## Connective Tissue Points

In the view of osteopathic medicine, the connective tissue points are to the right and left of the xiphoid process.

## Scarring

Thoracic expansion may be restricted by large scars (e.g., burns).

> In neural therapy, scars are considered interference fields and should receive special consideration.

## Locomotor System

The composition and structure of the lungs changes with increasing age. In terms of intrapulmonary changes, the lung architecture becomes lax, and there is diminished capillary circulation as well as a decrease in the alveolar surface area. Extrapulmonary changes can occur with atrophy affecting the diaphragm as well as intercostal, abdominal, and back muscles.

Further contributing to impairment of respiratory mechanics are osteoporotic and degenerative changes to the vertebral bodies and costovertebral joints as well as calcification of the costal cartilages. This leads to stiffening of the bony thorax and a rounded back. The diminished flexibility of the thoracic wall and the reduced strength of the respiratory muscles are especially relevant. The ossification of the cartilage attachments of the ribs reduces their pliancy and leads to greater dependence on abdominal and diaphragmatic muscles to ensure sufficient ventilation.

Thoracic wall pain, without impaired breathing, may occur with malalignment of the thoracic vertebral bodies. If thoracic spine blockages persist for a longer period of time, additional blockages of the ribs are possible. Intercostal neuralgia is thus often not a true neuralgia, but rather is caused by primary or secondary rib blockages.

One should also take into account that the articulation of the head of the rib, including its surrounding ligaments, has a close connection to the motion segments of the thoracic spine. For this reason, if a rib is blocked, the physical therapist must treat the motion segment at the same level in order to prevent the disorder from recurring. The reverse is also true: in dysfunction affecting the thoracic spine, the ribs should be treated as well.

The internal organs can cause thoracic pain that may be attributed to the thoracic spine. If the results of the examination show that the problem does not lie in the thoracic spine, then intrathoracic organ disease should be considered. The "reverse" may also be true. Motion-dependent pain is suggestive of a problem affecting the locomotor system (e.g., rib/vertebrae connection), while motion-independent pain tends to indicate a disease affecting the internal organs.

These examples show that it is worthwhile examining the thoracic spine and the costovertebral joints closely. This depends, of course, on the knowledge and the education of the physical therapist. Examination schemes from *manual therapy* procedures may be used.

In the previous sample examination of breathing (pp. 200–204), movements are often performed "separately" on a general level. Yet, during bending of the thoracic spine, sidebending also always occurs with accompanying rotation in the *same direction*, and during extension of the thoracic spine, sidebending and rotation occur in the *opposite direction*.

In "painful" findings in the upper thoracic spine region, the physical therapist should perform an examination of the cervical spine and cervicothoracic junction. If there is irritation of the C3–C4 nerve root, diaphragmatic abnormalities may be the cause. Under the "locomotor system" the respective examination scheme from orthopedics or gynecology may be used.

In recent years, the importance of peripheral muscle strength has gained attention (primarily in COPD patients). It should therefore also be examined and taken into account during treatment.

### Measuring Thoracic Circumference (Breathing Measurement)

In the supine or sitting patient, measurements are taken in centimeters at the following sites:
- Under the axilla
- At the tip of the sternum
- Five cm below the tip of the sternum
- At the height of the navel

The patient should inhale (record the measurement) and exhale deeply. The difference between maximum inhalation and maximum exhalation is the breathing measurement.

The patient must be able to forcefully inhale and exhale. This examination is thus inappropriate for patients with severe obstruction or for ill patients, who cannot make use of inspiratory reserve volumes. Measurements of 1 cm or less can occur, for example, in patients with Bechterew disease.

The degree of breathing depends on the expandability of the thorax, the mobility of the costovertebral joints, and the ventilatory ability of the patient. It is difficult to determine normal values; hence, breathing measurements must be seen in their individual context.

> *To document the results, record the starting position to ensure that it is identical when the examination is repeated.*

## Cardiopulmonary Function and Exercise Capacity

These are expressed by heart rate, blood pressure, and respiratory rate. Additionally, any signs of *strain* should be identified. Results from physical therapy stress tests are available. (See Büsching and Hilfiker 2009.) Physical therapy estimates of exertion, which are used in acute care (*walking on a level surface and climbing stairs*), have not been verified or validated. Scientifically based exertion tests conducted in acute care hospitals can usually only be determined using ergometric tests performed by a physician.

Some physical therapists try to convert steps per minute or movement exercises in the sitting patient into workload in terms of watts. This is only a rough estimate of capacity, however. The reader is referred to **Table 5.7** as an aid.

### Example: Six-minute walking test
This test is available for rehabilitation clinics and outpatient treatment units focusing on sports medicine. Because walking is an everyday activity, it is easier for the patient to use this familiar movement function.

The test is especially important for patients with progressive disease (e.g., COPD, cystic fibrosis, or fibrosis). The test is valid if it is performed a repeated number of times, and it provides both the patient and the therapist with feedback on the course of disease.

- *Necessary material:*
  - Walking distance about 30 m long, without any distractions
  - Stopwatch
  - Continuous pulsoximetry
  - Ten-point Borg scale
  - Blood pressure cuff
  - Stethoscope
  - Aids (e.g., walker, chair along the pathway).
- *Performing the test:*
  - Before beginning the test, blood pressure, pulse, oxygen, perception of respiratory distress (based on the Borg scale), medications, oxygen intake, and aids are registered.
  - Medication use is as usual.
  - If the patient normally uses an oxygen device, the physical therapist should carry it.
  - The patient should select his or her own tempo and may take a break at any time.

**Table 5.7**  Physical (watts) and biological capacity (metabolic turnover) when walking or running on a level surface in a man weighing 70 kg

| Tempo | | | Bicycle ergometer | Metabolic turnover (approximation; working turnover, i.e., baseline turnover is subtracted) | |
| --- | --- | --- | --- | --- | --- |
| Steps/min | km/hr | Descriptor | Watts | kJ/min | kcal/min |
| Walking | | | | | |
| 60 | ca. 1.6 | Very slow | 10–15 | 4.2 | 1.0 |
| 80 | ca. 2.8 | Slow | 25 | 6.3 | 1.5 |
| 100 | ca. 3.6 | Normal | 50 | 12.6 | 3.0 |
| 120 | ca. 4–5 | Fast | 75 | 18.8 | 4.5 |
| Running | | | | | |
| 140 | ca. 5.5 | Jogging | 100 | 29.3 | 7.0 |
| 150 | ca. 7.0 | Running | 125 | 31.4 | 7.5 |

Source: Based on Spitzer and Hettinger (1969); Rost (1980); Teichmann (1980).

**Table 5.8**  Adapted Borg scale for assessing subjective exertion

| Value | Exertion |
| --- | --- |
| 0 | Not fatiguing |
| 0.5 | Very, very easy |
| 1 | Very easy |
| 2 | Easy |
| 3 | Quite easy |
| 4 | Somewhat strenuous |
| 5 6 | Strenuous |
| 7 8 9 | Very strenuous |
| 10 | Very, very strenuous Maximum |

– During the test, oxygen saturation, pulse, respiratory distress, and exertion are recorded based on the Borg scale (**Table 5.8**).
– Symptoms and statements made by the patient, as well as how often he or she needs a break and for how long, should be documented.

> If the patient experiences significant symptoms during the test, stop immediately!

– After the test, the same parameters as those described above are recorded.
– The test takes a total of 6 minutes, including breaks.
– The total walking distance, and the time needed for breaks, should also be recorded.

## 5.1.4   Example of Examination

---

**Case Study: Mr. Pulmo, 67 years old, Chemical Worker**
1. Diagnoses:
   a) Chronic-obstructive pulmonary disease
   b) Coronary heart disease
   c) Cardiac insufficiency
2. Diagnosis at time of admission: Respiratory insufficiency
3. Current diagnoses:
   a) Pneumonia, bilateral
   b) Pleural effusion, bilateral

Mr. Pulmo was hospitalized with respiratory insufficiency and physical exhaustion. The patient has a history of COPD. He was taken to the hospital by ambulance and was already intubated.

His $O_2$ saturation was 73%. Despite increasing the dosage of his medication and supplying oxygen, his improvement remained unsatisfactory. The patient, still intubated, was moved to intensive care. Along with the pulmonary crisis, he had a complication consisting of intermittent atrial fibrillation. He refused to undergo coronary angiography after extubation.

The patient stated that he had had "problems breathing" for more than 10 years; this led to early retirement. In his job as a chemical worker he was exposed to harmful vapors. He also smoked 2 packs of cigarettes a day for 45 years. He quit smoking 2 years ago.

Mr. Pulmo lives with his wife on the first floor of their building. He can only manage to climb the 16 steps with great difficulty. Slowly walking around the apartment is still possible; he needs his wife's to dress and wash. He has been using an oxygen device for 2 years for long-term oxygen therapy.

At present, the patient's physical capacity is extremely reduced; simply changing positions in bed leads to respiratory distress.

*Physician Report*
1. Ultrasound: Pleural effusion, bilateral
2. Chest x-ray: Infiltrates, bilateral
3. Ultrasound cardiography: Moderately impaired left ventricular function
4. Laboratory values: Leukocytosis

Current medication: Antibiotics, ACE inhibitors, digitalis, beta blockers, 25 mg/daily systemic corticosteroids, corticosteroid inhalation, diuretics, long-acting beta-sympathicomimetics, anticoagulation, 2 to 4 L oxygen.

The patient appears to be emotionally unstable and cries frequently. His cooperation varies according to his mood swings; the focus of his life is his wife, who is caring for him. A psychologist will be consulted.

Currently, Mr. Pulmo experiences respiratory distress at rest, during and after physical exertion, when speaking, and with emotional agitation. He is afraid of not being able to get any air and suffocating. Occasionally, he has a productive cough with a white, runny secretion.

Even at rest he breathes through his mouth. His resting respiratory rate is 26 breaths per minute. He alternates between deep and flat breathing; there is no end-expiratory pause. Breathing movements are primarily thoracic, and occur in a cranial and lateral direction; there is significant diaphragm–thoracic-wall antagonism and inspiratory retractions are visible on the ribs. He also has paradoxical respiratory movements with retraction of the abdomen during inspiration and protrusion during expiration. Even at rest he uses the accessory muscles of respiration during inspiration and expiration; he cannot tolerate application of even the slightest resistance against the ribs and abdomen. He prefers to lie supine during treatment, with a strongly elevated. He holds onto both trapeze bars firmly. He automatically uses pursed-lip breathing. If he focuses his attention on it, respiratory distress occurs.

The patient has lost a significant amount of strength. There is generalized atrophy affecting all muscles. He weighs 58 kg and is 1.78 m tall. Between the time of hospitalization and the physical therapy examination (5 days), he lost 4 kg.

His facial expression is one of anxiety and suffering. His movements are slow, deliberate, and targeted. His resting heart rate is 60 beats (measured for 1 minute at the carotid artery). His blood pressure is 140/80.

He has slight cyanosis about the lips and acral regions. In terms of his upper body, he has a barrel chest and kyphosis of the middle thoracic spine. Both shoulders are elevated and protracted. The trapezius muscle, pectoralis muscle, and sternocleidomastoid muscles are shortened bilaterally with hypertonicity, while on the upper body the tissue tends toward hypotonicity.

---

Continued ▷

---

**Case Study: Mr. Pulmo (Continued)**

Due to the patient's diminished physical capacity, a specific examination of the thoracic spine and ribs was not performed. A manual therapy examination was ruled out because in recent years the patient had taken several courses of high-dose systemic corticosteroids.

Although the results of osteoporosis tests are not yet available, they will presumably be positive.

The patient is no longer on strict bed rest; he can walk around his room and hallway without ventilator assistance; climbing stairs is not yet permitted.

The patient hopes that physical therapy will help him increase his physical ability to an extent that will allow him to live in his apartment.

---

# References

Bänsch P. Prävention, Diagnostik und Therapie des chronischen Atemversagens. Z Krankengymnastik. 1989;41

Bänsch P. Atemtherapie bei neuromuskulären Erkrankungen. Z Krankengymnastik. 1992;44

Bauer PC. Chronisch obstruktive Atemwegserkrankungen—Therapeutische Strategien bei geriatrischen Patienten. Pneumologische Notizen. 1998;13

Bienstein C, Klein G, et al. Atmen. Die Kunst der pflegerischen Unterstützung der Atmung. Stuttgart: Thieme; 2002

Brocke M. Aktuelle Atemtherapie in der Physiotherapiepraxis. Munich. Pflaum; 2003

Bungeroth U. Pneumologie BASICS, 2nd ed. Munich: Urban & Fischer 2010

Büsching G, Hilfiker R, et al. Assessments in der Rehabilitation. Band 3: Kardiologie und Pneumologie. Bern: Hans Huber; 2009

Dautzenroth A, Saemann H. Cystische Fibrose. Stuttgart: Thieme; 2002

de Coster M, Pollaris A. Viszerale Osteopathie. Stuttgart: Hippokrates; 1995

Edel H, Knauth K. Atemtherapie. 6th ed. Munich: Urban & Fischer; 1999

Ehrenberg H. Aufgaben und pathophysiologische Grundlagen der krankengymnastischen Atemtherapie. Z Krankengymnastik 1983;35

Ehrenberg H. Atemtherapie in der Physiotherapie/Krankengymnastik. 2. Überarb. Auflage. Munich: Pflaum; 2001

Ehrenberg H, Siemon G. Zur Beobachtung und Beurteilung der Atmung in der Krankengymnastik. Z Krankengymnastik 1979;31

Fischer H, Fischer W. Die einfache Lungenfunktionsprüfung in der Praxis. Pneumologische Notizen. Munich: Gedon & Reuss; 1990

Göhring H, ed. Atemtherapie—Therapie mit dem Atem. Stuttgart: Thieme; 2001

Gross R, Schölmerisch P. Lehrbuch der Inneren Medizin. Stuttgart: Schattauer; 1987

Holle D. 6-Minuten-Gehtest. Z Physiother 2001;53: 1146–1149

Inhalative Kortikoide bei Asthma und chronischer Bronchitis. Glaxo Atemwegstherapeutika

Johnson NM. Erkrankungen der Atmung. Stuttgart: Fischer; 1991

Kirchner P. Physiotherapeutische Techniken in der Atemtherapie. In: Hüter-Becker A, Schewe H, Heipertz W, eds. Physiotherapie—Lehrbuchreihe. Band 4: Untersuchungs- und Behandlungstechniken. Stuttgart: Thieme; 1996

Kisner C, Colby LA. Vom Griff zur Behandlung. Stuttgart: Thieme; 1997

Lauber B. Chronische Bronchitis. Berlin: MEDICUS; 1996

Mang H. Atemtherapie. Stuttgart: Schattauer; 1992

Neurath M, Lohse A. Checkliste Anamnese und klinische Untersuchung. Stuttgart: Thieme; 2002

Reimann P. Befunderhebung, 2nd ed. Munich: Urban & Fischer; 2002

Rutte R, Sturm P. Atemtherapie. Berlin: Springer; 2003

Schacher Ch, Worth H. Mein Asthma habe ich im Griff! 2nd ed. Cologne: Deutscher Ärzte Verlag; 2009

Schildt-Rudloff K, ed. Thoraxschmerz. Innere Erkrankung oder Funktionsstörung des Bewegungsapparates. Berlin: Ullstein Mosby; 1994

Schmidt M. Zur Physiologie und Pathophysiologie der Atemmuskulatur. Z. f. Physiotherapeuten 2006;58:5

Schoppmeyer MA, Polte M. Innere Medizin. Dermatologie. Krankheitslehre für Physiotherapeuten und Masseure. Stuttgart: G. Fischer; 1998

Schuh I. Bindegewebsmassage. Stuttgart: G. Fischer; 1986

Schultz K, Stark J. Asthma bronchiale. Berlin: Medicus; 1996

Siemon G, Ehrenberg H. Leichter atmen—besser bewegen. 4. Überarb. Auflage. Balingen: perimed-Spitta; 1996

Sulyma MG, Klenke TG, et al. Asthma-Bronchitis-Emphysem von A bis Z. BYK Gulden Atemwegslexikon Band I–III. Munich: Medikon; 1990

Teirich-Leube H. Grundriss der Bindegewebsmassage. 12th ed. Stuttgart: G. Fischer; 1990

van den Berg F, ed. Angewandte Physiologie. Band 2: Organsysteme verstehen und beeinflussen. Stuttgart: Thieme; 2000

van den Berg F, ed. Angewandte Physiologie. Band 3: Therapie, Training, Tests. Stuttgart: Thieme; 2001

van Gestel AJR, Teschler H. Physiotherapie bei chronischen Atemwegs- und Lungenerkrankungen. Berlin: Springer; 2010

## 5.2   Examination of Cardiac Functions

*Andreas Fruend*

### 5.2.1   How Can You Determine Cardiac Capacity and Adaptability?

In internal medicine, movement therapy may be compared to medication use: overdosage, under-dosage, and exact dosages are possible.

If any medication could deliver all of the positive health effects of physical activity, it would probably be the drug of the century. Unfortunately, the physical law of inertia stands in the way of its use in actual life (Hollmann 2000).

The treatment goals form the basis for any therapy. The objectives of treatment should be geared toward the resources of the patient. Although physicians generally prescribe movement therapy, the important thing is the clinical examination. It should be performed repeatedly, and a new one should be done for each treatment. This includes information from the *general examination*, including strength, height, weight, ability, and expression. The World Health Organization (WHO 2001) has described these criteria in the International Classification of Functioning, Disability and Health (ICF). Every treatment should be based on these.

### 5.2.2   Preparing the Examination

**Patient History**

For patients who are hospitalized with cardiovascular problems, the therapist should prepare for the examination by first collecting the patient's history. This means interviewing the patient and also looking at his or her file.

The patient's records contain clues as to whether (and with what results) examinations have already been performed (e.g., radiograph, ultrasound).

> The therapist should note any important medications with effects that should be taken into account during the examination and that may influence the results of the examination (e.g., beta blockers, which lower the patient's pulse).

In addition, the patient's records indicate which examination methods are contraindicated, for example, ergometer stress tests immediately after infarction or in patients with angina pectoris (**Table 5.15**, p. 218).

In addition to personal data, such as name, date of birth, occupation, date of admission, diagnosis at hospitalization and current diagnosis, time and type of prescribed physical therapy, height, and weight, the therapist should gather information related to the cardiovascular system from the patient's family history, own history, and current health status.

- *Family history:*
  - Cardiac disease in grandparents, parents, siblings
  - Diseases impairing metabolic or respiratory function (e.g., coronary heart disease, diabetes mellitus, allergies, TB).
- *Own history:*
- Pulmonary diseases.
- In smokers, the therapist should ask what the patient smokes, how, and when he or she last smoked.
- In women: Beginning of last menstrual cycle and contraceptive use (e.g., pill).
- *Current history:*
  - Current disease course: When did the first symptoms or complaints occur and when was the first diagnosis made? What symptoms does the patient have at present?
  - General symptoms: Loss of appetite, fatigue, worry.
  - Disease-related symptoms: What symptoms does the patient have? When do they occur, where, and how severe are they?

Based on the information collected, the therapist should have an idea of the patient's current situation, their attitude toward disease, how they view the causes of their disease and prior therapy, and their willingness to cooperate. The treatment goals should be developed together with the patient and set out in a "treatment contract."

**Medication Influences the Examination Results**

Before beginning to examine the cardiovascular system in a given patient, it is important to know whether he or she takes any drugs for a heart condition and, if so, which ones; this will alter the results of the examination, which will not correspond to their actual situation (**Table 5.9**).

> Beta blockers lower the patient's blood pressure and heart rate.

**Table 5.9** Mode of action of important heart medications ( ⇑ ⇓ strong decrease/increase, ↑ ↓ weaker decrease/increase)

| Effect | Drug groups | | | | | | | | |
|---|---|---|---|---|---|---|---|---|---|
| | Positive inotropic drugs cardiac glycosides | Adrenaline | Anti-anginal drugs (NTG) | Beta blockers | Vasodilators (Xanef) | Calcium antagonists (Adalat) | Anti-arrhythmic drugs | Thrombocyte aggregation inhibitors | Fibrinolytics |
| Contractility | ⇑ | ⇑ | ⇓ | ⇓ | | | | | |
| Heart minute volume | ⇑ | ⇑ | ↓ | ↓ | ↓ | ↓ | | | |
| Afterload | | | ⇓ | | ⇓ | ⇓ | | | |
| Preload | | | ⇓ | | | | | | |
| Ca⁺⁺ inflow | | | | | | ⇓ | | | |
| Coronary perfusion | | | ⇑ | | | | | | |
| Inotropy | ⇑ | ⇑ | | ⇓ | | ⇓ | ⇓ | | |
| Chronotropic heart rate | ⇓ | ⇑ | | ⇓ | | ⇓ | ⇓ | | |
| AV conductor | ⇓ | ⇑ | | ⇓ | | ⇓ | ⇓ | | |
| Aggregation inhibitors | | | | | | | | ⇓ | |
| Thrombocyte metabolism | | | | | | | | ↓ | |
| Fibrin degradation products | | | | | | | | | ↓ |
| Sinoatrial node activity | ↓ | | | | | | | | |
| Blood pressure | | ↑ | ↓ | ↓ | ↓ | ⇓ | | | |
| O₂ consumption of the myocardium | ↑ | ↑ | ⇓ | ⇓ | ⇑ | ⇓ | | | |

If the patient is under physical strain during the examination, his or her heart rate will nevertheless remain stable or "low." Heart rate is thus no longer a criterion for excessive strain on the cardiovascular system.

If the patient is taking cardiovascular drugs (e.g., beta blockers, ACE inhibitors), during the examination the therapist must pay close attention to other signs of physical strain in order to ensure adequate stress without placing the patient at risk.

> Signs of excessive strain include breaking off sentences, respiratory distress, and increasing pallor.

### What to Discuss with the Patient's Physician before the Examination

The physician prescribes physical therapy measures and sets the individual level of stress in terms of *maximum watts (workload)* or a *therapeutic heart rate*. In some group sessions for heart patients, the presence of a physician is mandatory (e.g., outpatient heart groups). In a hospital setting, on-call urgent care is the norm (rehabilitation activity in heart groups).

### When to Interrupt the Examination

The examination places the patient's cardiovascular system under stress. Stop immediately if any of the following occur:
- Subjective complaints, angina pectoris, respiratory distress, dizziness
- Worsening arrhythmia
- ECG: Block
- ECG: Disturbance of repolarization
- Very high (250/120 mmHg) or low blood pressure (dropping during the examination by around 20%)
- Inadequate heart rate
- Myocardial insufficiency (e.g., pallor, blue discoloration of the lips or acral regions)

> Some examinations may not be performed under certain conditions. (For absolute and relative contraindications for an examination with an ergometer or a treadmill, see **Table 5.15**, p. 218.)

---

**Summary**
- Preparing the examination:
  - View the patient's medical records and note important information.
  - Determine which examinations are contraindicated.
  - Create a list of questions on the symptoms and disease course and determine suitable examination methods.

### Which Criteria are Relevant to the Physical Therapy Examination?

The patient's cardiovascular system may be assessed using *objective* and *subjective* criteria. Objective criteria are measurable (e.g., heart rate and pulse), while subjective criteria are *not* measureable, but can be described. For instance, the patient may rate his or her sense of well-being on a scale, or the therapist may report abnormal changes to breathing, facial color, or the acral regions.

### 5.2.3    Examining Objective Criteria (see Table 5.17)

### Heart Rate

The heart rate (number of heartbeats per unit of time; number of beats/minute) is typically measured using an ECG lead and then read from a monitor. To measure cardiac output, the patient can perform a physical stress test on a bicycle ergometer. For pulse rate as well, the main criterion is the duration of measurement (10, 15, 30 seconds or 1 minute). Modern equipment requires about 3 seconds for a precise analysis.

> Physiologically, the heart rate increases with physical stress. This is the body's normal response to increased oxygen and nutrient consumption by the skeletal and cardiac muscles (myocardium).

The normal resting heart rate in a healthy person is 60 to 80 beats/minute. People who have undergone endurance training may have heart rates of 30 to 45 beats/minute (e.g., cyclists and long-distance runners). Similarly low rates are also found in patients taking drugs that block the beta receptors (beta blockers), the receptors of the sympathetic nervous system that are necessary for increased stroke volume and heart rate.

> When measuring heart rate, the therapist must be certain about whether (and at what dosage) a given medication can influence the heart rate; this is to prevent errors in the exercise dosage and help avoid disastrous consequences (Kindermann 2004).

### Pulse Rate

The pulse rate is primarily measured to check the effects of cardiac output in the periphery of the body. It assesses whether the periphery of the body is being adequately supplied with oxygen via the cardiovascular system, so that the patient can perform physical activities (e.g., movement, climbing stairs). The pulse rate is important for regulating exertion level, especially in patients with pacemakers and mechanical circulatory assistance systems (artificial heart). Yet, false estimates can occur in patients with nonpulsatile pumps. The use of the Borg scale leads to better results. One must also carefully observe the pulse rate in patients with known or new arrhythmia under stress.

At rest, the heart is the largest consumer of oxygen in the body. This pumping organ uses about 30% of inhaled oxygen. As the pulse rate increases, so too does oxygen consumption. It is essential to avoid this in patients with a history of heart damage (e.g., cardiac infarction).

In patients who have had a heart valve replacement or myocardial infarction, attention must be paid to heart rate during the first year. High pulse rates are a possible indication of oxygen deficiency, a sign of inadequate oxygen supply to the myocardium.

> In young athletes, pulse rates of up to 210 beats/minute are completely normal during stress testing. In patients with a history of disease, rates exceeding 140 beats/minute should be viewed very critically. In most instances, stress testing should be stopped.
> In patients with an automated internal defibrillator, the programmed upper limit of the pulse should never be exceeded. Here, too, the effects of medication must be taken into account (e.g., beta blockers) (**Table 5.9**).

## Pulse Measurement

The patient's pulse is usually measured at a superficial artery (e.g., radial artery). To take the patient's pulse, the therapist should place his or her second to fourth fingers on the patient's left distal forearm on the radial artery (**Fig. 5.9a**). Only slight pressure should be applied. The pulse is also easily palpated at the carotid artery (**Fig. 5.9b**).

> Before taking the patient's pulse at the carotid artery, one should determine whether the patient has carotid stenosis. If so, syncope can occur (as a result of arrhythmia or disrupted arterial flow).
> Cardiac arrhythmias can be problematic when taking the patient's pulse; they are easily missed, especially in patients with low blood pressure. Care should be taken when measuring the pulse in a patient with cardiac arrhythmia.

An experienced therapist may also use palpation to develop hypotheses concerning the patient's blood

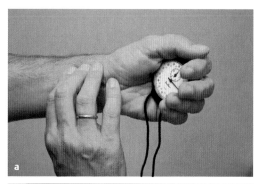
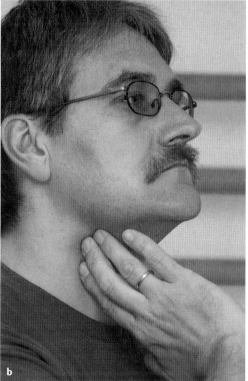

Fig. 5.9a, b Pulse measurement.
**a** Radial artery pulse.
**b** Carotid artery pulse.

pressure. For instance, systolic pressure may be roughly estimated based on tension (hardness) of the pulse. Tension depends on how much pressure must be applied to suppress the movement of the vessel (Witzleb and Lochner 1957).

> A conversion table may be used to determine the optimal heart rate (**Table 5.10**).
> The mean heart rate (MHR) is particularly important, as it should never be exceeded during stress testing (220 minus the patient's age).

**Table 5.10** Optimal heart rate

| Age | MHR (220 – age) | Stable health (50–60% of MHR) | Active fat metabolism (60–70% of MHR) | Improved fitness (70–85% of MHR) |
|-----|-----------------|-------------------------------|----------------------------------------|----------------------------------|
| 20  | 200 | 100–120 | 120–140 | 140–170 |
| 30  | 190 | 95–114  | 114–133 | 133–161 |
| 35  | 185 | 92–111  | 111–129 | 129–157 |
| 40  | 180 | 90–108  | 108–126 | 126–153 |
| 45  | 175 | 87–105  | 105–122 | 122–148 |
| 50  | 170 | 85–102  | 102–119 | 119–144 |
| 55  | 165 | 82–99   | 99–115  | 115–140 |
| 60  | 160 | 80–96   | 96–112  | 112–136 |
| 65  | 155 | 77–93   | 93–108  | 108–131 |

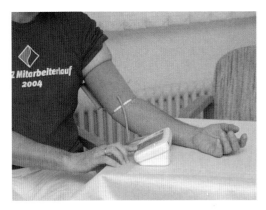

**Fig. 5.10** Blood pressure monitor.

## Blood Pressure

Blood pressure (pressure of the blood against the vessel wall) should be measured under calm, resting conditions. A distinction is made between systolic and diastolic blood pressure values. Systolic pressure occurs when the cardiac muscle contracts; diastolic pressure is when it is at its most relaxed (**Table 5.11**). A blood pressure cuff is placed at the level of the heart; this is the only means of ensuring comparability of values.

Given that blood pressure cuff inflation and deflation, as well as listening to the pulsation in the vessels, can vary greatly on an individual basis, this type of pressure measurement should really only be performed by highly experienced therapists. The use of a blood pressure monitor is at least equally effective and precise (**Fig. 5.10**).

**Table 5.11** WHO guidelines on high blood pressure

| Category | Systole (mmHg) | Diastole (mmHg) |
|----------|----------------|-----------------|
| Optimal | < 120 | < 80 |
| Normal | < 130 | < 85 |
| High normal | 130–139 | 85–89 |
| Hypertension, grade 1 (mild) | 140–159 | 90–99 |
| Hypertension, grade 2 (moderate) | 160–179 | 100–110 |
| Hypertension, grade 3 (severe) | ≥ 180 | ≥ 110 |
| Isolated systolic hypertension | ≥ 140 | > 90 |

Source: Deutsche Hochdruckliga 2014.

Measuring blood pressure is an essential part of the treatment of patients with heart valve defects and those who have undergone a heart or heart-lung transplantation.

> During the initial phase after surgery, in particular, excessively high pressure may damage the sensitive valves or transplant. This may even result in valve avulsion.

## Respiratory Rate

Especially when the exertion level is high for a given patient, precisely determining the respiratory rate may be difficult.

> At a breathing rate of more than 28 breaths per minute, one may assume that the exercise is mainly anaerobic, given that the amount of oxygen inhaled is no longer sufficient for sustaining aerobic metabolism.

### Body Plethysmography and Spiroergometry

> Precise measurements may only be obtained using body plethysmography and spiroergometry.

Body plethysmography measures all respiratory parameters. In spiroergometry, using an ergometer or treadmill, and specific exertion programs, the heart rate and exertion level can be determined with very high precision (**Fig. 5.11**). Both maximum performance as well as the individual anaerobic threshold (IAS) may be evaluated.

> Signs of excessive strain are evident clinically (e.g., if the patient's sentences are shortened), even without complicated diagnostic methods.

## Vital Capacity

Vital capacity is a measurement of how much air the lungs can hold. It is normally 3,500–5,000 mL and consists of breath volume and expiratory and inspiratory reserve volumes (**Table 5.12**).

### Spirometer

Vital capacity may be measured using a spirometer. If it is significantly diminished, the stress that the patient is placed under must be adapted accordingly, because the body's oxygen supply is inadequate (see the section on examination of the pulmonary system).

## Oxygen Saturation of the Blood

### Pulsoximetry

Pulsoximeters (small hand-held devices) allow one to measure the oxygen saturation of peripheral blood. As a rough guideline, values should be more than 90% (**Table 5.13**). Measurements may be taken at the fingertip or earlobe; in children, measurements may also be taken at the toes.

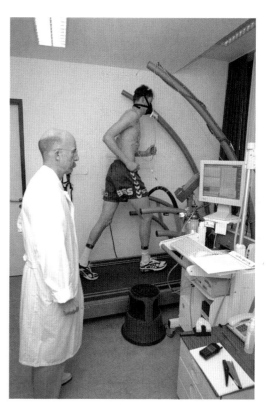

**Fig. 5.11** Spiroergometer.

> The measurements are only accurate in patients who have no vascular calcifications and whose blood pressure is sufficiently high.

### Spiroergometry

The most precise method for guiding training is *spiroergometry*. Under specific conditions of exertion, the body's ability to inhale oxygen and expel carbon dioxide is measured. Typically, the examination is performed using bicycle ergometry, although treadmill ergometry is increasingly popular and is ultimately closer to actual everyday stress.

Based on an analysis of the data, the aerobic threshold, the individual aerobic/anaerobic threshold (IAS), and maximum performance of the cardiovascular system may be determined. The training data may be used to guide circulatory training.

### Lactate Test

The lactate test is a common diagnostic test in "healthy" people (e.g., athletes). It is simple, but not nearly as valid as spiroergometry. One should avoid switching between devices to ensure precision in

**Table 5.12** Vital capacity

| Parameter | Abbreviation | Values in men | Values in women | Unit |
|---|---|---|---|---|
| Breath volumes | Vt | 450–650 (6 mL/kg body weight) | 300–550 (6 mL/kg body weight) | mL |
| Inspiratory reserve volumes | IRV | 2,200–4,300 | 1,500–3,600 | mL |
| Expiratory reserve volumes | ERV | ≈ 1,200 | 700–1,000 | mL |
| Residual volumes | RV | 1,700–2,100 | 1,200–1,600 | mL |
| Forced vital capacity | (F)VC | 4,100–4,800 (height [cm] × 25 mL) | 2,800–4,200 (height [cm] × 20 mL) | mL |
| Functional residual capacity | FRC | 2,400–3,300 (52 mL/kg body weight) | ≈ 2,300 (34 mL/kg body weight) | mL |
| Inspiratory capacity | IC | 63–72 | 63–72 | % of TC |
| Total capacity | TC | 6,000–6,500 | 4,300–4,500 | mL |
| Tiffeneau test | FEV1 | 70–75 (50–60 mL/kg body weight) | 75–80 (50–60 mL/kg body weight) | % of VC |
| Physiological dead space ($V_d$ × 0.33) | $V_d$ | ca. 150 (2 mL/kg body weight) | ca. 150 (2 mL/kg body weight) | mL |

**Table 5.13** Normal values for blood oxygen saturation in an adult with normal body temperature

| $O_2$ | Oxygen saturation in % |
|---|---|
| Arterial | 95–98 |
| Mixed venous | 70–75 |
| Source: Sirtl and Jesch (1989). | |

the examination situation. Attention must also be paid to the same food and liquid intake prior to the exertion test each time. Depending on the type of exertion (jogging or cycling), various lactate concentrations may be used as an indicator of IAS.

Lactate is generally taken in a mixed venous concentration from the earlobe. Various programs are available for determining the IAS in lactate assessment. In athletes, lactate measurements are often used as a field test with set running/walking speeds in a stadium (400 m track).

## Power Output

Physically, the power output (SI unit: watts) may be summed up in a simple formula. In simplified terms, 1 watt describes 1 joule (J) of work that is performed in the time (s) 1 second:

$Watt = m^2 \times kg \times s^{-3} = J/s$ (m = height of lift, kg = weight, s = time in which the work was done).

## Bicycle Ergometry

Despite its relatively simple definition, it is difficult to measure a patient's physical capacity. In Germany, most patients are evaluated using bicycle ergometry. A normed foot pedal with normed weight is moved along a circular path.

Depending on the patient's height and weight, the same patient may experience very different levels of stress (e.g., two patients of different weights experience different levels of physical strain when climbing stairs). Thus, specialists in sports medicine often use conversion tables that show exertion in watts.

**Example:** Walking, jogging, and running speeds (**Table 5.14**)

Spiroergometric values (watts) may be converted into walking or running speeds (in m/min). The numbers give an idea about how the measurement unit of a "watt," from physics, can be used in real-life everyday circumstances. For instance, a person weighing 50 kg who has a 150-watt power output

**Table 5.14** Walking, jogging, and running speeds

| | Body weight in kg | | | | | | | | | | | | | |
|---|---|---|---|---|---|---|---|---|---|---|---|---|---|---|
| Watts | 50 | 55 | 60 | 65 | 70 | 75 | 80 | 85 | 90 | 95 | 100 | 105 | 110 | 115 |
| 50 | 95 | 90 | 85 | 80 | 75 | 70 | 70 | | | | | | | |
| 60 | 105 | 100 | 90 | 85 | 80 | 75 | 75 | 70 | | | | | | |
| 70 | 115 | 110 | 100 | 95 | 90 | 85 | 80 | 75 | 75 | 70 | | | | |
| 80 | 125 | 115 | 110 | 100 | 100 | 90 | 85 | 80 | 75 | 75 | 70 | 70 | | |
| 90 | 135 | 125 | 115 | 110 | 105 | 95 | 90 | 90 | 85 | 80 | 75 | 75 | 70 | 70 |
| 100 | 145 | 135 | 125 | 120 | 110 | 105 | 100 | 95 | 90 | 85 | 80 | 80 | 75 | 75 |
| 110 | 155 | 145 | 135 | 125 | 115 | 110 | 105 | 100 | 95 | 90 | 85 | 85 | 80 | 75 |
| 120 | 165 | 155 | 140 | 135 | 125 | 120 | 110 | 105 | 100 | 95 | 90 | 90 | 85 | 80 |
| 130 | 175 | 165 | 150 | 140 | 130 | 125 | 120 | 110 | 105 | 100 | 95 | 95 | 90 | 85 |
| 140 | 190 | 175 | 160 | 150 | 140 | 135 | 125 | 120 | 115 | 110 | 105 | 100 | 95 | 95 |
| 150 | 200 | 185 | 170 | 160 | 150 | 140 | 130 | 125 | 120 | 115 | 110 | 105 | 100 | 95 |
| 160 | 205 | 190 | 175 | 165 | 155 | 145 | 140 | 130 | 125 | 120 | 115 | 110 | 105 | 105 |
| 170 | 215 | 200 | 185 | 170 | 160 | 150 | 145 | 135 | 130 | 125 | 120 | 115 | 110 | 105 |
| 180 | 225 | 205 | 190 | 180 | 170 | 160 | 150 | 140 | 135 | 130 | 125 | 120 | 115 | 110 |
| 190 | 235 | 215 | 200 | 185 | 175 | 165 | 155 | 150 | 140 | 135 | 130 | 125 | 120 | 115 |
| 200 | 245 | 225 | 205 | 195 | 180 | 170 | 160 | 155 | 145 | 140 | 135 | 130 | 125 | 120 |
| Walking | m/min | | | | | | | | | | | | | |
| Jogging | m/min | | | | | | | | | | | | | |
| Running | m/min | | | | | | | | | | | | | |

Source: Halhuber (1982).
Note: The blank spaces at the top right of the table show that people who weigh more must use more watts to begin moving.

on an ergometer/bicycle, would jog 175 m/min, while a person weighing 100 kg, with the same ergometer/bicycle output, would only be able to jog 95 m/min.

> *Walking on a level surface corresponds to about 25 watts; climbing stairs corresponds to about 75 watts. (This estimate was obtained in comprehensive control studies with healthy subjects.)*

## Calculations Using a Treadmill

Treadmill readings are a much more precise and reality-based method than bicycle ergometry. These allow an exact diagnosis and assessment of performance that tend to correspond to reality, given that the incline (angle of the treadmill) and body weight are determined.

A problem in terms of evaluating performance is the reproducibility of exertion level. Exertion may only be compared if the baseline situation is the same.

**Examples:**
- If an incline of 3% is being used for the treadmill, the same incline should be used for all controls.
- If exercise begins at 2 km/hour, the same speed should be used for all control tests.

Comparative measures can be particularly difficult if the patient is moved to another hospital. Measurements at various hospitals or rehabilitation centers often are done under different conditions. For this

**Table 5.15** Ergometer and treadmill checklist

| | |
|---|---|
| Criteria for stopping | • Subjective complaints: Shortness of breath, dizziness, angina pectoris<br>• Increasing arrhythmia<br>• ECG: Block<br>• ECG: Disturbance of repolarization<br>• Drop in blood pressure when transitioning from resting to exertion of around 20 mmHg<br>• Blood pressure exceeding 250/120 mmHg<br>• Bradyarrhythmia |
| Absolute contraindications | • Recent infarction<br>• Resting angina<br>• Aortic dissection<br>• New onset of ventricular tachycardia<br>• Acute inflammations |
| Relative contraindications | • Manifest cardiac insufficiency<br>• More extrasystoles<br>• Untreated hypertension<br>• Uncontrolled highly frequent supraventricular arrhythmia |

**Table 5.16** Weight classification and BMI (WHO)

| Weight classification | BMI |
|---|---|
| Ideal weight | < 25 |
| Overweight | 26–29 |
| Obesity | > 30 |
| Pathological obesity (Pickwick syndrome); in medicine scales are now used that use electric impulses to measure fat, muscle mass and water (impedance scales) | > 45 |

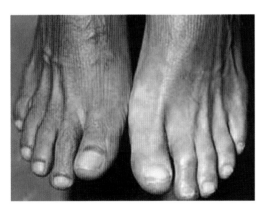

**Fig. 5.12** Ratschow test.

reason, evaluation of physical capacity is done using a bicycle ergometer, as it enables maximum standardization. **Tables 5.15** lists contraindications and reasons for stopping treadmill and ergometer measurement.

## Body Mass Index

The body mass index (BMI) is the most reliable quotient currently available for the relationship between height and weight (see section 2.1.3, Chapter 2).

■ $BMI = weight\ (kg): (height)^2\ (m^2)$

The BMI may be used to draw conclusions about a person's nutritional status (**Table 5.16**). A BMI between 19 and 25 is considered good. The higher the BMI, the more the cardiovascular system must work in order to move the larger body mass.

## Peripheral Circulation

### Ratschow Test

The most well-known function test was developed by Max Ratschow, the founder of angiology in Germany. It is primarily used in patients with peripheral artery occlusive disease (PAOD). In this classic stress test of the lower extremity the patient lies on his or her back with 90° hip bending and extension of the knee joints. Using the tempo of a metronome (30 beats/minute), they move their feet in alternation: dorsal extension/plantar bending in the upper ankle joint and extension/bending of the toe joints. The patient moves in this position for as long as it takes until their pain occurs or if, due to inadequate circulation, they can no longer perform the movement precisely (**Fig. 5.12**).

> The Ratschow test is difficult to perform in patients with peripheral diabetic neuropathy because they have abnormal pain perception. In such patients, peripheral circulation may be tested using the positioning test.

Afterward, the patient should sit up. His or her legs should be dangling freely, and in this position are observed for a change in color. Slight, initial pallor is followed by reddening, which is especially evident in the feet. If the venous system is intact, this is followed by filling of the veins with prominent veins in the feet. In healthy patients, this occurs within the first 15 seconds after sitting up. In occlusive diseases, the changes are delayed, depending on the severity of symptoms (more than 30 seconds).

> The examination also serves as training in patients with abnormal peripheral circulation.

### Positioning Test

This is basically a variation of the Ratschow test. The patient changes from lying down to sitting, letting his or her legs dangle. After changing positions, the therapist should observe capillary and venous filling. This provides information on the extent of the circulatory disorder: in patients with severe circulatory disturbances, there is a significant delay in capillary filling.

> Cold, nicotine, or agitation may lead to false-positive results.

### Allen Test

In patients with PAOD primarily affecting the arms, the Allen test may be performed. This stress test is comparable to the Ratschow test. While sitting, the patient lifts their arms overhead and performs fist-closure exercises until they have pain or until they can no longer perform the movements precisely. First, with the arms lifted, the degree of skin pallor is evaluated. Then the patient allows their arms to hang while the therapist records the time it takes until capillary and venous redness occurs.

### Modified Allen Test

In older patients who have difficulty performing the test, the following alternative may be used: a flat grip is used to stop the circulation in the ulnar artery and the radial artery until the hand loses color. Then the pressure is taken off one artery at a time.

If the hand reddens again only very slowly, this is suggestive of PAOD with primary arm involvement. Further diagnostic testing may be necessary.

## Endurance

### Walking Distance

The distance the patient is able to walk is measured for a set period of time. This may support information on cardiac and pulmonary endurance.

For an exact comparison of the walking distances, the same conditions must be set in terms of floor surface qualities, incline, and walking tempo. The walking speed (steps per minute) should be defined beforehand and practiced with the patient. In addition, the patient and therapist must agree on a clear criterion for stopping, for example, onset of pain or beginning respiratory distress. Only then can the results of treatment be objectively compared with one another.

> It can be difficult to evaluate the walking distance in patients with polyneuropathies (diabetic foot syndrome). Because of diminished pain perception, they lose their sense of when to limit their exertion. The criteria for stopping must be determined ahead of time (e.g., if the patient's gait becomes visibly worse, or if he or she can no longer roll down through the foot optimally or begins to limp).

### Six-minute Walking Test

The patient is asked to walk about for 6 minutes. They should walk as quickly as their own assessment of their ability indicates. The pathway should have an even surface and be as straight as possible, without many turns. The test measures the distance covered in 6 minutes. The therapist is only there to ensure the patient's safety; he or she should indicate to the patient every time 1 minute has passed; he or she should be present without supporting, encouraging, or accompanying the patient.

Using conversion tables, endurance may be determined based on walking speed. If the patient covers a distance of less than 300 m, one may assume that they are at serious risk. Studies on patients with heart disease have shown a fatality rate of 80% within 5 years among such patients.

## Cooper Test

The Cooper test of endurance (developed by Dr. Kenneth Cooper in the 1960s) is a simple procedure. The test simply measures how far the patient can walk or run in 12 minutes.

> The reported normal values should be viewed with caution because they have not been updated.

The figures for adolescents have decreased since 1980 by up to 30%. In soccer referees, for whom the Cooper test is a basic assessment test, the values have continuously risen.

For initial testing of children and adolescents, the Cooper test has been replaced by the 6-minute run, because the majority of children and adolescents no longer appear to be able to run for 12 minutes without stopping.

## Muscular Endurance

### Harvard Step Test

The patients should step for 5 minutes, or until they are exhausted (i.e., they can no longer maintain the established frequency), up onto a bench or box about 50 cm high. A metronome is used to establish a speed of 30 steps/minute.

The patient's pulse is measured after 1, 2, and 3 minutes. It should continuously decrease: the quicker it drops, the better the fitness level.

> The test was originally designed as a test of endurance exertion. Yet it is primarily a test for estimating muscular endurance, given that exertion depends, among other things, on the patient's weight.

### Steep Ramp Test

The steep ramp test, based on Meyer (2000), lasts about 120 seconds. A modified test protocol begins on the first step with 25 watts and 30 seconds of ergometer training (http://www.escardio.org/communities/EACPR/about/EACPR-main-sections/Pages/EACPR-Sports-Cardiology.aspx). The test measures training intensity; 50% of maximum exertion is used for interval training. Stopping the exercise also allows one to determine maximum lactate mobilization.

The test and protocol begin with 25 watts of ergometer workload. Increase workload by 25 watts every 30 seconds and perform lactate measurement. The Lactate Scout analyzer offers a quick, reliable measurement system. The maximum lactate mobilization may be assessed when exercise is stopped (and after 1–3 minutes). The workload intensity is based on heart rate due to the basically linear relationship between heart rate and oxygen intake.

---

**Risk of Falling**

In older patients, lacking strength, and especially inadequate muscular endurance, increase the risk of a fall. In older patients, in particular, immobilization after a fall often leads to complications for subsequent treatment (e.g., risk of thrombosis). For prevention, strength and muscular endurance training are helpful due to improved coordination (movement control) as well as increased coarse strength.

---

## The Timed Up and Go Test

For this test (Podsiadlo and Richardson 1991), the therapist merely needs a watch with a second hand or a stopwatch. The patient should sit on a normal chair with their back resting against the back of the chair. Their arms should be relaxed and resting on the arms of the chair. Next, they should stand up, walk 3 m forward and then back to the chair and sit down again. They may use their usual walking aids (e.g., walker).

The therapist should measure the length of time from standing up until sitting down. The movement sequence should be performed within 7 to 10 seconds. If this is not possible, the patient has serious mobility problems, especially if they need more than 20 seconds. Geriatric examinations have shown that such patients have a high risk for falls.

> Some geriatric clinics are well experienced in prescribing hip protectors (undergarments with protective padding); these reduce the risk of a femoral neck fracture related to a fall by more than 90%.

### 5.2.4   Examining Subjective Criteria (Table 5.19)

## Exertion

### Borg Scale

Using the Borg scale, the patient can select from a list of adjectives to describe his or her perception of physical exertion after exercise (**Table 5.18**).

**Table 5.17** Objective criteria

| Physical therapy examinations | |
|---|---|
| Pulse rate | Pulse measurement |
| Blood pressure | Blood pressure measurement (monitor, cuff) |
| Vital capacity | see **Table 5.12** |
| Performance | • Bicycle ergometer<br>• Treadmill |
| BMI | see **Table 5.16** |
| Peripheral circulation | • Ratschow test<br>• Positioning test<br>• Allen test |
| Endurance | • Simple walking<br>• Six-minute walk/run test<br>• Cooper test |
| Muscular endurance | • Harvard step test<br>• Steep ramp test |
| Physician examinations | |
| Heart rate | • ECG<br>• Exercise ECG |
| Respiratory rate | • Body plethysmography<br>• Spiroergometry |
| Oxygen saturation | • Pulsoximetry<br>• Spiroergometry<br>• Lactate diagnosis |

**Table 5.18** Borg scale

| Index | Description of exertion |
|---|---|
| 5<br>6<br>7 | Very, very easy |
| 8<br>9<br>10 | Very easy |
| 11<br>12 | Quite easy |
| 13<br>14 | Rather difficult |
| 15<br>16 | Difficult |
| 17<br>18 | Very difficult |
| 19<br>20 | Very, very difficult |

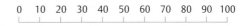

0   10   20   30   40   50   60   70   80   90   100

**Fig. 5.13** Visual analogue scale (VAS).

No pain          Worst possible pain imaginable
0                          10

**Fig. 5.14** Simplified pain scale.

**Table 5.19** Subjective criteria

| Physical therapy examinations | |
|---|---|
| Exertion | Borg scale |
| Pain | • Visual analogue scale<br>• Simplified pain scale |

> *After performing coordinative tasks, the patient's perception of physical exertion is often higher than his or her actual pulse. The reverse is true after familiar forms of exertion (e.g., walking); his or her actual pulse is higher than his or her perception of physical exertion.*

The index score is then multiplied by 10 to arrive at an approximate heart rate that would correspond to the level of exertion reported by the patient.

Index × 10 = heart rate

Various derivations of the original Borg scale, which simplify documentation, are also available.

## Pain

### Pain Scales

The simplest and most common pain estimate is done using the visual analogue scale (VAS; **Fig. 5.13**). A *0* means that there is no pain and *100* represents maximum pain.

A simplified form is a pain scale on a straight line measuring 10 cm long (**Fig. 5.14**), on which the patient marks his or her perceived pain.

Based on the results of the pain scale, the therapist may easily adjust treatment. For instance, treatment methods may be adapted to individual needs of the patient, if pain worsens consistently after treatment, for instance, or if it remains the same or improves.

Additionally, pain scales also help the patient with his or her pain diary.

## 5.2.5   Evaluation

In order to successfully treat the patient, and to bring treatment to a close, it is important to agree on treatment goals, which can then be assessed.

> *The treatment goals must be realistic and they must be achievable during the inpatient or outpatient course of treatment. This will help avoid disappointment for both the patient and the therapist and will help ensure continued patient satisfaction.*

## Better Quality of Life with Successful Therapy

### SF 36 Questionnaire

A questionnaire is a helpful tool for estimating treatment success. The SF 36 is an internationally standardized questionnaire that is used to assess quality of life. It is increasingly used in medicine to evaluate treatment success, for example, after hip joint replacement surgery, in pain therapy, and after heart surgery. The individual evaluation allows for a more complete picture of the patient beyond individual treatment measures.

**Summary**

The goal of the physical therapy examination is to determine whether skeletal and cardiac muscle are being adequately nourished by the cardiovascular system in accordance with exertion level (movement, body weight).

Before the physical therapy examination, the doctor should determine the maximum exertion level (watts) and heart rate in order to avoid cardiovascular complications.

The patient history gives the therapist important clues as to his or her current situation, physical capacity, and medication use.

The therapist must be aware of any medications the patient is using and their influence on the cardiovascular system.

Signs of heart strain should be identified promptly, regardless of pulse rate.

The examination distinguishes between objective (measured under standardized conditions) and subjective (patient reports) criteria.

## References

Büsching G, Hilfiker R, et al. Assessments in der Rehabilitation. Band 3: Kardiologie und Pneumologie. Bern: Huber Verlag; 2009

Halhuber C. Rehabilitation des Koronarkranken. Erlangen: Perimed; 1982

Hillegass EA, Sadowsky HS. Essentials of Cardiopulmonary Physical Therapy. Philadelphia: Saunders; 1994

Hornbostel H, ed. Innere Medizin in Praxis und Klinik. Band I. Stuttgart: Thieme; 1984

Kapit W, Macey R, et al. Physiologie Malatlas. Munich: Arcis; 1992

Kindermann W, Dickhuth H, et al. Sportkardiologie. 4th ed. Darmstadt: Steinkopff; 2004

Podsiadlo D, Richardson S. The timed "Up & Go": a test of basic functional mobility for frail elderly persons. J Am Geriatr Soc 1991;39(2):142–148

Schmidt RF, Thews G, eds. Physiologie des Menschen. Berlin: Springer: 1990

Sirtl C, Jesch F. Anästhesiologisches Notizbuch. Wiesbaden: Abbott: 1989

Witzleb E, Lochner W. Lungen und kleiner Kreislauf. Berlin: Springer; 1957

World Health Organization (WHO). ICF—International Classification of Functioning, Disability and Health. Geneva: World Health Organization; 2001

ZVK. Standardisierte Ergebnismessung, Physio-Akademie 2006

# Appendix

## Practice Questions on the Physical Therapy Examination as a Process and Clinical Reasoning

Review the material, deepen your knowledge, and prepare for the examination. (The page numbers in parentheses indicate where the appropriate answers may be found.)

Describe the relationship between the physical therapy actions *examining* and *treatment*. (pp. **3–4**)

Describe the physical therapy process. (p. **3**)

What is the definition of physical therapy according to the World Confederation for Physical Therapy (WCPT)? (p. **4**)

Which models of thought form the basis for physical therapy? (pp. **4–6**)

What is the definition of clinical reasoning? (pp. **8–9**)

On what levels do therapists make decisions in the clinical reasoning process? (pp. **8–9**)

Name three examples of different types of clinical reasoning. (p. **12**)

Which factors influence a physical therapist's clinical reasoning? (p. **11** and **14**)

What are the typical errors that may occur in clinical reasoning? (p. **16**)

Treatment hypotheses may be grouped into various categories. Name three common examples. (p. **19**)

What are the advantages and disadvantages of clinical patterns? (pp. **22–23**)

What is evidence-based practice? (p. **24**)

In the list of "best evidence" what level are reviews? (p. **25**)

Name phases in the physical therapy process. (p. **26**)

What are the goals of the physical therapy process? (p. **27**)

What is the value of reassessment processes in the treatment process? (pp. **31–32**)

## Practice Questions on the Examination of Structures and Functions of the Locomotor System

Review the material, deepen your knowledge, and prepare for the examination. (The page numbers in parentheses indicate where the appropriate answers may be found.)

What is the neutral zero position? (p. **39**)

How do you document your measurement results according to the neutral zero method? (p. **40**)

Right knee joint: Bending/extension 130/20/0. What does this measurement result mean? (p. **40**)

How do you measure movements in the hip joint? (p. **41**)

How do you measure movements in the shoulder joint? (p. **43**)

You are measuring dorsal extension of the ankle joint. How does the starting position of the patient differ between single-joint stretching of the gastrocnemius muscle and multi-joint stretching? (p. **46**)

Hand function: Name three hand-grasping shapes. (p. **48**)

Describe the muscle activity that occurs with fist closure. (p. **48**)

How can you measure spinal mobility? (pp. **48–51**)

What are the types of leg-length discrepancy? How do they differ? (p. **51**)

What do you pay attention to when measuring circumference? (p. **51**)

What are the different values measured during tests of muscle function? (pp. **51–52**)

What are the advantages and disadvantages of muscle function tests? (pp. **52–53**)

How do you conduct a test of muscle function? (p. **53**)

Test the extensors of the elbow joint. (p. **54**)

How do you calculate a person's body mass index (BMI)? What does the BMI indicate? (p. **60**)

Which criteria do you evaluate when you test active and passive joint mobility? (p. **63**)

Which principles do you take into account when you test active and passive joint mobility? (p. **63**)

When testing joint mobility, your patient has pain. When you re-test mobility, under altered conditions, how do you ask the patient about his or her pain? What do you pay attention to when querying the patient? (p. **63**)

What is the physiological reserve? (p. **64**)

Describe the physiological and pathological end-feel. (p. **64**)

What is the close-packed position of a joint? (p. **65**)

In which order do you test spinal mobility? (p. **66**)

How do you document hypomobility and hypermobility of spinal segments? (p. **65**)

How do you test a dancing patella? (p. **70**)

When is the neutral zone of a joint enlarged? (pp. **70–71**)

Describe how you can test the stability of the knee joint. (p. **72–73**)

What is a physiological passive insufficiency? (p. **74**)

Describe how you can examine the musculature. (pp. **74–76**)

Which factors may cause neurogenic disorders? (pp. **77–78**)

How can you measure subjective reports of pain and symptoms? (p. **79**)

Which findings are included in your examination of impaired mechanosensitivity of neural structures? (p. **79**)

When do you use sensitizing movements? (p. **80**)

What does a neural provocation test examine? (p. **82**)

Name examples of neural provocation tests? (pp. **83**)

Provocation test: What distinguishes a normal physiological pain response from an nonphysiological pain response? (p. **84**)

Name two examples of nerves in the upper extremity that you can palpate. Where can you palpate them? (p. **88**)

Name two examples of nerves in the lower extremity that you can palpate. In which starting position can you palpate them? (p. **90**)

Which aspects belong to a peripheral neurological examination? (pp. **xXXXx**)

How can you examine superficial sensitivity? (p. **94**)

Name the segment-indicating muscles of the upper and lower quadrants. (pp. **96–97**)

Which instruments can you use in order to test functions? (pp. **104–106**)

When do you use the Roland questionnaire? (p. **105**)

Which tests do you use if you wish to test the patient's self-care ability? (p. **106**)

Which instruments may be used to test muscle strength? (p. **106**)

# Subject Index

Page numbers in *italics* refer to illustrations; those in **bold** refer to tables